TWINS

Much has been written about twins. Very little, however, is about their everyday lives. In this fascinating new study, Alessandra Piontelli follows the development and behavior of thirty pairs of twins from their early life in the womb through to their third year as members of the community. She draws on detailed ultrasound observations and work with mothers and families in clinical and natural settings to trace the subtle ways in which various types of twins behave and interact with their unequally shared and unique prenatal and post-natal environments.

Piontelli shows how from very early on, distinctive and personal traits can be seen in the behavior of each member of a twin couple and how these traits continue to strengthen well beyond birth. At the same time, the 'couple effect' has an impact on their behavior even after birth when social interactions begin. The book describes not only the behavior of the twins, but the impact they have on the lives of their family and carers – what family members say, how they react and how the family changes.

Scientifically based, but warmly human in content, this unique longitudinal study offers new insights to professionals working with others and families of twins, and to researchers in human development across a range of disciplines.

Alessandra Piontelli is Visiting Professor of Child Neuropsychiatry and Researcher in the Department of Maternal/Fetal Medicine and Perinatology, University of Milan. She is the author of *From Fetus to Child*, also published by Routledge.

TWINS

From Fetus to Child

Alessandra Piontelli

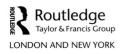

Routledge
Taylor & Francis Group

LONDON AND NEW YORK

First published 2002
by Routledge
11 New Fetter Lane, London EC4P 4EE

Simultaneously published in the USA and Canada
by Routledge
29 West 35th Street, New York, NY 10001

Reprinted 2004

Routledge is an imprint of the Taylor & Francis Group

© 2002 Alessandra Piontelli

Typeset in Sabon by Wearset Ltd, Boldon, Tyne and Wear
Printed and bound in Great Britain by TJ International Ltd, Padstow, Cornwall

British Library Cataloguing in Publication Data
A catalogue record for this book is available from the British Library

Library of Congress Cataloging in Publication Data
Piontelli, Alessandra, 1945–
Twins : from fetus to child / Alessandra Piontelli
p. cm.
Includes bibliographical references and index.
1. Twins–Psychology. I. Title.
BF723.T9 P56 2002
155.44'4–dc21
2001048410

ISBN 0-415-26227-5 (pbk)
ISBN 0-415-26226-7 (hbk)

To Luigi

CONTENTS

FIGURES

N.B. All figures read from top to bottom and from left to right. Twin 1 always indicates the twin on the left of the picture and Twin 2 the one on the right.

TABLES

ACKNOWLEDGEMENTS

Of the many people who have helped me throughout my work my deepest thanks are due to the following: to all the families who so generously let me share such an important part of their lives; to my friends at the Department of Maternal/Fetal Medicine: Alessandra Kustermann, Umberto Nicolini, Luisa Bocconi, Chiara Boschetto, Elena Caravelli, Sara Salmona, Beatrice Tassis, Laura Villa and Cinzia Zoppini. They have made possible the transition from Neurology and Child Psychiatry to other disciplines and to another working environment, and over the years have all put up with my innumerable requests with enormous patience; to the neonatologists, too numerous to mention, but especially to Chiara Vegni for her availability and support; to Anna Rambaldi-Piovella and Fabio Mairani for helping me with psychological testing and psychological and behavioral assessment; to Elizabeth Bryan and Ronald Higgins for commenting and advising me on several versions of this manuscript, and to Alan Fidler for his careful copy-editing of the final one; to Sergio Belfiore for assisting me with artwork; to Christopher Benton for so patiently and skilfully revising my English and for assisting me with computer work. Finally my deepest thanks are due to my editor, Edwina Welham, for always believing in me and being so ready to give me precious editorial advice. Ultimately the responsibility for what I say in this book remains mine alone.

INTRODUCTION

Describing primitive creeds surrounding natural phenomena, Sir James George Frazer wrote:

> A couple who have given proof of extraordinary fertility by becoming the parents of twins are believed by the Baganda of Central Africa to be endowed with a corresponding power of increasing the fruitfulness of the plantain-trees ... The Galalareese are of the opinion that if a woman were to consume two bananas growing from a single head she would give birth to twins. The Guarany Indians of South America thought that a woman would become a mother of twins if she ate a double grain of millet.
>
> (Frazer [1922] 1932: 137)

His work was aimed at documenting the development of 'primitive' ways of interpreting nature. Twins were not central to Frazer's studies. However, since such births were often regarded as extraordinary, even bordering on magic, twins were quoted by him along with other natural phenomena equally enshrouded in mystery and superstition.

Some of the above-mentioned tribes may well be extinct by now and science has dispelled many such superstitions or indeed religious creeds. However, not all superstitions and ancient beliefs about twins have been swept away by progress. Even certain branches of modern science are not immune from old tenets. Furthermore, contemporary myths are continuously being created around them.

For centuries midwives, and subsequently obstetricians, have dealt with these often hair-raising multiple births. Their endeavours, however, were not considered scientific, but merely the menial task of dealing with some of the many impurities of female biology.

Only in 1875 did Sir Francis Galton's work 'The history of twins as a criterion of the relative powers of nature and nurture' bring twins fully into the noble realm of inquisitive science. Since then innumerable studies have centred on twins as an 'experiment in nature' in an attempt to resolve the nature/nurture controversy: trying to tease out the relative strengths of the genetic, inherited make-up and the various environmental components in determining different characteristics of the individual.

Galton's methods have since been greatly refined. Virtually no aspect of the lives of twins has escaped close scrutiny. Geneticists and psychologists have become familiar figures in many twins' lives. However, the fundamental theory which Sir Francis Galton originally propounded has remained virtually unchanged. Behavioral genetics is a direct derivation of his nature/nurture approach.

Epidemiological and macro-genetic studies utilising twins have contributed to our understanding of the genetic nature of several diseases. However, all the disorders involved are single-gene diseases. When applied to behavioral or psychological phenomena these same studies have given far less satisfactory or unequivocal results (Hinde 1968; Bronfenbrenner 1972; Lewontin et al. 1984; Arnold 1987; Plomin 1990; Wahlsten 1990; Benson 1992; Billings et al. 1992; Michel and Moore 1995; Gould 1996). Behavior, even in its simplest form, is probably inextricably controlled by a multitude of genes as well as by an infinity of environmental factors. So far none of the alleged discoveries linking complex behavioral traits to specific disorders have been confirmed beyond doubt (Horgan 1999).

We are now facing a new wave of interest in twins which goes beyond Galton's heirs. In the last twenty years the Western world has witnessed a dramatic rise in twinning rates due to assisted reproduction, improved prenatal and perinatal care and widespread maternal postponement of childbearing. Many more twins are conceived, and many who were previously doomed now survive. In the 1980s twins accounted for one in 105 Caucasian births; this has now risen to about one in 72 (Machin and Keith 1999). This almost epidemic explosion does not concern all types of twins equally. It is confined almost exclusively to dizygotic twins. The overall rate of monozygotic twins has remained virtually unchanged. However, such a remarkable growth has naturally prompted a renewed interest in twins.

Twins have also captured the attention of many products of contemporary times. They have, for instance, become an infinite source for the ever-growing list of manuals written by 'experts' who aim to advise and shepherd us through the innumerable facets of our lives. A few of these primers are indeed excellent and could be really useful in helping often distraught parents with practical advice. When having to deal simultaneously with two screaming babies, frantic caregivers don't find it terribly helpful to be told that a given trait of the twins is 60 per cent inherited and 40 per cent environmental. However, having to reinforce 'positive thinking' makes many of these primers resemble travel guides. Beautiful pictures and idyllic descriptions largely mask many of the unpleasant or even potentially dangerous aspects. The predominant philosophy is that the trip is always worth while and will inevitably lead to enriching and mind-enlarging experiences for all the components of the venture.

Parents of twins, or twins themselves, have written the overwhelming majority of these survival guidebooks. Having been there and lived through 'it' fully entitles them to be experts in the field. It is impossible, however, to be very objective when talking about oneself or one's own children. A nostalgic and romantic mood strongly intertwined with 'family romance' tends to permeate this type of literature.

Besides guidebooks, twins nowadays make the headlines in various forms of media. Popular magazines sensationalise everything, of course. A deluge of futuristic scenarios from Dolly and cloning to 'build a twin for your own future transplant' are reported daily. Another favourite of the media are those rare higher multiple births which are products of fertility treatments. These 'super-parents' are often portrayed all smiles as they proudly hold six or seven tiny babies. Unfortunately very few articles mention the frequent long-term consequences and poor outcome of such events.

Long before magazines became widespread, twins often figured in higher literary forms, but would now appear to have fallen from grace, frequently featuring, as they do, in less 'noble' contemporary sources. They have become almost ubiquitous in science fiction, thrillers, and horror stories, and in the movies that derive from them. Replicants, body snatchers, black magic, indissoluble lethal entanglement, thought transmission, and more besides, are all associated with them nowadays. The dark 'neo-gothic' side of twinship is clearly on the rise.

Alongside these more popular sources of interest regarding twins, truly revolutionary aspects concerning them have been revealed. However, but for a few restricted scientific circles, these findings have remained more or less in obscurity.

Many scientists no longer consider genes as implacable blueprints. Concepts of plasticity, interaction and expression, to name but a few, are all replacing former inflexible associations between genes and ineluctable destiny.

Very rapid progress has also been made by obstetrics, embryology and various other disciplines connected with our origins. Twins have proved to be extremely important 'experiments in nature' in elucidating aspects of medicine and biology which are quite different to those that first brought them under the close scrutiny of science. What were once considered lowly and fairly repugnant aspects of female reproductive biology and physiology are increasingly in the forefront.

With such a plethora of multi-layered information on twins why yet another book about them?

This is the first study commencing before birth and taking into account the intrauterine environment and the behavior of the twin fetus from a very early stage of pregnancy. Thirty pairs of twins, fifteen monozygotic and fifteen dizygotic, were followed longitudinally from ten weeks gestation. The same twins were also observed within their natural habitats throughout the first years of their lives. Readers will become familiar with most of these twins as this work proceeds.

Twins have usually been studied in laboratory settings and at later stages. Adopting a naturalistic, longitudinal stance enables the observation of many subtle interchanges between the twins as well as with the people populating their world. These dynamics could easily be overlooked in more neutral and artificial environments. Besides which, from the very beginning of their first evoked movements *in utero*, twins influence each other's behavior. Whilst proper social interchanges only start in life after birth, by the time twins come to laboratories a complex network of mutual and external influences has usually already been built by them and by those caring and interacting with their lives. The formation of many similarities and/or dissimilarities, as well as the largely social and emotional construction of 'twinship', is often rooted within such an intricate system.

Prenatal factors and determinants are also probably the most neglected areas of twin research by the affirmed mainstream body of science. The intrauterine environment has for a long time been considered a neutral and 'equal' non-environment, and prenatal elements have frequently been regarded as constitutional (Scarr 1968; Piontelli 1989, 1992; Plomin 1990; Bryan 1993; Rutter *et al.* 1993).

This work does not intend to prioritise the relevance of the intrauterine environment in shaping the whole of twins' lives. However, confusion about different types of twins and their origins is widespread. All twins, but especially monozygotic ones, can have very unlike and unequal starts. Furthermore, their first environment is always unequally shared, often remarkably so, and leaves some twins scathed for the rest of their lives. Individual variation and individuality begin to be moulded in the womb.

In contrast with the relative silence of twin research, the interest of pseudo-science in prenatal life is growing to ever-greater dimensions. Possibly no other environment is subject to so many contemporary legends and esoteric myths as the intrauterine one.

In order to dispel some such myths, an outline will first be given of the essential findings regarding the origin of twins and their hazardous pregnancies. These notions, which derive from several and varied fields, are generally unknown to non-specialist readers; primarily they constitute an essential basis to understand many later phenomena. After this the behavior and development of the twin fetus will be described up to and including birth. Then the early years of post-natal life will be outlined.

Inequalities for twins do not cease at birth. A description of the subtle ways in which various types of twins live, behave and interact with their unequally shared and unique post-natal environments is still lacking. From before birth twins are hardly comparable, in many respects, to the rest of us. Their prenatal and post-natal environmental conditions are quite singular and unlike those of singletons.

Again, the focus on the early years of post-natal development is not intended to imply that this period is more important than later moments in life. Early experience is not unalterable by later experience as is all too commonly assumed (Kagan 1998; Bruer 1999).

Though this work is based on the above-mentioned longitudinal study of thirty pairs of twins, its contents go beyond the account of a particular investigation. Having worked as a researcher and consultant in the Department of Maternal/Fetal Medicine and in the Department of Perinatology of the University of Milan for the past ten years, many of the points examined are taken from other research work which focused on specific aspects of the intrauterine behavior of both singleton and twin fetuses. Besides proper research work, my background in neurology, child neurology and psychiatry, as well as psychoanalysis, was used by obstetricians and perinatologists alike for various forms of intervention. In particular, Chapters 3, 4 and 5 are based on a much wider experience which by now encompasses nearly five hundred twin pregnancies and relative immediate post-natal periods. However, obvious restrictions in time prevented the same detailed follow-up as described in the thirty selected cases. Therefore many elements described in those chapters stem from an active participation in both prenatal and post-natal clinical work, from observations within clinical and natural settings, and from countless contacts with young twins, their parents and those attending to their care during the early stages of their lives.

Since this work covers several areas of knowledge, encompassing notions from such varied fields as biology, obstetrics, neurology and developmental psychology, a fairly plain and discursive style is used in order to blend what are generally compartmentalised notions to render them accessible to the reader. In order to maintain a degree of fluidity, elements such as numerical data, exact composition of the sample, frequency of occurrence of described phenomena and the evolution of each single pair of twins are presented in the tables and their explanatory notes (see pp. 174–208) which can be read independently of the main body of the work by interested readers.

STUDYING TWINS IN DIFFERENT ENVIRONMENTS

PRENATAL RESEARCH

Setting

All the prenatal investigations mentioned in this work were carried out in the First Department of Maternal/Fetal Medicine of the University of Milan, a public structure belonging to the National Health Service. This is a highly specialised unit of the biggest (7,000 deliveries per year) maternity hospital in Italy and one of the largest in Europe. A special sub-unit for twin pregnancies is part of the Department. Between 100 and 120 twin pregnancies are followed each year. Women come to this division from a very large catchment area.

This setting does not offer the tranquillity characteristic of many laboratories of psychology, where neat experiments can be carefully designed and elegantly carried out. Most of the time one has the feeling of being flung onto a frantic and relentless firing line. Everyone is busy in urgent and highly demanding clinical work. Having to deal with recurrent emergencies tends to make things fairly hectic. Decisions have to be made on the spot, and the action to be taken frequently cannot wait. The study of fetal behavior is inevitably, and quite rightly, one of the last priorities to be met in a busy obstetric ward. Therefore one has to constantly adapt to these emergencies and the changing requirements of often dramatic circumstances. These and other problems frequently render research on fetal behavior painstakingly long. The 'ideal' case you have waited months for may simply volatilise, as other more essential matters have to be dealt with.

Furthermore, if you intend following individual behavior from prenatal to postnatal life, matters become even more complicated. Curiously, most obstetricians completely lose interest, or at best retain just a very superficial interest, in the child once it is born. Involvement and co-operation, therefore, can be very low for topics relating to developmental research which continues after birth.

Working in a special sub-unit dedicated to twin pregnancies accentuates all such difficulties. Pregnancies here are at greater risk and at times pose complex medico-legal and ethical problems. Competencies involved in working with at-risk pregnancies are highly specialised. The traditional figure of the paternalistic male obstetrician is rapidly being substituted by that of female doctors in their forties or even thirties. This generally favours a more relaxed dialogue between doctor and patient. However, all the medical staff tend to speak in technical jargon. Rationally this is done to speed up communication, to protect themselves against possible legal problems later, and to avoid transmitting suppositions and further anxieties to the patient before a firm conclusion has been reached. The resulting atmosphere closely resembles that of an initiatory clan. Mothers often feel excluded and worried by the flood of whispers and cryptic remarks. Doubts and suspicion often linger on even after a careful explanation has finally been provided.

Ultrasounds

The best procedure so far available for unobtrusively observing the behavior of the human fetus is ultrasounds. Their use in scanning the fetus within the watery medium of the intrauterine environment has revolutionised the medical approach to pregnancy. Fetal Medicine is now an autonomous and rapidly expanding field.

Besides strictly clinical applications ultrasounds have opened the unprecedented possibility of studying the behavior of the human fetus within its natural habitat by non-invasive means. Studies of human fetal behavior have begun to emerge from the mist of anecdotal evidence, and a wealth of data on fetal competencies is now available and rapidly accumulating. Ultrasounds, however, also have limitations, some of which are greater in the case of twins. After the twentieth week only very global or very focused behavioral studies are possible.

Thanks to their advent we now know when a human fetus begins to move, what movements it can perform and at what age, how its behavior changes with passing time – and much more besides. It is impossible for reasons of space to go into detail of all the behavioral knowledge that has been gained through ultrasounds. These topics could fill a book in their own right, and indeed have.

Parallel to ultrasound recordings all clinical and several psychological parameters were also registered.

Subjects

Northern Italy has one of the lowest birthrates in the world. Pregnancies are usually planned well in advance and the carefully programmed children are generally regarded as extremely precious. A lot is 'invested' in terms of emotions, time and money in the few children most couples eventually decide to have. Twin pregnancies are increasingly the result of lengthy, laborious and costly fertility treatments and are therefore frequently regarded as particularly priceless. Furthermore, all twin pregnancies, whether spontaneous or not, carry with them greater risks and discomforts of various kinds. Twin pregnancies have to undergo more frequent, sometimes continuous, check-ups. Therefore prospective parents of twins are particularly eager for information and anxious for reassurance. Parents hang on to the obstetricians' every word and to any nuance in their voice. Doubts may well be explained but, nonetheless, many fears, questions and simple curiosities inevitably remain unanswered.

During ultrasound examinations their 'precious' twins are necessarily dealt with efficiently, fairly quickly and rather anonymously. Often all that parents get are just some rather confused images of the particular sections of the fetal body measured to ascertain regular growth.

All parents attending the unit are generally impressed with the competence of the medical management of the pregnancy, but they all seem to wish for more. Most parents come expecting to be treated as something fairly exceptional, with cries of wonder and special interest. They soon discover that twin pregnancies are not the exception but the rule within the unit. Here they are just part of the herd. The long line of women with monumental abdomens waiting their turn for an ultrasound examination overawes many.

When planning this study prospective parents were approached once the first ultrasonographic examination was over. This examination is carried out to establish correct initiation and continuation of pregnancy, accurate gestational age and proper implementation. In choosing the appropriate subjects the following criteria were used: (1) placental appearance; (2) early gestational age; (3) vicinity to the hospital (so as to make post-natal visits feasible); (4) general maternal good health. The reasons for the first two points will become clear in Chapters 2 and 3. The final composition of the sample is reported in Table 1.

Ten new cases were enrolled each year and the study was spread over three years. Whilst all twins are at least four years old at the time of writing, most are five and beyond.

After introducing the question of fairly lengthy (half-hourly) observations to be done on a regular basis (usually once a fortnight), the study and its objectives were explained in detail.

Parents' faces invariably lit up when they were asked to participate in a behavioral study. Someone was finally taking a special interest in their precious twins.

The observations, it was explained, were to be recorded on cassette for retrospective and independent analysis to guarantee objectivity to the whole procedure. Parents were informed that they would receive a free copy of all the material after the delivery. This also felt like a special bonus and thrilled most. Formal, written, though not binding, permission was then obtained.

During the observations the atmosphere was fairly relaxed. Questions and curiosities could be answered. Anatomical details and physiologic functioning were explained. In addition, after recording was over, it was often possible to choose particularly pictorial sections of the fetal body for the parents to see in more detail. Parents usually asked if they could bring one or two relatives along next time, and soon entire families were added. All this was conducive to an atmosphere of friendliness and trust.

It should come as no surprise that there was never any difficulty in enrolling mothers for fetal behavioral research.

The thirty couples approached for the prenatal and post-natal study of twins whose observations form the main part of this book were all extremely pleased. The observations were to be extended to the family environment once the twins were born, and as far as possible would also include the delivery itself. Parents felt greatly reassured knowing that someone would assist them throughout the pregnancy and after. In fact, once the news spread around the Unit many more women than any one person could realistically follow volunteered to participate in the study. In-depth longitudinal studies can give us unique information. Furthermore, they can be conducive to hypotheses formation and consequently to more focused research later on. However, such investigations are enormously labour and time consuming.

POST-NATAL RESEARCH

The main prenatal and post-natal research forming the substratum of this book took place in Milan. Milan is the financial and industrial capital of Italy. Save for certain inevitable differences between any two countries, the kind of upbringing found in Milan and the rest of northern Italy is certainly comparable to that of any other developed part of Europe. Therefore the post-natal rearing practices described here may well be considered as typical of any Western country.

The delivery

As birth is generally regarded as a dramatic change, if not a complete caesura, from the former prenatal environment, I always tried to include it in my observations. In twenty-eight cases I observed the delivery and documented it with a video camera. The babies were videotaped a few minutes after birth, once they had been handed over to the neonatologist in charge. In addition medical parameters such as birthweight, need for reanimation, neurological examination, and so on, were also recorded.

The delivery, as well as being a dramatic event in itself, also represents a notable change in the setting and methods of investigation. These changes are clearly familiar to anyone working in the field of infant research and therefore only a few particular points will be highlighted here.

Purely descriptive methods are unacceptable, not only to obstetricians but also to most developmental researchers. They are also regarded with increasing suspicion by the parents themselves who want to be sure of your objectives and intentions. The use of videotape, as well as being an extremely valuable tool in itself for studying preverbal children, also gives a scientific halo and a clear focus to research work, making it more acceptable to parents. Furthermore, videotape, with the possibility it gives of calmly looking at the images over and over again, is especially useful when you have to concentrate on two children simultaneously – and even more so during a particularly frantic and emotionally charged event such as childbirth. Independent viewing and microanalysis of videotapes by different researchers, based on a shared definition of various selected behavioral activities, also guarantees objective judgement.

Unfortunately, however, video cameras are generally an unwelcome intrusion for the various professionals attending the delivery of twins! Legal questions render this type of documentation potentially fraught with danger. Besides, obstetricians, paediatricians and midwives tend to voice their anxieties and to comment loudly and freely during the first care of the babies and do not like the idea of someone recording their actions and remarks. An atmosphere of suspicion and hostility, therefore, is often tangible.

On the other hand, mothers (and fathers) find having someone there that they have known for several months an important support. In addition mothers find the idea of videotaping the birth of their newborn twins particularly important as they frequently have to undergo Caesarean sections. A sense of loss usually accompanies women who have had to be anaesthetised and have not been able to participate in the event at all or, in the case of an epidural, only partially.

In twenty-eight cases initial encounters between the babies and their parents were also filmed. This, as will be explained in Chapter 5, proved to be of great value in retrospect.

The Neonatal Intensive Care Unit

Several twins have to spend a more or less lengthy stay in the Neonatal Intensive Care Unit (NICU). The NICU is particularly hard on parents who find themselves in daily contact with grief, distress and alarm. In this environment the babies are monitored constantly by paediatricians and nurses. Though the emotional needs of babies and parents are taken into account more and more nowadays, the prevalent sensation still tends to be one of activity. Videotaping may seem frivolous and mundane compared to the life-and-death struggles often occupying the minds of paediatricians and parents, and whilst daily visits were clearly a solace to them, filming had to be handled sensitively. Nevertheless, despite the problems, all cases involving a period in this harsh environment were filmed there. Besides the spontaneous behavior of the twins, parental reactions and parental handling were also videotaped. Clinical parameters, as well as paediatricians' and nurses' comments, were also registered.

The home environment

After discharge from the hospital, twins were visited at home. The observations took place once a fortnight during the first year, once a month during the second year, once a term during the third year and once a year afterwards. Each observation lasted at least one hour, but generally extended well beyond. At least half an hour was dedicated to filming, while the rest of the visit was left fairly unstructured. As the visits became less frequent observations became longer (up to three to six hours) and filming was extended to at least one hour.

Given the previous extended prenatal contact, acceptance into the household did not pose any relevant problems. At this stage mothers were generally full of anxieties about their twins, their health, and their capacity to deal with their care. They were also very lonely and keen to have someone ready to listen to them. The presence of an observer was eagerly awaited and regarded as a great help by most of them.

Videotaping in the home setting

Whilst video cameras would have been unwelcome in the home setting only a few years ago, by now most families have one or are at least familiar with them. However, mothers are understandably very sensitive about their children and like to show them in a good light. In most instances during the home visits the twins were wearing their best clothes, as if ready for a formal portrait. If the twins were crying desperately or were frantic and inconsolable their mothers easily became irritable. Occasionally it proved necessary to stop the recording procedure. Parents were inclined to talk to the observer when the videotaping was going on. As an observer I tended to say as little as possible, but they did not easily tolerate total silence. Complete naturalness was difficult to attain. Mothers tended to overact in trying to show themselves in their best possible light. When the recording was over, this was usually accompanied by a sigh of relief and a return to more spontaneous behavior.

In addition babies and young children are not good at posing. They are also acutely aware, almost from the very beginning, of the strangeness of the video camera and tend to look at it in amazement. Their tropism for the human eye renders them capable of distinguishing something discordant almost from the start. Setting the focus on them without looking directly into the viewfinder helped.

Despite these limitations, which render them a not entirely 'neutral' tool, video cameras are invaluable in the study of infant behavior, of mother/infant pairs and in the case of twins of intrapair relationships.

Video, however, cannot replace what is particular to the human eye: the perception of subtle interpersonal, emotional dynamics as well as a deeper and broader view of behavioral phenomena (Bick 1964; Harris 1969; Miller *et al.* 1989). As soon as the recording session was over, mothers started freely voicing their concerns, fantasies, projects, and so on, as they would in normal encounters. They also started to act out all sorts of dynamics towards the observer. These were often a pleasure, but at times they were also a real strain. Given their extreme isolation and fatigue some mothers tended to become excessively dependent upon the observer. Demands and unexpressed needs were such as to be impossible to satisfy. This occasionally resulted in feelings of resentment, a lack of collaboration, and missed appointments.

Many mothers, also understandably, did not want to be considered 'cases' and tried to transform the quality of the relationship from friendliness to pure friendship. Invitations to stay on for dinner or to go out for a walk, leaving the twins behind with another caregiver, had to be handled carefully. At times mothers did not collaborate with the 'scientific' part of the observation, as if trying to deny the real nature of the contact. Lights were dimmed or even switched off, twins were put down to sleep, or were placed in a playpen in another room whilst their mother chatted on. One of the greatest strains was avoiding being forced to take sides in marital disputes or in blatant inequities in the handling of the twins.

Laboratory settings, by introducing a fairly aseptic atmosphere, tend to screen an observer from most of these feelings.

Photographs

Photography was not part of my initial plans. The request for pictures of the children came from many of the mothers, who were enthusiastic about the video material that had been given to them. Therefore, to begin with only a few photographs were taken – simply to satisfy parental requests. However, many subtle interchanges can be captured with this technique. Since children are not good at being still most pictures were done in series. Photographs beautifully capture glances, minute facial expressions and small changes of position, which can easily be overlooked in the overall movements offered by tapes. Therefore, though this was not properly part of the research, photographs became a fairly constant feature. Several of the illustrations in this book are taken from these photographs. They clearly offer a better resolution than stills from videos and are therefore particularly well suited to this purpose. Their intrinsic value goes well beyond editorial questions, however.

Developmental, environmental and psychological tests

Parallel to my regular visits as observer, a psychologist with no prior knowledge of the prenatal and perinatal history of the children visited the families and administered developmental tests (Bayley 1969) at six months, one year, two years and thirty months. At one year an independent assessment of the home environment and of the quality of the care of the children was also carried out using a standardised testing procedure (Caldwell and Bradley 1984). The same assessment was repeated independently for each twin when they were three years old. Since many of the items evaluated in this testing procedure are family items such as toys this permitted an evaluation of possible non-shared environmental components. Finally, a session specifically devised to test the twins' attachment to their mother and to each other was carried out. The parents were always given a copy of any material.

CONCLUDING REMARKS

This book endeavours to describe how twins live and behave within their first natural environments. The statistical/mathematical emphasis which usually permeates studies of twins has been deliberately avoided and, instead, the kind of descriptive language in common use in human ethology has been adopted throughout the text (Blurton-Jones 1972; Hinde 1982, 1983; Richards 1974; Eibl-Eibesfeldt 1975; Bateson 1991).

The use of descriptive language in recounting observations in the home environment of urban families can pose problems. Investigations on human beings so close to ourselves are much more complex, and debates about them are likely to be more heated. We are studying subjects – not just from our own species but from our own culture. They could be our neighbours, families or friends. We can all identify ourselves in at least some aspects of them. This could inevitably elicit strong and often irrational reactions in us all. When studying the realm of 'innocent' childhood and of 'sacred' maternity, one inevitably has to expect increased emotional disruption and dispute.

Visiting families is far from being an 'aseptic' procedure. Though most house-holds were indeed very amiable, family life can also be complex, messy and far from the 'rosy' picture presented by so many publications on infancy (Blaffer Hardy 1999). Naturalistic observations involve professional hazards.

These can represent particularly touchy issues with families of young twins. Childcare and education may indeed be sub-optimal in these circumstances, given all the hardships, strains and turbulence caused by the twins' birth. This does not mean that twins are destined to doom. The overwhelming majority move on to lead normal, contented lives. Flawless, 'optimal' education is never possible, but families with twins feel doubly at fault for not providing it and are therefore particularly sen-sitive to any potential judgement. The majority of parents of young twins easily fall victim to an acute sense of guilt. Obviously this problem is not limited to them alone. Most families in our Western society seem to seek a certificate of spotless, almost inhuman, perfection, though the problem is easily amplified in the case of twins.

In this book the sensibility of the subjects is taken into consideration and their anonymity has been guaranteed by various means, though detail has not been sacri-ficed; a shallow, stifled, over-optimistic or too general and aseptic a description of how twins live and behave would not help us, or indeed help future twins and those who will care for them, to better deal with the difficulties which may arise from their birth.

CHAPTER 1

BIOLOGY OF TWINNING

In recent years such diverse fields as placental studies, embryology, molecular biology, genetics and many others have deeply altered the way we understand the remote origins of twins. Complexity and variance have replaced previously fairly simplistic views. Twins have proved to be extremely important 'experiments in nature' when looked at from a fresh angle. They have helped us to elucidate different features of our beginnings with far-reaching implications well beyond the nature/nurture debate (Nussbaum and Sunstein 1997).

ORIGINS

A fertilised egg is called a zygote. Twins can derive from two different ova or from a single fertilised ovum. The terms monozygotic and dizygotic twins thus indicate whether the twins derive from a single zygote (monozygotic) or from two (dizygotic). Other very rare varieties of twins have been shown to exist, such as blood chimeras (individuals that appear to be a mixture of cells from two genetically different sources), whole body chimeras (or completely fused fraternal twins) and boy–girl monozygotic twins possibly having a dispermic monovular origin (Dunsford *et al.* 1953; Benirschke 1972; Muller *et al.* 1974; McLaren 1976; Bieber *et al.* 1981; Hall 1996; Benirschke and Kaufmann 1995).

For reasons of simplicity, only dizygotic and monozygotic twins will be referred to in this book,[1] and since the mechanisms which lead to their formation are fundamentally different they will be treated separately.

DIZYGOTIC TWINS

Dizygotic twins (also commonly referred to as fraternal or non-identical twins) derive from two different eggs fertilised by two distinct spermatozoa. This gives origin to separate and genetically diverse embryos.

Genetically speaking, dizygotic twins are like ordinary siblings. They can be of the same or opposite sex and their appearance can display varying degrees of similarity or dissimilarity.

Causes of dizygotic twinning

Though most dizygotic twins are conceived during the same menstrual cycle, share the same pregnancy and are born at the same time, this is no longer the rule.

New fertility treatments have entirely revolutionised the circumstances leading to the genesis of ever-growing numbers of twins. Dizygotic twins can now be 'induced' by hormones not produced by the body of the woman who will give birth to them (Wyshak 1978a). The eggs can be fertilised artificially in aseptic laboratories, not just by natural intercourse. Furthermore, zygotes, no matter how obtained, can also be frozen, thawed and implanted at will, thus rendering fertilisation independent of the initiation of pregnancy. Once the embryos are frozen (or 'cryopreserved') gestation can be started at a later, convenient date. This also opens up the possibility of 'twins' being implanted at different times and thus being born from diverse pregnancies. Consequently one twin could theoretically be older or younger than its co-twin. In addition, for the first time in the history of mankind the old dictum 'mater semper certa est' (you always know who the mother is) no longer proclaims a universal truth. Egg donation can lead to embryos being hosted in the uterus of a woman who is not their genetic mother. All this, of course, applies to singleton pregnancies as well. However, fertility treatments quite frequently result in twins, especially, but not exclusively, dizygotic ones (Derom *et al.* 1987). Therefore all these new possibilities and combinations have a particular relevance in their case. They also, in turn, open up new semantic and conceptual problems, such as the criteria for being a twin. Is it a shared conception or a shared pregnancy? New developments inevitably open up new dilemmas.

Genetic and environmental causes

However, getting back to old-fashioned spontaneous methods, the release of two or more ova has been found to be triggered by many influences. Dizygotic twins originate from both genetic and environmental causes (Gedda 1961; Liebermann *et al.* 1978; Nylander 1978; Parisi *et al.* 1983; Wenstrom and Gall 1988).

Whatever the primary cause, this usually acts on the level of particular hormones secreted by the hypophysis or pituitary gland, and principally on the so-called follicle stimulating hormone (FSH). A rise in the circulating levels of FSH has the consequence of producing increased ovarian stimulation (Benirschke and Kim 1973; Nylander 1975; MacGillivray 1986). Clomiphene citrate (Clomid), one of the most used 'fertility drugs', also operates in this way.

Dizygotic pregnancies present wide variations of rate of occurrence in different racial groups. These estimates are frequently being revised due to new reproductive technologies. However, dizygotic twinning rates are especially high in African populations (from 1:63 to as high as 1:11 births) and very low in Asiatics (1:330 births). Caucasians stand in the middle (between 1:125 and 1:80 births) (Bulmer 1970; Little and Thompson 1988; Bryan 1992; Segal 1999). Such differences seem to be linked principally to genetic factors. It is frequently said that twins 'run in the family', and a genetic predisposition has indeed been found to exist (Allen 1978).

Higher or lower levels of FSH have been described in women belonging to ethnic groups with respectively elevated or infrequent incidence of dizygotic twinning (Milham 1964; Martin *et al.* 1984). Dietary influences on hormonal levels have been documented as well (Nylander 1975, 1978). Amongst those interested in the biology of twinning (as well as in anthropological–cultural aspects related to twins) the Nigerian Yoruba ethnic group is particularly famous. Women belonging to this large group have very high twinning rates. Approximately one in every eleven Yoruba is a twin. Higher levels of FSH were found to be present in the blood of these women (Nylander 1973, 1978).

However, when Yoruba women migrated to urban areas – with a consequent change of diet – their twinning rate decreased. This would indicate that besides endogenously produced levels of FSH, dietary components containing some hormone-stimulating substance could also account for this especially high incidence of twins.

Other factors influencing dizygotic twinning

Older women and women who have already had children are more likely candidates for having dizygotic twins (MacGillivray *et al.* 1988). Probabilities increase up to 35–37 years of age and rapidly decline thereafter (Campbell *et al.* 1974; Allen and Parisi 1990). This may be due to an increased ovarian activity before the changes heralding menopause begin to set in (Nylander 1975; Schwartz *et al.* 1980).

Taller and strongly built women are also more predisposed to having dizygotic twins (Nylander 1971; Campbell *et al.* 1974), and so are women with short regular menses and an early menopause (Wyshak 1978b, 1981).

Seasonal variations, too, have been described as having an influence on dizygotic twinning rates (Cheng *et al.* 1986; Nakamura and Miura 1987). Summer months, with increasing daylight, may induce increased hormonal production.

However, several of these factors influencing twinning rates still await a conclusive explanation, and it may be that many other determinants contribute to dizygotic twinning.

Common beliefs

It was once thought that the transmission of a propensity for twinning was only matrilineal. Though the main genetic determinant of twinning is certainly transmitted directly through the female line, nevertheless a paternal role, albeit still unclear, appears to exist as well (Gedda 1961; Parisi *et al.* 1983; Wenstrom and Gall 1988).

Another common belief is that twins only occur in alternate generations. However, this is far from being a general rule. Family studies have shown that the genetic determinant for dizygotic twinning may not be expressed in every generation, which occasionally, but not constantly, causes the omission of a generation.

The common belief that the release of two eggs is easily triggered by the suspension of contraceptive pills has not been demonstrated either (Braken 1979; Campbell *et al.* 1987).

Superfecundation

On rare occasions dizygotic twins may be the result of superfecundation. Separate ova are fertilised during two different intercourses occurring within the same menstrual cycle. The same partner, or two different ones, may cause the two fertilisations. Superfecundation has been demonstrated in man by DNA techniques (Teraski *et al.* 1978; Majiskys and Kout 1982; Bsat and Seoud 1987; Monga and Reid 1992). Until quite recently (and probably even now) in several parts of the world twins were inevitably thought to be the result of adultery. This belief often had grim consequences both for the mothers and for the twins. Modern science has proven that while this could be so, it remains only a remote possibility. However, superfecundation brings with it other questions which go beyond the realms of mere matters of cuckolding. For instance, we don't know if the follicles releasing the ova have synchronous maturation or indeed if the ova are released simultaneously. Whether an egg is 'aged' or has a delayed maturation is not an irrelevant triviality. It could have an influence on the egg's quality, thus rendering it at risk (Bomsel-Helmreich and Papiernick 1976; Al Mufti and Bomsel-Helmreich 1979; Boklage 1990).

Superfetation

Though superfetation has never been proven in human beings (Baldwin 1994), it often gets mentioned. Superfetation implies that separate ova have been fertilised during different menstrual cycles within the same pregnancy. Even professionals occasionally still take weight differences as evidence of superfetation. Weight discrepancies are in fact very frequent in all twin pregnancies, including monozygotic ones (Blickstein *et al.* 1987; Storlazzi *et al.* 1987; Blickstein and Lancet 1988; Tchobroutsky 1991). If superfetation does indeed ever occur in humans, however, it must be an extremely rare event.

MONOZYGOTIC TWINS

Monozygotic twins derive from the fertilisation of one egg by a single sperm. This combination forms a zygote which then splits into two (or more) embryos sharing the same genetic endowment.

Real frequency of monozygotic twins

The frequency of monozygotic twins is calculated to be 1:250 live births, about one-third the dizygotic rate. This ratio is fairly constant all over the world, showing no racial or environmental component as with dizygotic twinning (Bryan 1992).

However, the birthrate of monozygotic twins is not representative of their effective incidence. Though prenatal demise can also affect dizygotic twins, it overwhelmingly concerns monozygotic ones (Robinson and Caines 1977; Boklage 1990; Baldwin 1994). About one in eight of all natural pregnancies begin as twins (Boklage 1995), but only 2 per cent of these will result in the delivery of twins. Both fetuses will die before ten weeks gestational age in one-third of cases (Baldwin 1994).[2] The death of just one fetus is also quite common. An early scan may show two gestational sacs each containing a fetus or an embryo. A few weeks later another scan can reveal that just one fetus is alive. This phenomenon, which has been given the eerie name of 'The Vanishing Twin Syndrome' (Jeanty *et al.* 1981; Landy *et al.* 1986), possibly occurs in as many as 50 per cent of all twin gestations (Levi 1976; Robinson and Caines 1977; Bryan 1992; Boklage 1995). Though this affects mothers to varying degrees emotionally, the other fetus is usually not harmed by the loss of its co-twin and is eventually delivered as a singleton child.

Embryonic or early fetal death is usually linked to chromosomal anomalies as well as to a variety of malformations (Baldwin 1994). However, fetal loss can take place at any stage during twin pregnancies. Whilst up to twenty weeks various abnormalities seem to be the main cause of demise, obstetric complications prevail near birth (Adams and Chervenak 1992).

Different timing of the twinning event

The process leading to monozygotic twinning is not a temporally fixed event (Benirschke 1998). The division of one embryo into two distinct ones can take place at any stage during the first fourteen days following fertilisation, but no later (Moore 1996). When the fertilised egg reaches the uterus and implants within its lining the placenta begins to develop. This essential and exclusively prenatal organ is made up of maternal and fetal components. Its function is to allow the transfer of nutrients and waste products between fetal and maternal circulations. Such exchanges occur at the level of minute finger-like protrusions of fetal origin called 'villi', which are bathed in the mother's blood. The fetus is attached to the placenta and hence to the maternal circulation through its umbilical cord. In addition the fetus is contained within a fluid-filled sac usually consisting of two membranes. The outer one, whose villous component forms the fetal part of the placenta, is called the chorion. The inner membrane is called the amnion. According to the timing of the cellular division leading to the formation of monozygotic twins some components will already be formed, others not. Those already assembled will not undergo further division. Variation in respect to timing brings with it differences in the type of placentation and fetal membranes the twins will acquire (Hamilton *et al.* 1978; Bomsel-Helmreich and Al Mufti 1995).

(1) When the division takes place within the first seventy-two hours after conception, the resulting embryos will have separate placentas and, since amnion and chorion have not yet formed, they will also have a complete set of individual membranes (Hall and Lopez-Rangell 1996). Hence the twins being contained within their own amnion and chorion will be called dichorionic–diamniotic. A thick four-layered septum with two layers belonging to each membrane will separate them. All

dizygotic twins are dichorionic–diamniotic and roughly 30 per cent of all monozygotic twins belong to this group (Bryan 1992).

Early separation allows for greater independence (Moore and Persaud 1993, 1998). Not only is the septum dividing the two amniotic sacs considerably thicker, but also each embryo can be implanted at a different location within the uterine cavity.

However, if they are implanted close together the two separate placentas will be adjacent and become, as they say, 'fused' (Baldwin 1994). These may have the macroscopic appearance, but not the structure, of a single placental mass. No vascular connection will exist between them. The absence of blood-vessel links will spare dichorionic twins from frequently fatal repercussions.

(2) Division of the zygote between day 4 and day 8 will give rise to two embryos sharing the same placenta and having a single chorionic sac. By this time the placenta and the chorion are already formed and cannot undergo further division. Since the amnion is not yet assembled the embryos, although contained by the same chorion, will be harboured within two different and separate amniotic sacs. Consequently these twins are called monochorionic–diamniotic. The septum dividing them will be translucent, considerably thinner and two-layered, only containing amniotic membranes. A common placenta frequently implies some type of vascular connection between its two fetal circulations (Baldwin 1994; Benirschke 1998). Over two-thirds of monozygotic twins belong to this group (Keith *et al.* 1995).

(3) Division between day 8 and day 13 will further reduce the autonomy of the two embryos. These will share the same placenta and both chorion and amnion. Such twins are called monochorionic–monoamniotic. Monochorionic–monoamniotic twins account for less than 3 per cent of all monozygotic twins (Folgman 1976).

(4) If separation takes place later, duplication of the cells forming the embryo may be incomplete. The outcome will be conjoined or so-called Siamese twins, as well as a host of other anomalies. Conjoined twins are estimated to occur in one in every 50,000 twin pregnancies (Benirschke 1998).

Knowing the type of placentation and of fetal membranes is not only valuable for indicating the timing at which the twinning event occurred, but can also serve to determine whether the twins are derived from one zygote or two (Benirschke 1961; Bryan 1986; Derom *et al.* 1991). All monochorionic twins are monozygotic. Although refined DNA analyses have revealed very rare exceptions (Perlman *et al.* 1990; Yokata *et al.* 1994; Machin 1996), all opposite-sex dichorionic twins are considered dizygotic. However, dichorionic twins of like-sex can be either monozygotic or dizygotic. Even though the majority of these twins will be dizygotic, all will require further analyses to ascertain their zygosity (Bryan 1986; Derom *et al.* 1991). It is still frequently assumed that only monozygotic twins have a shared placenta and that all twins with separate placentas are dizygotic.

Correct ascertainment of zygosity is important for parents, and indeed for the host of researchers usually present in most twins' lives. Parents, and later the twins themselves, understandably want to know if the twins are monozygotic (Machin and Keith 1999). Besides psychological implications, however, correct assessment of zygosity is significant for another reason. Should one of the twins need an organ or a tissue transplant in later life, a monozygotic co-twin would be the ideal donor. A transplant of tissues between monozygotic twins (a so-called isograft) would not be subject to the manifold problems of rejection that all the rest of us 'allografts' can undergo (Sumethkul *et al.* 1994). However, the prenatal assessment of placentation, chorionicity and amnionicity is first and foremost of primary and immediate clinical concern (Fisk and Bryan 1993). This will be discussed in greater detail later on, but suffice it to say here that monochorionic–diamniotic pregnancies can undergo specific, often fatal, complications and monochorionic–monoamniotic ones have an extremely high mortality rate. Both warrant special clinical management and very careful and frequent monitoring.

Ultrasound diagnostic advances have made prenatal classification of placentation possible. Though it should always be confirmed at birth, ultrasonographic distinction between monochorionic and dichorionic twins is now 100 per cent accurate if it is performed by expert hands by the twelfth week (Kurtz *et al.* 1992; Benacerraf 1998). Various parameters, such as placental appearance, thickness, number of layers and mode of implantation of the membranes are used to reach a diagnosis (Barrs *et al.* 1985; Hertzberg *et al.* 1987; Bromley and Benacerraf 1995; Scardo *et al.* 1995; Hill *et al.* 1996; Sepulveda *et al.* 1996; Wood *et al.* 1996).

Monozygotic twinning is a random event that can have different causes

Monozygotic twins can have different and varied starts. No single explanation of the monozygotic twinning phenomenon has yet been given. Different theories convincingly explain specific aspects of it, but probably no single causal factor is involved. Furthermore, since the incidence of monozygotic twins does not vary with race or maternal age, and no known environmental components or recognised hormonal factors appear to be implied, monozygotic twinning, unlike dizygotic twinning, appears to be a random event. Nor are mothers of monozygotic twins any more likely to have another set of twins in a subsequent pregnancy (Bryan 1992). Monozygotic twinning appears to be a random event in other species too. The armadillo is the only exception to this general principle. In this much-studied animal monozygotic twinning is a constant, perfectly timed, programmed event (Storrs and Williams 1968).

Causes of dichorionic–monozygotic twinning

Though both types of twins can have separate placentas, the mechanisms underlying their origin are completely different. Dichorionic–monozygotic twins probably derive from an incomplete split of the zona pellucida, the elastic membrane surrounding the ovum. The embryo hatches progressively through this small fissure, thus attaining an hourglass shape. A tearing of the thin tissue joining the two halves then occurs, leaving each of them to develop independently (Malter and Cohen 1989; Bryan 1992).

Causes of monochorionic–monozygotic twinning

Two main theories have been put forward to explain the start of monochorionic–monozygotic twins (Baldwin 1994). According to the splitting theory the developing embryo undergoes a division and the two halves then continue to grow as separate individuals. According to the multiple axis theory, after fertilisation duplication of the inner cell mass occurs (Bomsel-Helmreich and Al Mufti 1995). Instead of a single embryonic mass, which subsequently undergoes splitting, two cellular aggregates form and develop independently within the same matrix, the embryonic plate. This then undergoes a division.

Either, or possibly even both, of the theories may be correct. Many studies also tend to agree in viewing the twinning phenomenon itself as a malformation. This only means that an original weakness may lie at the basis of its genesis. Animal studies have shown that delayed fecundation of the egg provokes an 'ovopathy' or 'over-ripeness' of the ovum (Boklage 1981) leading, by whatever mechanism, to the formation of monozygotic twins. This could explain the unexpectedly high proportion of monozygotic twins resulting from IVF and assisted conception (Derom *et al.* 1987). The procedure itself may damage the zona pellucida or may lead to a delay in implantation that predisposes the ovum to monozygotic twinning. In fact, the majority (90 per cent) of 'assisted' pregnancies result in dizygotic twins. However, it still remains that very often IVF and fertility treatments are associated solely with dizygotic twins.

Over-ripeness would also take into account another particular characteristic of the human species – the possibility of performing intercourse independently from ovulation. Conception could occur when the ovum is already 'old', thus predisposing it to twinning. Other factors, such as oxygen deprivation or the sub-optimal intrauterine environment at the basis of the original fertility problem, may predispose to the division of the zygote (Bryan 1992). Other adverse environmental conditions could also be responsible.

The possibility that the twinning phenomenon in itself is a form of malformative, 'teratogenic' event occurring early in development could explain the unusually high rate of mortality and of chromosomal and congenital anomalies amongst monozygotic twins (Myrianthopoulos 1975; Bryan *et al.* 1987; Little and Bryan 1988).

The likelihood of hereditary factors in the initiation of monozygotic twinning has recently been put forward. More than one genetic component would seem to be implied (Bomsel-Helmreich and Al Mufti 1991). Some constituent would seem to act on the characteristics of the cell membrane, with subsequent cascading effects on cell aggregation (Wolpert 1991, 1994; Wolpert *et al.* 1998). However, it is well beyond the scope of this book to go into detail about the ever-growing list of different and compound causes which may contribute to the origin of monozygotic twins. Suffice this brief exposition to give an idea of the extent of diversity and complexity surrounding the origin of so-called 'identical' twins.

Similar, not identical

It was once assumed that the splitting which gives rise to the twinning phenomenon was an equitable, impartial one. Monozygotic twins were taken to be identical almost to the minutest detail. More and more sophisticated studies reveal that things may not be as simple as is generally assumed. Let it suffice to illustrate just a few points here.

First of all so-called identical twins can indeed have discordant chromosomes. Monozygotic twins with different karyotypes are a reality, albeit a rare one. During early separation, for instance, chromosomal components can be lost, leading to numeric chromosomal aberrations. Monozygotic twins discordant for the genetic disease known as trisomy 21 (commonly called Down's syndrome) are an example of this case (Rogers *et al.* 1982).

Although differences in genetic sex are thought to be antithetic to monozygosity, monozygotic twins discordant for genetic sex have been described. Other chromosomal errors and mechanisms such as translocation, segregation, inactivation of the X-chromosomes, existence of fragile sites on chromosomes, all leading to different syndromes and various manifestations, are also possible and have been described (Lewin 1997).

Besides which, chromosomal expression is also influenced by environmental components. Therefore not even identical chromosomes are necessarily a guarantee of identical outcome.

Chromosomal discrepancies and aberrations occur during early splitting of the zygote. When the splitting takes place after many cell divisions this results in unequal distribution of cells and cellular material (Bomsel-Helmreich and Al Mufti 1991). The splitting of a zygote is more akin to a tearing apart than to a microsurgical precision operation. Besides chromosomes, which are contained within the nucleus, cells are made up of various other components. It is highly unlikely that these could be divided equally to the minutest detail amongst the two embryos. More cells and unequal cellular components are generally allotted to one embryo, thus creating inherent discrepancies. One embryo can be bigger from the start, have a greater portion of placental surface and generally benefit from better physical and environmental circumstances.

Furthermore, with late splitting, in the period between conception and division, environmental components of various origin may intervene giving rise to further dissimilarities between the embryos. All of these factors could account for the considerable rate of discordance in anomalies and malformations of monozygotic twins (Benirschke and Kaufmann 1995; Baldwin 1994). They could also explain the high percentage of twins with discordant growth rates and development, as well as what are sometimes striking differences in appearance.

Though in practice most people will continue to talk of 'identical' twins, most experts prefer to use the term 'monozygotic' twins, realising that for many reasons these twins are not truly 'identical' (Bomsel-Helmreich and Al Mufti 1991).

CHAPTER 2

TWIN PREGNANCY AND THE TWIN FETUS

Twins represent a disproportionate share of prenatal and perinatal mortality. This clearly renders multiple pregnancies highly 'at risk'. Monochorionic pregnancies are particularly exposed to such dangers (Machin 1993; Adams and Chervenak 1992; Fanaroff and Martin 1992). Furthermore, certain aspects of perinatal pathology are met solely in these pregnancies. Prenatal and perinatal components can and do affect twins for the rest of their lives.

EARLY RISK

Complications may start very early on indeed for twins and, overwhelmingly, it is pure chance which determines whether they do. The size of their placentas is usually smaller than those of singletons. Furthermore, the two placentas are rarely equal. The single placenta of monochorionic twins is not only relatively small for sustaining both but is also unequally shared between the two. Placental size correlates with fetal growth and therefore has a cascade effect upon fetal development. Also, umbilical cords containing a single artery instead of two are four times more frequent in twins. This again is associated with increased poor outcome (Baldwin 1994). In addition, anomalously inserted umbilical cords are more frequent in twins and doubly so in monochorionic ones. A number of problems ranging from an increased rate of abortions to prematurity and decreased fetal weight can derive from what is an entirely fortuitous circumstance.

Survivors still have to face many intrauterine hazards. Again monochorionic twins are more affected than dichorionic ones, being subject not only to the general risks all twins have to encounter but also to those which are specific and unique to a shared placenta.

Monochorionic–monoamniotic twins

The highest prenatal mortality rate is to be found in those very rare monozygotic twins who also share the same amniotic sac. As many as 50 per cent of these will not reach birth alive. Mutual entanglement of the umbilical cords, with resulting asphyxia, is largely the cause of this high mortality rate (Carr *et al.* 1990). Death usually occurs before twenty-four weeks and is very rare after thirty-two weeks (Benirschke and Kaufmann 1995). Nevertheless, the risk of mutual strangulation, though reduced during the later stages of pregnancy, never completely ceases. Up to mid-gestation both fetuses are freer to move and general body motions are largely prevalent (Prechtl 1984), which possibly favours complex knotting. In addition, the absence of any barrier between the twins seems to render them particularly subject to the disruptive effect of intrapair stimulation on their cycles of rest. This causes more frequent bursts of activity which could, in turn, increase the likelihood of further entanglement. Increased hazards also occur during the delivery. One or both cords may be expelled prematurely (prolapse), thus cutting the twins off from their vital lifeline. In order to avoid this, monoamniotic twins are commonly delivered by elective Caesarean at around thirty-four weeks. These twins then have to face the consequences of their prematurity. Far from having the idyllic effects imagined by many, close proximity and the absence of barriers frequently exposes them to a merciless fate.

Monochorionic–diamniotic twins

Though spared the risks of entanglement which come from sharing the same amniotic sac, monochorionic–diamniotic twins can also undergo specific, potentially lethal complications. Roughly 15 per cent (Benacerraf 1998) will suffer from a particular condition, which has been given the deceptively altruistic-sounding name of 'Twin-to-Twin-Transfusion-Syndrome' (Achiron *et al.* 1987; Bendon and Siddiqi 1989; Danskin and Nielson 1989; Urig *et al.* 1990; Benirschke 1992; Bajora *et al.* 1995; Lopriore *et al.* 1995; Sharma *et al.* 1995; Machin *et al.* 1996). The mortality rate amongst twins affected by this syndrome is very high. Each year in the United States alone about 2,200 fetuses die from it (Benirschke and Kaufmann 1995). However, mortality is influenced by gestational age: the earlier the onset of the condition, the greater the risk. The syndrome commonly starts after mid-gestation. Onset before twenty weeks means a very poor prognosis: 90 per cent of such twins will die. Onset after this age gives a survival rate of approximately 30 per cent (Benacerraf 1998). The exact dynamics of this complex condition are still unclear. Artery-to-vein connections within the shared placenta of the twins seem to lead to an imbalance between the two. As a consequence the so-called 'donor' twin will show severe lack of amniotic fluid. At times such scarcity is so extreme as to leave it 'stuck', so tightly wrapped by its amniotic membrane and adherent to the uterine wall as to be hardly able to move (Mahony *et al.* 1990; Reisner *et al.* 1993). The 'recipient' twin, on the contrary, will have a massive excess of amniotic fluid. The unidirectional exchange of blood will also lead to anaemia, dehydration and growth retardation in the 'donor' and to a plethora of blood in the 'recipient', with sub-sequent hypertension and swelling of all organs. The distension of the bladder and the thickening and enlargement of the heart of the recipient are often impressive. Heart failure can, in fact, be one of the lethal consequences for the apparently favoured twin. Aggressive and repeated amniocentesis of the 'recipient' are usually undertaken (Elliott *et al.* 1991; Wax *et al.* 1991; Saunders *et al.* 1992; Weiner and Ludomirski 1994). Often this can reduce, albeit temporarily, the imbalance. Large quantities of amniotic fluid may have to be drained week after week. However, this procedure does not guarantee the survival of either twin. In addition, when one twin dies the co-twin also risks dying. The vascular placental communications between them may lead to a massive perfusion of blood from the living twin to the other. The survivor can literally bleed to death in the vascular bed of its deceased co-twin (Benirschke and Kaufmann 1995). The survival of just one twin is often fraught with grim long-term repercussions. The survivor may later show permanent neuro-logical sequelae, brain damage due to the acute hypotension provoked by the flow of blood towards the dead twin (Hagay *et al.* 1986; Patten *et al.* 1989; Jou *et al.* 1993; Lopez-Zeno and Navarro-Pando 1995).

Generally this syndrome is a chronic and progressive condition, but it can also occur acutely. Acute, quickly reversed and clinically undetected forms of Twin-to-Twin-Transfusion-Syndrome may account for the otherwise inexplicably high rate of cerebral palsy which is five times more common in this type of twin (Asher and Schonell 1950; Alberman 1964; Petterson *et al.* 1990; Benirschke and Kaufmann 1995).

Recently, laser treatment with occlusion of selected superficial vessels has been used in an attempt to stop the potentially lethal exchanges between twins from occurring (De Lia *et al.* 1995). However, a purely 'hydraulic' explanation of the syn-drome is not sufficient. Other unknown factors are probably involved.

Acute polyhydramnios

Acute polyhydramnios, an excess of amniotic fluid, although rare, is another compli-cation almost exclusively confined to monozygotic pregnancies, regardless of chorion type (Bryan 1992). This condition needs to be distinguished carefully from the Twin-to-Twin-Transfusion-Syndrome. A huge amount of amniotic fluid usually forms in both amniotic sacs, causing enormous uterine distension. Acute polyhydramnios develops rapidly and generally causes premature delivery. The uterus responds to its massive stretching as if it had reached term (Besinger and Carlson 1995).

Complications common to all twin pregnancies

The only complications common to all twin pregnancies, but not encountered in singletons, are those due to fetal crowding. Two fetuses in a uterus that is ideally meant to host just one may result in various deformations, particularly of the limbs and skull. Most of them are reversible; some are not (Baldwin 1994).

Other complications

The majority of the complications which affect twin pregnancies are common to singletons, but will be much more severe. It is sufficient to look at some comparative data on the two main complications to get an idea of the proportion of risk involved in starting life as a twin.

Prematurity and intrauterine growth retardation are the main causes of the increased perinatal mortality of twins. The probability that they will die after reaching viability is nine to twelve times higher than for singletons (Adams and Chervenak 1992).

Prematurity: term and pre-term

Twins are generally considered to have reached term three to four weeks before singletons (Bryan 1992). By this time the capacity of the placenta and of the intrauterine environment in general to sustain their growth adequately has usually come to a halt. A series of events follow this situation, only a few of which will be mentioned here.

Fetal urine production decreases, with a consequent reduction in amniotic fluid volume. This in turn increases the likelihood of umbilical cord compression and, therefore, of acute fetal hypoxia and of consequent sudden death (Chauhan and Roberts 1996). Failure of intrauterine growth, which may have started before, now accelerates and leads to a loss of subcutaneous fat and dehydration.

Twins also have an 'ideal' birthweight, which is lower than that of singletons. Paradoxically, for reasons which remain unknown, twins who do not fail to thrive can be in greater danger. A birthweight above 3,000 g brings with it an exponential rise in neonatal mortality (Papiernick-Berkauer and Richards 1991). Consequently by 36–37 weeks the advantages of being delivered far outweigh the disadvantages of not waiting until what is normally considered term.

However, many twins do not make it even to this natural deadline. Premature delivery is three times more frequent in twins (Bryan 1992), who account for 10 per cent of all premature births (Adams and Chervenak 1992). Eleven per cent of all twins are born earlier than thirty-one weeks (Besinger and Carlson 1995). Twenty-eight per cent of twins born between twenty-nine and thirty-two weeks, and 67 per cent of those born between twenty-five and twenty-eight weeks, will die of complications linked to prematurity. The lower limit for survival is currently 23–24 weeks, and both the immediate and the long-term risks associated with such untimely births are enormous.

At any stage, however, prematurity can lead to well-known, often enduring and distressing complications.

Causes of prematurity specific to twin pregnancies

Most of the causes of prematurity are still unclear. Apart from the factors which apply to all pregnancies, two determinants specific to twin pregnancies further increase the risk of an untimely birth. Uterine contractility is higher and gradually increases with advancing gestation. In addition uterine overdistension, as mentioned earlier, predisposes the activation of the mechanisms responsible for the initiation of labour (Besinger and Carlson 1995). Uterine overdistension is evident in most twin pregnancies. In many twins a frequent excess of amniotic fluid in one or both sacs further increases stretching, and consequently the probability of a premature birth. At times pre-term labour is also heavily influenced by the presence of chorioam- nionitis, an inflammation of the fetal membranes with consequent infection of the amniotic fluid (Naeye 1992; Benirschke and Kaufmann 1995). Monozygotic– monochorionic twins in particular have a greatly increased risk of being born pre- maturely (Bryan 1992). Monoamniotic twins, as already stated, are usually delivered by elective Caesarean section at around thirty-four weeks as soon as lung maturity is attained.

Growth retardation

The other main cause of perinatal complications and death in twins is growth retar- dation. Roughly two-thirds of twins show some sign of growth retardation at birth, and more than 50 per cent of all twins are born weighing less than 2,500 g (Chauhan and Roberts 1996). Factors which contribute to low birthweight include overcrowding of the uterus and insufficient blood supply, as well as the inability of the mother to provide sufficient nourishment for the satisfactory growth of two fetuses (Monteagudo et al. 1997). Growth retardation intervening during the last trimester is almost the rule and generally less serious. However, it can start much earlier. In addition most twins show a more or less marked discrepancy in their growth. Such discordance is not determined by sex and increases in monochorionic twins (Baldwin 1994).

MATERNAL COMPLICATIONS

Twins are not the only ones to suffer during pregnancy; their mothers too are at increased risk.

Pregnancy-induced hypertension is 2–3 times more frequent in women bearing twins, one-third of twin pregnancies being affected (Kochenour 1992). Pregnancy- induced hypertension is indeed dangerous, primarily for the mother, and is probably the commonest cause of maternal death. However, it also has cascade effects upon the fetuses, increasing growth retardation.

The incidence of gestational diabetes and of urinary tract infections is also higher in twin gestations (Skupksi and Chervanek 1996).

Anomalous insertion of the placenta (*placenta previa*) or its premature detachment (*abruptio placentae*), which both lead to sudden massive bleeding as well as post-partum haemorrhage, are encountered more frequently in twin pregnancies (Crowther 1999).

Physiological adaptations of the maternal body to pregnancy are also greater (Gardner and Wenstrom 1996). When a pre-existing pathology, such as maternal heart or kidney disease, is present, this may pose significant increased risk (Pridjian and Chin-Chu 1993).

However, even minor ailments such as breathlessness, difficulties in digestion and in sleep, backache, frequent micturition, swelling of feet and legs, and uncontrollable itching all contribute to make the later stages of twin pregnancy very hard and full of discomfort for the mother.

This chapter might sound very grim. However, most parents enter a twin pregnancy completely unaware of its risks. When, if and to what extent prospective parents should be informed of all the potential perils, especially of monochorionic twin pregnancies, poses complex medico-legal questions as well as important psychological problems which are open to debate (Jacoby 1988; Hay *et al.* 1990).

Unfortunately, what is even more serious is the fact that only too often the very professionals involved, unless specialists in the field, seem to be unaware of the risks entailed in a twin gestation. As a consequence mothers are frequently only referred to a specialised unit once problems have occurred; by then a point of no return may well have already been reached.

Getting back to the specific scope of this book, it is clear that the hazards of the intrauterine life of all twins are not to be ignored. Their unequally shared, complex, and often adverse intrauterine nurture is not irrelevant or neutral for their future existence.

CHAPTER 3

INTRAUTERINE BEHAVIOR

FICTION

The disquieting alikeness encountered so frequently in monozygotic twins is clearly one of the main reasons why twins in general have always been so intriguing. However, twins, unlike ordinary siblings, also share a most important environment – the uterus. This joint sojourn, during what is usually a solitary nine months pregnancy, is undoubtedly another essential element accounting for the distinctive enchantment surrounding them. Many myths, legends and popular beliefs have flourished around the intrauterine activities of twins (Gedda 1961; Corney 1975; Gélis 1991; Lévi-Strauss 1991; Pison 1991; Frontisi-Ducroux 1992; Sergent 1992; Savary and Gros 1995; Farmer 1996). Sharing pregnancy and intrapair stimulation have often transformed their prenatal life in the collective imagination into a lively, social affair. Fights abound, but we also hear of twins stimulating each other in all sorts of ways and being generally involved in 'adult', sophisticated, interpersonal interchanges, culminating in the popular belief of incest between brothers and sisters occurring within the narrow intrauterine space. There are still many such myths and legends surrounding the beginnings of twins' lives. Some apply to singleton fetuses as well, but are doubly strong in the case of twins. Others are specific to twins. Therefore, before dealing with the reality which technological and scientific advances have confirmed, some of the main reasons why such fables linger on will be sketched out. This digression will hopefully be of value in helping the reader to understand otherwise apparently irrational behavior.

Miniature adults

The behavior of the fetus, and doubly so of the twin fetus, is more easily studied during the early stages of pregnancy. Simultaneous visualisation of both fetal bodies in their entirety is only possible till about fifteen weeks' gestational age. From then to about the twenty-second week twins can only be observed separately, and the field of observation only includes those parts of the co-twin which come into contact with the one being observed. After the twenty-second week only a part of a single fetal body can be observed at any one time.

Early fetuses, for various reasons, some still unknown (Gandelman 1992), move a lot. From the onset of movement at 7–7.5 weeks (de Vries *et al.* 1982) they alternate rapidly and continuously between rest and activity cycles, short spells of inactivity followed by brief intervals of intense and turbulent motion (Robertson *et al.* 1982; Robertson 1988; de Vries 1992a). If a fetus is in a state of rest, usually only a few minutes pass before dramatic activity starts again. As gestation advances, periods of inactivity become progressively longer whilst periods of activity are gradually condensed and clustered (de Vries 1992b). Whole body motions involving frequent changes of position, predominant at early gestational ages, become less frequent as well as more difficult to perform. The 100–200 movements per hour which can be detected in a first trimester fetus drop to a mean of fifty-three by week twenty-four (Nasello-Patterson *et al.* 1988; Manning 1995). However, it is only towards the end of pregnancy that 'behavioral states' comparable to the neonate's various phases of sleep begin to appear. Particular variables start to act in concert, in fixed and temporally stable ways (Nijhuis *et al.* 1982). In other words, the presence or absence of body movements combined with eye movements, as well as specific heart-rate patterns, tell us that the fetus is in a particular state. State concomitants, regular or irregular so-called fetal breathing movements and mouthing movements, albeit episodically, also join in. If a fetus 'breathes' or mouths, however sporadically, in a characteristic way, this also tells us that it is in a specific state (Nijhuis *et al.* 1984). Earlier these same elements occurred briefly and disjointedly.

Despite all these rapid developmental changes, most people refer to 'the fetus' in general, quite independently of gestational age. Growth and evolution are extremely accelerated and concentrated in fetal life. We are often talking about days and weeks rather than months or years, as in post-natal life. Therefore, what is appropriate to ascribe to a certain gestational age may clearly not be equally pertinent to an earlier or later phase. A fetus approaching birth is undoubtedly quite different from a first trimester one.

However, the image of the fetus which most readily comes to the public's mind and is most commonly depicted is that of the early, active, first trimester. A third trimester fetus, and even more so a third trimester twin fetus, only visible in segments, is clearly less glamorous and therefore less prone to be illustrated in non-specialist publications and other media.

The lively activity of the early fetus is all too often equated with wakefulness, which is then automatically regarded as identical to intentionality and consciousness. As will be explained later, an active fetus may not be awake at all. Furthermore, though wakefulness is a prerequisite for consciousness, the two do not necessarily coincide. Anencephali, malformed fetuses born without the cerebrum, cerebellum and flat bones of the skull, can be periodically awake and display several behavioral patterns of ordinary newborns (Peiper 1963). Activity does not even necessarily imply awareness (LeDoux 1996).

Superior brains

There is another reason which also helps account for the 'miniature adult' mystique. Animal studies and post-mortem examinations of fetal and neonatal human brain tissues have shown an overproduction of neurons during fetal life. All cortical neurons are generated in massive quantities during the first seventeen weeks of gestation (Otake and Schull 1984). At birth the number of neurons is more or less that of an adult brain. Furthermore, neuronal cells of certain areas of the fetal brain have been shown to 'branch out' an overabundance of axons.[1] An excess of synapses is also produced (Rakic 1978, 1991; O'Kusky and Colonnier 1982; Sidman and Rakic 1982; Provis *et al.* 1985; Rakic *et al.* 1986; Huttenlocher and de Courten 1987; Herschkowitz 1988; Huttenlocher 1990).[2] In rhesus monkeys synapses are denser and more numerous during infancy than in adulthood, and the phase of high synaptic density lasts throughout adolescence (Rakic *et al.* 1986; Zecevich and Rakic 1991; Bourgeois and Rakic 1993; Bourgeois *et al.* 1994). An equal number of nerve cells, and a greater number of axons and synapses, has often been taken to mean equal or superior functions. In fact before reaching adult functioning the brain will undergo profound changes – particularly in terms of interconnections between neurons, development of receptors and development of the chemical systems that mediate synaptic transmission (Rakic 1991). Changes will continue throughout life.[3]

In the perinatal period neurons and axons projecting to incorrect or aberrant targets begin to undergo massive death and elimination. The reasons for such extensive 'trimming' are certainly physiological and functional (Hamburger and Oppenheim 1982; Rakic *et al.* 1986; LaMantia and Rakic 1990; Oppenheim 1991). A large component of cell death may be simply pre-programmed. However, one function of selective cell death is to refine projections and to eliminate misrooted axons (Blakemore 1991). These 'competitive interactions', which result in a massive elimination of nerve cells, axons and synapses, are most probably under the impact and control of inputs from the periphery (Rakic 1991). Besides other effects, this grants our brains considerable plasticity. Furthermore, in monozygotic twins it ensures substantial differences in neural organisation thus freeing them from becoming mere blueprints of their 'identical' genes (Edelman 1987, 1992).

Neuronal or axonal death and competitive elimination of synapses clearly cannot be ascribed to the 'superior' functioning of a fetal brain progressively losing its 'extraordinary' capabilities when approaching birth. Amongst other things, incomplete regional neuronal cellular demise could possibly lie at the basis of several neurological disturbances (Volpe 1987; Rakic 1988; Aicardi 1992).

Religious and anti-abortion issues, however, tend to foster and strengthen views of superior fetal capabilities. Economic and academic interests, too, are not immune from this attitude. Various forms of 'fetal therapy' and programmes of 'fetal enrichment' have started to flourish and the first 'fetal universities' have been opened, the rationale behind them all being to stop the little-understood neuronal death, axonal 'pruning' and synaptic 'trimming'.

Terminology borrowed from the vegetable kingdom has also added to the confusion amongst the lay public. Brains are depicted as functioning and developing like plants. Inundate the brain of your fetus, therefore, with the right kind of stimuli and it will blossom; unless you add plenty of 'enriched' soil it will wither; immerse it in highly exclusive and sophisticated inputs and your fetus will turn into a genius. Its 'competitive' synapses will beat all future rivals, and so on.

If any benefits are in fact derived from such attempts to retain and foster the imagined faculties belonging to a highly idealised stage, they are probably mediated through reinforcement of parental attention and bonding (Klaus and Kennell 1970).

However, followers of fetal fiction are reaching epidemic numbers and there are often no limits to their unreasonableness. Programmes of fetal 'enrichment' have even been activated in some underdeveloped countries where children are then left to starve in the streets.

Communicative partners

All this mythology is more than doubled in the case of twins. The 'mystical' union so often ascribed to them is frequently considered to date back to prenatal life. Intrapair stimulation, which is indeed unique to them, is taken to mean various forms of communication. Twins are regarded as particularly interactive partners, relating to each other in all sorts of complex and sophisticated ways. Even quite recently kissing and fighting have been 'scientifically' described. Apart from any other consideration, it is difficult to envisage how elaborate behavioral and emotional patterns such as kisses can be carried out across the membranes which in 99 per cent of all twin pregnancies separate the two different amniotic sacs (Baldwin 1994). These activities, like all truly social and complex emotional patterns, clearly only belong to later stages of post-natal life. In reality a behaviorally active fetus, save during short spells in the advanced stages of pregnancy (Parkes 1991), is not awake at all, but possibly just in a different phase of some vegetative state clearly more akin to oblivion than to alertness and wakefulness.

The turbulent motions of early fetal life have some important, though as of yet unspecified, role in neural development (Prechtl 1984). Animal experiments seem to indicate that fetal motion may be essential for the development of the musculo-skeletal system. Paralysed chicks display anomalous development in this respect (Drachman and Coulombre 1962; Drachman and Sokoloff 1966; Moessinger 1983). Fetal crowding certainly produces mechanical effects on the growth of bones and joints of some twins, with consequent permanent deformities.

However, when it comes to demonstrating the function of early motility, both for motor and neural development, matters become extremely complicated. Experimental data cannot be extended to mammals as immobilisation can be produced only for a relatively short time and in any case does not appear to affect neural activity (Prechtl 1984; Provine 1986; Michel and Moore 1995).

Nevertheless, it is not unreasonable to postulate that the constant sensory-motor feedback provided by early fetal motions may be of importance for neural development. Rest activity cycles could be more than a mere epiphenomenon due to the immaturity of the young fetal nervous system (Gandevia and Burke 1994; Arbib *et al.* 1998). Prenatal behavior is possibly one of the 'sculptors of the organism' (Hofer 1988). The incredible amount of activity of the early fetus would not make sense otherwise, if only for the expenditure of energy involved.

Intrapair stimulation, unfortunately, frequently seems to be used solely to uphold the belief that twins are highly intercommunicative partners. As a consequence all fetuses are regarded as potentially open to communication. Thus twin fetuses now fly the flag of the new era of the fetus.

The premature infant is in many ways simply a fetus removed from its natural environment. Though certainly not insensitive to various forms of stimulation, including human contact (Als 1994), in the wake of an almost fanatical belief in 'extraordinary' fetal competencies many tend to overlook the fact that it clearly does not have an intense and lively 'social' life. Most of the time it lies inert and hypotonic (Amiel-Tison and Korobkin 1993), crushed by gravity, dormant and scarcely responsive to any of the commotion surrounding it. This cannot be ascribed solely to the fact that it may be suffering various consequences linked to a premature delivery. Furthermore, the extremely premature infant, unable to breathe and feed independently and too weak to move, may even be disturbed by forms of supposedly 'enriching' stimulation.

Unrestrained meaning

Another reason for ascribing sophisticated, emotional exchanges to the intrauterine life of twins derives from the universal tendency to attribute meaning to everything. During an ultrasound session, as soon as the image of a fetus appears on the screen, it is almost inevitably accompanied by cries of wonder. Everybody in the room starts to comment on its actions. Most remarks allude to the apparent temperament of the fetus and, in the case of twins, to their 'relationship'. Whilst it is true that not all fetuses behave alike (de Vries *et al.* 1988) and not all twin fetuses react to intrapair stimulation in the same way (Piontelli *et al.* 1999), when this tendency to attribute meaning is taken to its extreme, twins end up being regarded as already having a well-defined character and being intensely bonded as if they were miniature adults right from the beginning of their lives. Meaning attribution is an essential mechanism in life after birth which helps us to care for our infants (Hinde 1988; Plutchick 1990) and to deal with the complex nuances of social relations in general (Kelley 1971; Johnson-Laird and Byrne 1991; Hinton 1993). An inability to attribute meaning to social/emotional interchanges may lay at the basis of autism (Wing and Gould 1979; Rutter and Schopler 1987; Wing 1988; Frith 1989; Baron-Cohen *et al.* 1993; Hobson 1993; Trevarthen *et al.* 1996).

Long before ultrasounds were invented mothers already had the tendency to give some kind of meaning to the perceived motions of their fetuses. Mostly they tried to imagine what the future temperament of their children would be like. These conjectures largely belonged to the realm of fantasy. However, such daydreaming also helped them to gain consciousness and to get acquainted with the fact that an independent life was unfolding within their bodies. Ultrasounds have laid bare what was sheltered by nature during the nine months of pregnancy. By allowing us to observe the real motions of the fetus they have opened up a visual dimension which normally only starts at the neonatal stage. Such premature unveiling has, amongst other things, caused the phenomenon of complex meaning attribution to be applied to the physiologically concealed motions of the fetus. Attributing the meaning connected to neonatal manifestations to the behavior of the fetus is understandable but, particularly when applied to an early fetus, is neither a functional nor a pertinent phenomenon.

Tabulae rasae

Though technical and scientific advances render this attitude less common, at the other end of the spectrum we find those people who still regard fetuses as complete *tabulae rasae*: amorphous, senseless beings unable to interact with their environment. Hard-wired, pre-programmed intrinsic forces or all-powerful extrinsic ones are thought to drive their development, leaving them marked for life. Maternal emotions are perhaps the most overpowering of the external forces which are presumed to permanently imprint totally malleable fetuses. This will be dealt with separately in the next chapter.

Underlying many twin studies is the common assumption of a totally shared and completely identical intrauterine environment. The macroscopic effects of environmental variations cannot be denied, as in the case of the differences in birthweight affecting the majority of twins. However, behavioral consequences are scarcely considered and are thought to be 'washed away', leaving intrinsic pre-programmed drives free to emerge again in all their true power in later life.

Fetal life also tends to be overlooked by many researchers in the developmental and behavioral fields. Neonatal capabilities are thought to spring up at or soon after birth without any prior history. Birth clearly represents a major environmental change and as such brings with it new and emergent vital adaptations. Whilst it is true that several fetal capacities are adapted solely to the unique conditions of intrauterine life, fetuses do have anticipatory and preparatory functions as well (Oppenheim 1984; Provine 1993; Lecanuet *et al.* 1995). For instance, as gestation advances fetuses smile (though unintentionally) and begin to display a limited repertoire of facial expressions which, after birth, will be associated with specific emotions by their caregivers, thus favouring their care. If a twin is touched on the chin by a kick of its co-twin after mid-gestation it begins to show the so-called rooting response, turning its head towards the stimulus and opening its mouth. Later this response will help the infant to find the breast. The dramatic discontinuities brought about by birth often make us overlook the essential continuities with prenatal life. More and more sophisticated tests and experiments reveal that infants, far from being Lockian *tabulae rasae*, come into this world well equipped with a wealth of sophisticated competencies which enable them to adapt to the complexities of postnatal life. Many of these have been acquired and prepared during prenatal life (Robinson and Smootherman 1987; Smootherman and Robinson 1988; Bekoff *et al.* 1980).

Oceanic merging and the 'fusional' stage

Newborns are sometimes still assumed to lack any sense of boundaries with their environment. The existence of a 'fusional' stage has been postulated (Mahler *et al.* 1975).

Some bodily sense probably begins to originate in the early prenatal days. Twins, with their mutually evoked motions, beautifully illustrate this. All fetuses in their frequent tossing and turning repeatedly touch the uterine wall. When at rest their body does not float freely in the amniotic fluid but usually lies against some part of the uterus, thus granting further bodily contact with an external surface. In addition fetuses frequently touch the umbilical cord and other constituents of their intrauterine space, which affords a wealth of contacts with extrinsic elements and an abundance of sensory-motor feedback. After the first 14–15 weeks fetuses push their feet against the placenta with increasing force and with alternating 'steps'. Infant-stepping at birth, in fact, has a long history dating from prenatal life. Amongst other things stepping is increasingly important for changing position. Interestingly, fetal feet are enormous compared to the rest when the first alternating leg movements begin. They are bigger than the fetus's thighs.[4] Big feet, besides perhaps providing a large surface available for sensory-motor feedback, may also be necessary at this stage to exert sufficient force to turn the fetus around. Self-touching is also very common. Fetuses very frequently cover or stroke their faces with their hands. Some bodily sense or proto-self (Damasio 1999) may have already begun to emerge by then. Bodily sense, as will be explained, does not mean any complex form of awareness or even perceiving. Even lowly organisms are capable of fairly complex motions and of withdrawing from or approaching various kind of stimuli. 'Spinal' frogs, whose nervous systems have been transected immediately above the spinal cord and therefore only function at a spinal level, are capable of generating the 'wiping reflex' – a complex sequence of movements to remove a noxious stimulus applied to the skin of their legs (Bizzi et al. 1994). 'Spinal' cats walk (supported) on a treadmill with a nearly normal stepping pattern. If their limbs come into contact with an obstacle they display a 'stumble corrective reaction', allowing their limbs to clear the obstacle (Grillner and Shik 1973; Forssberg 1985; Rossignol et al. 1988). Early fetuses could almost be considered as 'spinal' creatures in the sense that they function mainly at the level of the spinal cord and of the brain stem.[5] Their motor patterns are generated within these structures and modulated by sensory inputs.

However, a 'fusional oceanic merging' possibly never subsists in the human fetus. Twins react to each other's blows almost from the beginning. Mere bodily sense possibly exists from very early on in pregnancy. This would enable the organism to adapt to changing internal and environmental conditions. Later in gestation mere body self could probably evolve into the dawning of a 'core self' (Damasio 1999) or 'perceptual and motor self' (Fuster 1999). These are mere hypotheses. It is not possible to take a 'quantum leap' from observable behavior alone. The early twin fetus, however, may well contribute to clarify the big 'consciousness conundrum' (Horgan 1999) by showing what a young human organism can do and react to without being at all conscious.

FACTS

With various limitations, ultrasounds have given us the unprecedented possibility of studying the spontaneous behavior of the human fetus within its natural environment.[6] Several 'developmental milestones' (Birnholz et al. 1978) have now been established and a wealth of data on fetal sensory-motor development is rapidly accumulating. Nevertheless, twins have generally been neglected by research on prenatal behavioral development. Difficulties in enrolling adequate numbers at comparable gestational ages, and other technical obstacles, probably account for this lack of attention.

Beginnings of intrapair stimulation

Whilst fetal movements start becoming evident between 7–7.5 weeks, intrapair stimulation before the tenth or eleventh week can be considered a fairly exceptional event (Piontelli *et al.* 1997). Twins are usually too distant, the space within their amniotic sacs too big, the membranes dividing these sacs too thick and their movements too weak for them effectively to reach their co-twin. Ideally one would have to observe monoamniotic twins from as soon as fetal motions begin, but they are extremely rare, representing only 1 per cent of all monozygotic pregnancies. Nevertheless intrapair stimulation can occasionally be noted as early as nine weeks. Whether its beginning in humans coincides with the onset of fetal movements still remains an open question.

From 11–13 weeks intrapair stimulation can be observed as a progressively more frequent event in monochorionic twin pregnancies. Presumably the nearness brought about by sharing the same placenta and the thinness of the membranes dividing the two amniotic sacs favour earlier contact.

From 12–13 weeks onwards intrapair stimulation begins to be noted in dichorionic pregnancies as well. This delay can be accounted for by the fact that the separate placentas of dichorionic twins can be implanted in different and quite distant sites. More importantly, perhaps, the membranes dividing the amniotic sacs are considerably thicker, rendering early contact of a sufficient strength fairly improbable (see Figure 3.1).

With advancing gestational age twins grow rapidly in size, with a corresponding increase in the vigour of their movements. This results in a greater likelihood of contact between them. Soon contact becomes inevitable. Growing proportions and increasing strength also lead to 'quickening', commonly at around 18–20 weeks.

By fifteen weeks intrapair stimulation is already a constant and, up to twenty-two weeks, an increasing feature of all twin gestations. From the occasional contacts that could be noticed at ten weeks, reactive movements come to represent almost one-third of all movements by 20–22 weeks. Therefore intrapair stimulation appears to be an important, consistent and unique determinant in the intrauterine behavior of all twins from late first trimester/early mid-gestation. It is also an active and important part of the intrauterine environment of the twin fetus.

Each twin has an influence on its co-twin. In addition to the countless intrauterine environmental factors affecting any fetus, the twin fetus is also influenced by interactions with its co-twin. Mutual influence extends well beyond behavioral aspects and can affect fundamental features of the intrauterine life of twins. However, twins would stand apart from singletons if only for the existence of intrapair stimulation.

By 15–16 weeks the motor repertoire of the fetus may be considered complete (de Vries *et al.* 1982). By then the fetus is capable of performing all the movements that will be found at later gestational ages and at birth (Prechtl 1984). Further maturation of the brain does not mean the introduction of new movements but rather a different organisation or combination of the same (Nijhuis 1999). Despite the dramatic

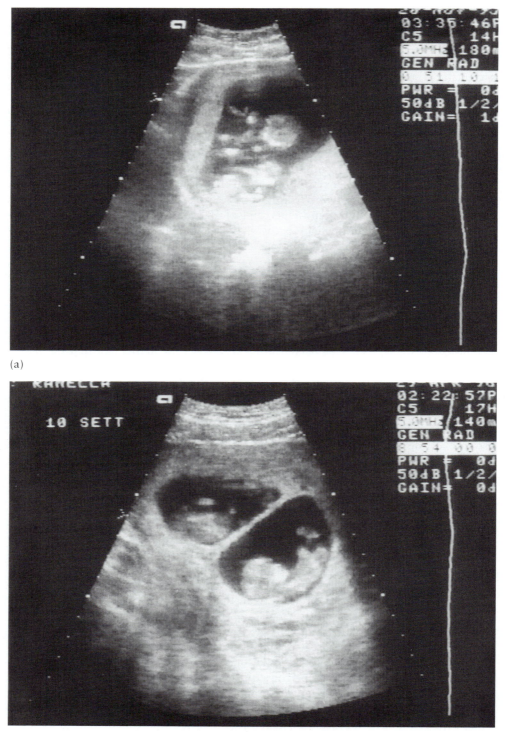

(a)

(b)

environmental changes brought about by parturition, neonatal movements, possibly due to the increased impact of gravity, will only show qualitative changes (Prechtl 1984). However, several quantitative changes take place as gestational age advances (Manning *et al.* 1979; de Vries *et al.* 1984, 1988). The rate of occurrence of hiccups, for instance, declines after thirteen weeks, whilst head movements increase up to nineteen weeks; so-called breathing movements steadily increase throughout gestation only to decrease near parturition (Patrick *et al.* 1980a).

The same variety of movements observed in spontaneous motion (de Vries *et al.* 1984) is also found in responses to intrapair stimulation. No specific stereotyped response is either always or necessarily elicited (Piontelli *et al.* 1999). However, evoked movements also change with advancing gestation. Total responses involving general body movements are observed as almost the only evoked responses up to eleven weeks. From then on an increasing complexity and variability of reactions may be noted. Legs, arms, feet, hands, heads and even buttocks join in. Advancing gestational age, with the increased crowding this entails, may indeed bring about some most bizarre combinations.

Nevertheless, intrapair stimulation does not mean complex interchanges. Sensing, the receiving of information about the external environment, including the environmental component represented by a co-twin, and perceiving, a more complex operation involving interpretation of the sensations to give them meaning, may not coincide in the fetus (Hepper 1992). An early fetus is possibly quite different from a mature one in this respect. An active early fetus may just sense what a mature one can by then perceive.

Fetuses do not live in a state of sensory numbness, nor do they inhabit a stimulus-free environment. Others have demonstrated the functioning *in utero* of such sensory modalities as hearing (Birnholz and Benacerraf 1983; Busnel *et al.* 1986, 1992; Lecanuet *et al.* 1989; Hepper *et al.* 1991), taste (De Snoo 1937; Bradley 1972; Liley 1972; Mistretta and Bradley 1986), smell (Alberts 1981; Pedersen *et al.* 1983; Hepper 1990), vibration (Gagnon 1989), pain (Anand and Hickey 1988; Anand and McGrath 1993; Giannakoulopoulos *et al.* 1994) and temperature (Timor-Tritsch 1986). Possibly only vision (Polishuk *et al.* 1975) and vestibular sensitivity (Visser *et al.* 1983) do not become fully activated until after birth.

Twins can in fact be used as a perfect 'experiment in nature' to demonstrate the functioning of two other sensory modalities which would otherwise be impossible to verify in the fetus within its natural environment. Intrapair stimulation, with responses to touch and pressure originating from the other twin, proves *per se* that so-called tactile and proprioceptive sensitivity (that is, touch and muscular/body sense) are operative *in utero* (Piontelli *et al.* 1997). The simple fact that a reaction is

Figure 3.1 Monochorionic and dichorionic twin pregnancies, 10 weeks gestation

(a) Monochorionic twins. Their single placenta is visible on the left. The septum dividing the two amniotic sacs is extremely thin and barely visible. Discrepancy in fetal size is already evident. The upper twin is considerably bigger than the other. Amniotic fluid is unequally distributed between the sacs, being more abundant in that of the bigger upper twin.

(b) Dichorionic twins. The twins have a fairly equitable intrauterine environment. Two separate placentas are visible at upper left and lower right. The septum is quite thick. Its insertion looks like the Greek letter λ and is hence called the 'lambda sign'. This sign is considered one of the distinctive indications of a dichorionic placenta.

produced in a twin when it is pushed by its co-twin adds to our knowledge of the sensory capacities of all fetuses.

Finally, twins may constitute an important 'experiment in nature' in another respect. From the outset of intrapair stimulation twin fetuses are not always responsive to it. Periods can be noted when they appear to be impervious. During these moments they are clearly stimulated by their co-twin, but their body is passively displaced within the amniotic fluid and they show no response. After being dislodged – often quite far from their original position – they fall back unperturbed into an inactive state. These periods of non-responsivity may well help us to better understand the largely unexplained rest/activity cycles so strikingly dominant during intrauterine life. Rest/activity cycles are not so chaotic and disorganised as commonly thought. The existence of distinctive periods of non-responsivity testifies that these cycles cannot be all lumped together. Precursors of later and differently organised behavioral states could be embedded within them (Piontelli *et al.* 1997). An infant immersed in deep sleep can be quite impervious to any but the strongest stimulation (Wollf 1966, 1973, 1984). Mothers know that gentle shaking may only arouse a comatose infant momentarily. They are also aware that infants need to be sleeping soundly before they can stop rocking and finally put them into their cot. Though several weeks separate these two events a temporarily insensitive twin fetus not responding to the vigorous motions of its co-twin could be linked to the neonate which cannot be aroused from its equally impenetrable, though much deeper and differently organised, state of sleep.

Similarities/differences

Until fairly recently the investigation of aspects of twin behavior *in utero* more properly linked to traditional twin research was limited by the fact that zygosity could only be determined in sets of twins of opposite sex, and hence clearly dizygotic. Modern diagnostic refinements now allow zygosity to be determined reliably *in utero*, even when the placenta is monochorionic (Benacerraf 1998). Prenatal determination of zygosity has allowed twin research to start *in utero*. The possibility of diagnosing monochorionic placentas with a fair degree of accuracy, apart from its primary clinical relevance, has also made it possible to compare the behavior of two populations of twins: monozygotic–monochorionic and opposite-sex dizygotic *in utero*. Though ideally one would eventually like to be able to evaluate the behavior of all types of twins, prenatal uncertainty regarding zygosity would mean observing an enormous population of twin pregnancies. Furthermore, since the majority of monozygotic twins share the same placenta, these are the most representative subgroup of the entire population of monozygotic twins. It may well be that some behavioral characteristics of monozygotic twins found by twin studies are related specifically to this type of twinning.

Intrapair similarities in levels of spontaneous activity and reactivity are initially greater in monozygotic than in dizygotic twins. However, monozygotic twins are never behaviorally identical and show important differences in motor activity from the start. Furthermore, these differences exhibit a tendency to increase progressively with advancing gestation. By 20–22 weeks they have almost reached the same level of diversity as dizygotic twins (Piontelli *et al.* 1999). Rough estimates from after twenty-two weeks seem to indicate that there are no further differences in the amount of activity between monozygotic and dizygotic twin fetuses as they grow older.

Complications, though, may alter these trends. For instance, marked discrepancies in amniotic fluid volume can develop. Due to scarcity of amniotic fluid one twin can become constrained in its movements, whilst the motions of the other may be enhanced by an abundance of liquid. More severe complications can have more dramatic effects and, indeed, some of the most dramatic behavioral differences may be observed in monozygotic twins discordant for particular major malformations.

By the time behavior becomes observable, the fetus is already 7–7.5 weeks old (de Vries *et al.* 1982). Though it may sound like a joke to an adult, a day (and even more so a week) is an enormous amount of time by embryological standards. By the time twins begin to move a lot could have already happened to set them on behaviorally distinct paths. In fact, as explained in Chapter 1, embryology and molecular genetics tell us that monozygotic twins are never identical right from the start (Bomsel-Helmreich and Al Mufti 1995). All this throws a new, less deterministic light on the lives of so-called identical twins. This new knowledge allows space for diversity, even genetic diversity, within apparent homogeneity and identity.

Though we are still far from being able to link overt behavior to molecular events, a chain of enormously complex and largely unpredictable circumstances has already been set in motion to make each twin a unique individual by the time it begins to move.

Behavioral individuality

Fetuses are behaviorally quite independent. They show differing levels of activity, preferential positions, and fairly distinctive favoured movements (Nathanielsz 1992). This is even more evident in twin fetuses, which provide a unique opportunity to observe a fetus and compare its behavior and that of its co-twin simultaneously.

As explained above, monozygotic twins become increasingly different and consistent in macroscopic features such as activity and reactivity levels, indicating clear behavioral autonomy. Nevertheless, when one gets down to analysing individual movements, the larger behavioral differences initially found in the activity and reactivity levels of dizygotic twins are no longer noted. Examined in detail, both monozygotic and dizygotic twins tend to merge together behaviorally and become indistinguishable (Piontelli *et al.* 1999). They also show individual prevailing movements. Some move their legs more, some their arms, some their hands or their heads, some swallow larger quantities of amniotic fluid, some cover their faces almost continuously, others frequently touch their legs, others hang on to their cords. In other words, each fetus, regardless of its zygosity, has its own fairly distinctive way of acting and reacting.

As in life after birth, monozygotic twins may be considered behaviorally alike at a macroscopic level of analysis, but can never be considered identical upon detailed examination (Piontelli 1998). Furthermore, without the interference of the often strikingly similar post-natal appearance of monozygotic twins, dissimilarities in behavior can be observed clearly during prenatal life. All fetuses can only perform certain activities and functions at given gestational ages. However, not even monozygotic twins carry them out in exactly the same way.

Coincidence/non-coincidence of rest–activity cycles

Another means of investigating behavioral difference and autonomy in twin fetuses is to determine whether their rest-activity cycles coincide in time.

From the beginning, variance and autonomy control these factors (Piontelli 1995). Only at 10–11 weeks do rest–activity cycles appear to be slightly more concomitant in monozygotic twins. After then, rapid alternations between turbulent motion and quietness become neither more, nor less coincident than those of dizygotic twins. In all twin fetuses rest–activity cycles are sometimes in phase and sometimes not. In the early stages of pregnancy rest–activity cycles alternate so rapidly that coincidence or disparity are more or less equally likely to occur. With advancing age, as cycles become more defined and clustered, coincidence becomes less pronounced.

A fetus emerging from a rest cycle usually first shows some isolated sign of activity signalling that it is coming out of this phase. A slight movement of one leg, hand or arm, a slight stretch of its head, a clonus or a twitch heralds the change. Quite frequently 'startles', sudden and brisk movements similar to 'jumps' involving the displacement of the entire fetal body, anticipate and precipitate the change.

If some kind of stimulation from one twin reaches the other when motor signs begin to indicate that it is entering into an activity cycle, the change of phase is accelerated. In other words, intrapair stimulation can be regarded as a potential environmental perturbator (Piontelli et al. 1997). Intrapair stimulation can precipitate the entry into an active cycle when a fetus is near a point of change. It has no effect when occurring at a time of stability (Glass and Mackey 1988; Kelso et al. 1986; Thelen and Smith 1994).

The occasional, irregular coincidence of rest–activity cycles in twin fetuses also tells us that an internal autonomous 'clock' regulates each twin. Monozygotic twins have therefore this added element of 'autonomy' and non-identity. This is particularly relevant in the case of those twins who share the same placenta. When monochorionic twins have vascular communications through their common placenta the often serious complications described in Chapter 2 can follow. Furthermore, should one twin die for any reason, the surviving twin is also likely to die. This aspect clearly links the majority of monozygotic twins in terms of life and death during their intrauterine existence. However, paradoxically, this same condition of extreme mutual dependence also demonstrates further behavioral autonomy. Through vascular communications substances could be exchanged between monochorionic twins, theoretically triggering more coincident behavioral cycles. The fact that rest–activity cycles are no more in-phase in monochorionic twins than in dizygotic ones disproves this and further underlines prenatal behavioral individuality and autonomy.

CHAPTER 4

ANTECEDENTS AND FORERUNNERS OF POST-NATAL LIFE

BEGINNINGS OF TEMPERAMENT FORMATION?

Besides showing the beginnings of behavioral diversity, ultrasounds also allow us to catch a glimpse of the dawning of individual dispositions. Albeit in a very rudimentary, embryonic form these tenuous initial inclinations could be considered the first small signs of later, more complex and structured traits. Individual propensities can be discerned in the variety of repeated fetal movement patterns, of preferred postures and activities. Within general broad similarities, each fetus moves differently and has slightly different rhythms, adjustments and clock times. Some are more active than others, some seem to need more startles before showing signs of activity. Some appear more jerky in their movements, and some react more strongly to co-twin stimuli. Some push their legs more, others go back to sitting in the yoga position as soon as they enter into a new cycle of rest. Some constantly rub their eyes, others touch their legs and feet all the time. One may squat, while another may try to turn upside-down. A preference for a particular posture could be favoured both by crowding and by purely structural environmental differences. Inequalities in space may leave one twin unable to lie horizontally, while another may be able to rest more easily in a cephalic version. Though spatial constrictions due to crowding are not relevant when fetal motions first begin, even apparently minor initial environmental variations would appear to prompt differential behavior. The placenta may have a lump or a small gorge. One fetus may roost on the edge of this gorge, while another may just dip its arms in. These diversities are always minute if measured against the environmental variety and complexity of behavior encountered in life after birth. Neither space nor behavioral maturation allows more apparent manifestations. When talking about movement, particularly during the first half of pregnancy, we are normally referring to short cycles of activity of the duration of several seconds rather than the several minutes of a mature fetus or neonate. Nevertheless, even in these initial brief periods of activity some minute differences begin to emerge. Time generally shows that this very tenuous first thread progressively takes on the qualities of a slightly more defined path (Piontelli 1995; Piontelli *et al.* 1999). Defined, however, does not mean definitive. We can speak of tendencies and inclinations perhaps, but clearly not of well-determined characteristics. Furthermore, the preceding chapters have explained how fraught with perils and variations the intrauterine sojourn of twins is. In life after birth an individual may be changed, hardened, softened, or bent by the fortuitous circumstances of life (Plomin and Dunn 1986; Hill-Goldsmith *et al.* 1987; Emde *et al.* 1992; Kagan 1994). It is not difficult, therefore, to imagine how the risks and hazards that crowd in upon the intrauterine life of twins may change and alter what is only a tenuous, unfolding trend. Nevertheless, all twins, including so-called identical twins, emerge from the troubled time of pregnancy as unique individuals with fairly distinct inclinations and behavioral manifestations. Individuality and uniqueness are shaped during gestation and are evident by the time the twins are born.

COMPARING TWO DIFFERENT WORLDS

In the prenatal period the twins' activity and reactivity levels are scrupulously measured and their behavioral patterns are carefully classified and quantified. All these procedures can then be compared with similar behavioral parameters after birth. Often continuity is found to exist. The less active twin frequently remains less active, the more reactive continues to be so, and vice versa (Piontelli *et al.* 1999).

However, the basic difficulty remains of comparing two different environments, each with its own particular demands. Although many prenatal functions progressively anticipate post-natal ones, some are uniquely adapted to the particular circumstances of intrauterine life (Kagan *et al.* 1978; Oppenheim 1981, 1984).

When classifying prenatal activity we may be measuring a different category from that pertaining to post-natal life. Activity means something before birth, and something else after. Except, perhaps, for brief periods during the later stages of pregnancy, prenatal activity is more akin to deep sleep than to wakefulness. After all, while they are sleeping babies continue to be active and to toss and turn.

On the other hand, reactivity is not only more consistent – the more reactive twin fetus tends to remain more reactive than the other throughout pregnancy – but could possibly also express a true initial disposition. After birth reactive twins continue to display a lower threshold towards stimuli of various kinds. 'Torpid' twins remain so, 'jittery' ones remain jittery, and easily 'excited' ones retain their initial characteristic (Piontelli 2000).

Enormous methodological problems remain, however. To mention but one, it is impossible to reproduce and classify the kicks and knocks of highly unruly twins in an active state. Some blows may be hard, others quite weak. How do we establish where the threshold to stimulation lies? Some twins may be reactive to the slightest touch, others may require violent blows. Twins *in utero* are not in neat and orderly laboratories. It may be impossible to convincingly demonstrate that the reactivity of undisciplined twins *in utero* begins to represent an inclination. However, this unique aspect of twins' intrauterine behavior warrants particular attention and may, hopefully, stimulate further research.

Other aspects of the intrauterine behavior of the twin fetus may be less relevant. Besides its constrictions and different physical requirements the intrauterine milieu is devoid of social exchanges, and is meant to be so. Although the fetus is rapidly and progressively preparing to enter into a social world, this prelude is geared towards the different stimuli and the more 'mature' human beings that it will come into contact with in the external environment. Fetuses are not equipped for complex social interactions with other fetuses. Twins are no exception to this. Though they happen to share the same prenatal habitat, they cannot be considered as already living in society. Prenatal life can have fundamental consequences, including social ones, on the later lives of all twins. Complex human interchanges, however, are alien to it.

This does not mean that a fetus is not already a unique human being long before emerging from its first habitat. It may help us to avoid excessive flights of fantasy if we remember that the fetus is uniquely adapted to its intrauterine milieu and is only gradually being prepared to enter into a wider, different and truly social world. Recognising that the intrauterine environment is not neutral, but favours and shapes individual differences, may further encourage us to look at so-called identical twins as behaviorally distinct and unique human beings from the start.

MATERNAL PERCEPTIONS DURING PREGNANCY

Until fairly recently twins were often a surprise pertaining to the delivery room. Nowadays a mother may know that she is expecting twins as early as her sixth week of pregnancy. Ultrasounds have clearly meant that maternal (and paternal) awareness of fetal life now comes much earlier than before. They have also brought forward prenatal attachment to a much earlier gestational age, as well as greatly enhancing it (Campbell *et al.* 1982; Kemp and Page 1987; Langer *et al.* 1988; Villeneuve *et al.* 1987; Heidrich and Cranley 1989). 'Quickening' has in fact lost much of its formerly emotionally charged quality. However, from around mid-gestation, when it normally begins, direct maternal perceptions start to play an ever-increasing part in the discrimination of differential movements (Lerum *et al.* 1989). As crowding increases and the consequent spatial arrangements of the twins become even more complex many mothers cannot tell which is which, but some report differences in the perceived movements of their twin fetuses. Maternal perceptions can at times be very accurate. They become extremely accurate when more serious matters are at stake. Alarm at changes in the perceived movements of their twins can often be tragically justified. When it comes to judging behavioral–temperamental intrapair differences, however, matters become more complicated. Some mothers, particularly those who have been told that they are expecting monozygotic twins, seem to be constantly on the lookout for differences between them. Their traditional image of 'identical' twins seems to make them fear that they won't be able to tell one twin from the other. Ultrasounds, with their grey tones and visual enhancement of particular tissues, bring out individual appearance only slightly more than an ordinary X-ray picture would. On the other hand, modern equipment reveals many developmental differences. Size and growth of the twins may be quite discordant, their amniotic fluid may be unequally distributed, and their blood-flows may announce asymmetrical suffering – to mention but a few of the more obvious.

Frequently a split between a 'good' and a 'bad' twin is already determined *in utero*. The bigger twin is sometimes ascribed bloodsucker qualities. The one moving freely in its abundant fluid may be regarded as the lucky one enjoying a more comfortable and freer life. The more active twin may be regarded as more 'intelligent' or as a 'pain in the neck'. The more reactive may be considered quarrelsome or more sensitive. Most mothers not only look for behavioral differences but also often tend to polarise them. This is occasionally reflected in the choice of names. The latest soap operas on the television are a common source of inspiration. However, one also hears more classically evil or outlandish names such as Cain, Morgana or Pantagruel. The less-favoured co-twin often becomes the bearer of a saint's name or one implying innocence, such as Abel, Ophelia or Bernadette. This splitting and heightening of differences particularly applies with monozygotic twins. However, male–female pairs are not immune to a kind of early 'sexing'. Females are frequently attributed flirtatious, seductive intentions and can be referred to as fetal Lolitas or Emmanuelles. Equally, boys get ascribed 'macho' qualities ranging from athletic dispositions to super-stud inclinations possibly to some extent due to the physiologically disproportionate size of their genitals during the fetal stage. On the other hand, some prospective parents seem to want to erase any differences whatsoever between their twins, effectively 'twinning' them from before birth. This, again, is often reflected in the choice of names, which in these cases may be confusingly similar.

Nevertheless, the temptation of 'twinning' the children is largely a post-natal phenomenon. The vast majority of these prenatal preconceptions will be renegotiated at birth. A few, however, will not. Contrary to the newborn baby, the fetus is only a passive participant in the interchanges taking place around it. The neonate will bring with it the impact of the visual dimension connected to its aspect. It will also bring with it its initial temperamental endowment (Kagan 1994) and its ability to sustain, initiate, reject and modulate social interchanges (Richards 1974; Papousek and Papousek 1975; Murray and Trevarthen 1986). In other words, whilst the neonate has a direct impact on its caregivers, the fetus does not. They are free to inscribe their thoughts, worries, fantasies and desires upon it as if it were a blank page waiting to be written upon.

MATERNAL EMOTIONS DURING PREGNANCY: BREAKING THE NEWS

When mothers are told that they are expecting twins their reactions can be very different (Bryan 1992; Noble 1995). Some are elated, some may want to abort, some may say that they had dreamt about having twins just the night before. The reaction to the news is very different according to family circumstances (Spillman 1985). Twins may be the result of a long and costly struggle to become pregnant. They may be an unplanned addition to a family which already has children. They may be accepted with resignation in a family with strong religious convictions. Usually twins born to couples with fertility problems are regarded as a blessing (Macfarlane *et al.* 1990) and their arrival is frequently over-idealised. Couples with no other children are also generally thrilled. Mothers often feel 'special' and fathers very proud. The reaction to the gender of the twins can also be quite different. Although most parents prefer a male–female pair, this being seen as a 'once-and-for-all' solution, some may wish to have just males or just females. The past history of both parents plays a significant role in this. Once gender is known (normally not before 15–20 weeks), most parents adapt quite well to reality. Overtly they frequently maintain that as long as the twins are healthy, their sex doesn't matter. However, in reality, sex may not be quite so irrelevant. When mothers come for the so-called morphologic scan, performed at around twenty weeks (the best time for detecting possible malformations), often the first thing they ask is whether it is possible to know the sex of their twins. Their disappointment is frequently quite great when one or both twins just won't open their legs. Whether they are expecting two boys, two girls, or a boy and a girl often seems more important than being told that their hearts and spines appear to be all right. Only a few parents want to have a surprise and put off knowing whether they are boys or girls until the delivery.

Changing emotions

Maternal emotions vary throughout according to the various stages of pregnancy (Leifer 1977; Reading *et al.* 1984; Birksted-Breen 1981, 1986; Raphael-Leff 1991, 1996; Stern and Bruschweiler-Stern 1998). Initially they range from simple acceptance to sheer elation. As described, elation prevails in childless couples, whether they have had fertility problems or not. Anxiety for the well-being of the twins is present from the very beginning in all parents, but particularly in those who have had to undergo various forms of assisted reproduction (Mazor and Simons 1984; Liebmann-Smith 1987; Williams 1988; Newton 1990). These have often had lengthy counselling beforehand and clearly know that their initial success may well end in failure. They are enormously relieved when the risk of early pregnancy loss is past. However, a strong sense of anxiety usually accompanies them throughout the pregnancy. With advancing gestation all mothers realise that their pregnancy is not so simple for the twins; they also begin to fear for their own personal health. At around 24–25 weeks their bellies start to reach increasingly huge proportions. Discomfort is normally considerable. Often their companions look at them with a mixture of disbelief, apprehension and embarrassment. As term approaches many women begin to voice the hope that the twins will be delivered early so as to alleviate their suffering. When reminded about pulmonary maturity, most somewhat unwillingly resign themselves to what they call their 'martyrdom'. The delivery itself also becomes the centre of their worries. Strangely, many mothers insist that they would like to have a Caesarean. No amount of explanation seems to convince them that a double delivery does not mean double suffering or a prolonged labour. Quite often, however, the twins then make the 'choice' themselves, by both being in an unfavourable presentation.

Suspended emotions and fetal death

Inevitably, from the moment they are given the news, parents begin to regard themselves as the mothers and fathers of twins. Even the most reluctant soon begin to cherish the reality of having two infants (Spillman 1985).

Things are generally more complex for those women expecting monochorionic–monozygotic twins. Once the various risks entailed in this type of pregnancy begin to sink in, some mothers seem reluctant to form too strong a bond with their twins. They withhold from rejoicing, fantasising or making future plans in the all-too-vain hope of escaping potential agonising pain should something go wrong. These women often postpone making preparations even though they are at an increased risk of premature delivery. Names are only decided upon very near term. Shopping for prams, baby bouncers and baby clothes is often delayed for as long as possible – sometimes until the twins are safely born. The thought of going back empty-handed to a home all prepared for the two newcomers is too intolerable for them to even contemplate.

The despair of mothers when something does go seriously wrong makes us realise how superficial and illusory such seeming detachment actually is (Piontelli 2000).

It is often difficult for mothers to accept the elusive, uncontrollable reality of intrauterine life. Pregnancy is frequently experienced as the gift of life par excellence, an exclusively life-giving condition and therefore essentially death-free. Many women seem to hang on to the illusion that they have the power to change the pre-natal fate of their infants. Though this clearly belongs to mystical realms, the deceptive fantasy of protecting the unborn with one's body often contributes to make gestation a particularly blissful state.

When something does go wrong, mothers are frequently completely taken aback. Many feel guilty about not having immediately taken to their beds. Could this have prevented prematurity? Others blame themselves for not 'eating for two'. Surely this could have favoured a more satisfactory growth of the twins. Still others, when told of an excess of amniotic fluid in one or both sacs, ask if this is the result of their having drunk so much liquid in order to prevent constipation or cystitis. Most women are quite surprised to hear that the amount of amniotic fluid or the prevention of prematurity are way beyond their control. The fact of not being able to shield one's children from the moment of conception is hard to accept.

Any fetal death, particularly after mid-gestation, can be a devastating blow (Bourne 1968; Lewis 1976; Kirk 1984; Leon 1986; Zeanah 1989; Friedman and Gradstein 1992; Gilbert and Smart 1992). The physical union of pregnancy inclines most women to experience fetal death as a very intense loss. However, the death of one or both twin fetuses is particularly distressing (Bryan 1992; Woodward 1998; Piontelli 2000).

After one twin dies the apprehension for the other holds no bounds. In addition, the survivor will often continue to be regarded as a twin, especially by the mother. The death of one of the twins poses special problems in monochorionic pregnancies. As explained before, such a demise often leads to the death of the other twin due to the vascular placental communications between the twins. Should one twin survive, the risks of neurological compromise are high. Sometimes neurological damage quickly becomes evident in macroscopic structural alterations of brain tissues and components. This is not always so, however. Unfortunately, an apparently intact brain is no absolute guarantee of a positive outcome later on. Anxiety will continue to pervade the lives of such parents for many months, and, indeed, sometimes for years, after the birth of the survivor.

Should both twins die certain feelings are the same as those experienced in any fetal demise. For instance, going through the delivery and all the physical pain connected with it only to give birth to death is seen as a particularly cruel trick of fate. As a mother whose twins had died the day before the delivery was programmed to take place said: 'I feel like a grave. Please spare me all this useless pain!'

Besides the suffering inherent in any fetal loss, women whose twins die *in utero* are exposed to unique facets of desolation. Twin pregnancies are generally a very public event, being easily discernible not only to relatives, friends and colleagues but also to shopkeepers and other casual acquaintances. Everyone knows and constantly asks how it's going and share some witticism. Having to explain death is particularly loathsome after all the excitement (Rizzardo *et al.* 1985). One woman declared, 'Passing from this hubbub to an embarrassed silence is very harsh.'

Furthermore, women expecting twins are particularly liable to continue carrying the signs of pregnancy after delivery. Leaking breasts and protruding bellies are then experienced as a cruel and sterile joke.

In addition, these women know that the chances of having another twin pregnancy are generally low – practically nil in the case of monozygotic twins. This 'exceptional' event will probably never happen again. Should they conceive again it will be just an 'ordinary' pregnancy. Changing status can in itself be a blow.

A few polaroids from the ultrasounds are generally the only enduring evidence of the 'exceptional' event which crossed their lives. In some cases giving birth to twins can be felt as 'the event' of an otherwise obscure and inconspicuous existence.

Impact of maternal emotions on the fetus

Before dealing directly with the possible impact of maternal emotions on the twin fetus a few words about the impact of maternal emotions on all fetuses may be opportune. It is not possible here to review all the growing literature on this controversial topic and interested readers should refer to the reviews of Ferreira (1965) and Carlson and Labarba (1979), and to the critical evaluations of Joffe (1978), Wolkind (1981), Reading (1983), Istvan (1986) and Van den Bergh (1992).

The creed that maternal emotions can influence the well-being of the fetus and its future development is age-old and universally widespread. Since ancient times maternal fantasies and emotions have been regarded as moulders of fetal temperament and health. For centuries women were told to think solely of their husbands during intercourse or they would have babies resembling their lovers instead of their legitimate spouses. Equally they were encouraged to satisfy even their most bizarre cravings during pregnancy or risk the birth of deranged and deformed infants. It is doubtful if any women still really believe that strawberry marks are due to an unfulfilled desire for the fruit of that name. It is true, on the other hand, that only too many mothers continue to worry that they may be hurting their children by worrying about them.

The study of the impact of maternal emotions on the behavior of the fetus is fraught with enormous and, for the moment, probably insurmountable methodological problems (Van Den Bergh *et al.* 1989; Van Den Bergh 1992).

Our knowledge of the physical substrata of emotions, for example, is still limited (Kopin *et al.* 1989; McNaughton 1989). Our understanding of placental crossing is also limited, and that of the mechanisms regulating fetal behavior is virtually nil

(Dawes 1984, 1986; Prechtl 1981). In addition, the overwhelming majority of the experimental information available necessarily comes from animal studies with all the difficulties of extrapolating these to man (Joffe 1978; Moyer *et al.* 1978; Peters 1984, 1986).

All fetuses are linked to maternal physiology. Constantly fluctuating states of mind continuously produce changes in the maternal substratum that can, in the end, reverberate on the fetus. In this sense all maternal emotions could have an impact on the fetus. However, maternal emotions are generally regarded as fairly fixed. Furthermore, certain emotional states such as anxiety or maternal daydreaming are often privileged over others. Besides changing moods, mothers have circadian and ultradian rhythms. The first recur in cycles of twenty-four hours, while the latter are more frequent. For instance they sleep, display fluctuations of uterine contractility or of glucose and circulating hormones, such as cortisol (Arduini *et al.* 1986, 1987), estriol and melathonin at certain times of day or night (Roberts *et al.* 1978; Patrick *et al.* 1980a, 1980b, 1982). Since the physical substrate of emotions is still largely unclear, how can we, for example, distinguish between fluctuations occurring normally and variations due solely to emotions?

In addition, the placenta has important endocrine functions, and there is a continuous exchange between placenta and fetus (Jones 1988, 1989). Placental metabolism effectively provides a barrier to maternal catecholamines, as it does for a range of other substances (Jones 1993). The placenta filters the components sent to the fetus, shielding it from, amongst others, maternal 'stressors'. There is convincing evidence that most maternally released catecholamines, generally considered the most important 'stressors', do not cross the placental barrier (Saarikoski 1974; Kittinger 1974; Artal 1980). Interestingly, contrary to catecholamines, melathonin rapidly crosses the placenta and possibly conveys information about various maternal and fetal endocrine rhythms and synchronises the light–dark cycle, thus possibly preparing the fetal circadian system to meet the prevailing post-natal environmental photoperiod (Longo and Yellon 1988).

Catecholamines are autonomously produced and released into its circulation by the fetus (Jones *et al.* 1989). Fetal adrenal secretions are especially important for lung maturation and for setting off labour. Catecholamines have also been demonstrated to play key roles both in the fetus and in the neonate in the adaptation of the organism to extrauterine life (Slotkin and Seidler 1989). A release of 'stressors' into the fetal circulation near delivery is responsible for the acute cardiovascular, respiratory and metabolic responses which are all necessary to survive birth. In fact, fetuses have enormous adrenals. At term a human fetal adrenal weighs almost as much as an adult's and is twenty-five times larger relative to body weight. The so-called fetal zone – a large component of the fetal adrenal gland – undergoes rapid involution immediately after birth (Casey and MacDonald 1993). Fetal metabolism is active in other ways too. Not all elements reaching the fetus do so in an unmodified form. Many are broken down, changed, or removed by the fetus itself to suit its needs. The fetal liver also plays an important role during prenatal life in removing maternal hormones (and other substances) before they enter fetal arteries (Moll 1988).

Nor are the fetus and placenta passive in coping with the effects of reduced uteroplacental bloodflow. For instance, in the case of pregnancy induced or chronic hypertension a protective chain reaction is set in motion (Jones 1986).

A distinction should also be made between the ordinary anxieties accompanying our daily lives and the acute, intense anxieties connected with particularly stressful, shocking events. Though some authors have described increased fetal activity in the presence of maternal anxiety (Lederman *et al.* 1978, 1979, 1981; Carlson and Labarba 1979; Ianniruberto and Tajani 1981; Talbert *et al.* 1982; Benson *et al.* 1987), it is automatically confused with fetal anxiety and therefore regarded as detrimental. As pointed out earlier, fetal activity is possibly a condition more akin to sleep and therefore not analogous to anxiety-driven hyperactivity states after birth. Furthermore, increased fetal activity may not be detrimental at all. Even assuming it were, it might be so only during certain stages of pregnancy and not others. Fetal activity may have different functions at different gestational ages.

Even these few simple facts illustrate that the feto-maternal unit is far from being a simple one-way system whereby the mother merely pours anything and everything into the fetus. This popular misconception is yet another version of the *tabula rasa* myth.

Too many questions regarding the impact of maternal emotions upon the fetus remain open-ended, and until we can answer many of the basic ones we'll be unable to produce any convincing or conclusive evidence of the impact of these emotions upon the fetus. This topic clearly warrants further investigation, even though such evidence may take a long time to acquire.

Maternal emotions and the twin fetus

Twins have been thought of as a possible 'ideal model' or yet another 'experiment in nature' to appraise the impact of maternal emotions on the fetus (Arabin *et al.* 1995). According to this model, if both twins are equally and systematically affected by the same maternal emotion or by the same by-product of an emotion, this proves *per se* that the alteration has been caused by the emotion.

Furthermore, twin pregnancies are highly subject to complications leading to alterations which have been postulated as possible mediators of maternal emotions. Again, the underlying assumption is that twins inhabit and share exactly the same intrauterine environment. Even assuming that maternal 'stressors', of whatever origin and kind, can reach the fetus, twin fetuses would only receive the same quality, but never the same quantity, of such substances.

Pregnancy induced hypertension is quite frequent in twin pregnancies. This is not known to have any causal relation to maternal anxiety. The opposite may well be true. Furthermore, pregnancy induced hypertension does not affect both twins in the same way. Twin fetuses have different umbilical cords as well as an unequal distribution of placental mass. At the very least, then, they have differing bloodflows.

Uterine contractility is particularly elevated in twin gestations. Uterine contractions as a result of maternal anxiety and stress have been postulated to increase fetal motion by applying pressure on the amniotic sac. Increased tension would be perceived as disruptive by the fetus, which would then start to move more. However, even assuming that this 'increased pressure' hypothesis were true, the vast majority of twins are contained in separate amniotic sacs; also, the amniotic fluid is unequally distributed between the two. Additional pressure on sacs which are different from each other may well act differently on each twin.

Twins are hardly an 'ideal model' for research on the impact of maternal emotions on the fetus.

Twin gestations, due to the various complications associated with them, are anxiety-provoking pregnancies. High-risk monochorionic pregnancies are filled with even greater apprehension. Until there is conclusive evidence demonstrating that maternal emotions could be potentially harmful to the fetus, already overanxious mothers of twins should be spared the additional burden of having to try to suppress their often uncontrollable emotions. Exercises to combat stress such as listening to Mozart or undergoing exotic forms of massage, whilst pleasurable in themselves, may do nothing to guarantee the future happiness and well-being of their twins.

PATERNAL EMOTIONS

Fathers of twins usually get pushed into parenthood sooner and harder than fathers of singletons. Once the initial elation (or dismay) has passed, many follow their companions closely during their frequent check-ups. This would have been unusual even only a few years ago, but is now virtually the norm. The visual dimension of ultrasounds allows fathers to participate more in the pregnancy (Weaver and Cranley 1983; Stainton 1985; Mercer *et al.* 1988). In an ordinary singleton gestation there may well be no more than two or three ultrasound examinations. For twins frequent scans are the rule. In some extreme circumstances twins may even be scanned daily. This clearly has an impact on fathers as well. Some simply stay in the background. They may hold their companion's hand, look at the screen, and ask a few questions, but otherwise they do not intervene very much. Others, however, want to hog the limelight. They ask all the questions. They stand next to the obstetrician during the examination and keep pointing at the screen. They demand precise statistics and impossible explanations. Some even go as far as talking about their own aches and pains. Nevertheless, with advancing gestation all fathers-to-be seem to be overwhelmed – if only by the sheer dimensions of their companions. Furthermore, if any complications set in most feel guilty, tired, confused or unnerved. Initial states of bliss and intense feelings of pride soon cease and many fathers, perhaps quite rightly, begin to fear that a series of uncontrollable changes are starting to take over their lives.

LONGING AND LOSS IN THE TWIN FETUS

The tragic event of fetal loss always has a deep impact on parents. The blow hits them differently according to gestational age and the circumstances that cause it.

This brings us to the question of when and how a twin fetus could 'long for' the presence of the other in cases of prenatal death. So far we have only anecdotal evidence of this, mainly from children or adults reporting a sense of loss which they can only explain in terms of a yearning for reunion with their dead co-twin fetus (Woodward 1998). However, in such cases it is impossible to ascertain how much of this longing is derived from real recollections of the sensations felt *in utero* and how much is the result of later constructions belonging to post-natal life alone. The yearning for a double, an ideal companion who understands us even without words, is fairly universal amongst adults and children alike. The abundance of 'doubles' in mythology and literature down through the ages testifies to this universal desire. In addition, it is not difficult to imagine how the parents' terrible sense of loss could be transmitted to the surviving twin. Here again we ought to make a distinction about the time and the circumstances in which such a loss occurs. Much has been made about the so-called 'vanishing twin' phenomenon (Landy *et al.* 1986), the not infrequent finding of another gestational sac during an early first-trimester scan. It is hard to imagine that an early fetus could 'miss' something that it has never felt. Intrapair stimulation usually only starts when such a 'vanishing twin' would have already ceased to exist.

A later fetal loss, whether spontaneous or by choice, is quite a different matter for a mother (Bryan 1989, 1994; Bryan and Higgins 1995). By 'choice' one means selective fetocide and fetal reduction, the procedures by which a malformed or genetically compromised twin fetus is selectively terminated (selective fetocide), or a higher multiple gestation is reduced to just twins (fetal reduction) in order to give the remaining fetuses a better chance of survival. Fetal reduction evokes a giddy sense of randomness and precariousness in all those involved. It is almost always perceived by parents (and by those performing it) as a cruel kind of 'Russian roulette'. No matter how rationally this painful decision is made, a sense of agonising guilt persists. It gives each and everyone the feeling that he or she is a near miss, a product of pure chance, that had our parents simply made love on a different day we may not have existed at all. Any fetal loss, however, as described above, is always a deep wound once the parents have got used to the idea of twins. When it occurs near term it is often devastating. Nevertheless, only when intrapair stimulation has become a consistent feature of the intrauterine environment can one postulate that a surviving twin might feel some kind of sense of 'loss'. This sentiment could presumably increase in intensity with advancing gestational age as fetal crowding renders regular contact inevitable. In any case, one should not forget that the overwhelming majority of twins are separated by a 'septum'. Therefore what a twin fetus might 'miss' would clearly not be a whole, distinct person, but just the stimulation, however strong, arising from the other twin (Piontelli 1999). Though intrapair stimulation is certainly an important factor in the intrauterine life of twins, the evidence is far too scanty and unconvincing, for the time being at least, to allow us to judge whether it remains forever embedded in the unconscious of a surviving twin.

CHAPTER 5

STILL IN HOSPITAL: BIRTH AND SOON AFTER BIRTH

BIRTH

Delivery route

In Chapter 2 we saw that twins are usually born earlier and smaller than most singletons. Pregnancy is considered to be complete three weeks earlier, but many twins are born even before this term.

Those twins who finally reach delivery are frequently at risk due to an anomalous presentation (Keith *et al.* 1995; Chauhan and Roberts 1996). Labour in itself is not more prolonged for twins, but only in 40 per cent of cases will both fetuses be in the favourable vertex presentation (Chervenak 1995). However, not even both twins in the vertex position is an absolute guarantee of delivery without complications. When the first twin is born the second is suddenly confronted with a hugely increased amount of space. Therefore it can easily turn round, sometimes rendering a spontaneous delivery impossible.

Presentations which are less favourable than vertex lead to an increased incidence of instrumental deliveries and Caesareans (Chauhan and Roberts 1996). Many twins are Caesarean births (Cetrulo 1986; Acker and Sachs 1989; Fleming *et al.* 1990). Besides presentation the mode of delivery is also determined by estimated birth-weight. Ultrasound measurement of several anatomical parameters provides a fairly accurate prediction of fetal weight. If this is assessed to be too low, or if a sponta-neous premature delivery starts, a Caesarean is usually performed in order to avoid potential risks. If prematurity is not an issue, provided that the first presenting twin is in the vertex position, there is no absolute impediment to a spontaneous delivery. However, once the first twin is born the second may show signs of acute intrauterine suffering.

Though nowadays more obstetricians, aware of the problem of an excessive use of Caesarean deliveries, suggest a natural birth it is often the mothers themselves who refuse this option. Nothing can convince them that a Caesarean is more painful once the effects of the anaesthetic have worn off or that post-operative pains are going to last for a long time. Apart from plain fear, however, for most mothers the thought of enduring all the pains of labour for the first twin, whilst there is the risk, albeit remote, of a subsequent Caesarean for the second, is all too appalling to consider. Therefore, despite continued efforts to make the birth of twins a more natural event (Chevernak 1986; Rabinovitch *et al.* 1987), many mothers end up on the operating table.

Unequal risks

Unequal risks do not cease during delivery. Though the inequality between first-born and second-born twins is now much less than it used to be, thanks to better fetal monitoring, hazards are still greater for the second (MacGillivray and Campbell 1988). Second-born twins are more likely to suffer from anoxia and the various complications linked to malpresentation, to suffer from respiratory problems, to be intubated, and to need resuscitation (Prins 1994; Monteagudo *et al.* 1998). In addition, if the first cord is not properly clamped massive haemorrhaging of the second twin can occur.

Twins and their parents often attribute a relevance to birth order long after the event of birth. They may well be right. Few twins like to be the second-born (Hay and O'Brien 1987). When they can finally speak many refer to birth order as a higher or lower status. However, this does not mean that the second born is 'younger' than its co-twin.

A well-planned event

Though twins can be born without warning, in the vast majority of cases their delivery is a carefully programmed event. Contrary to singletons, it is not customary to simply let nature run its course. Several weeks before reaching term most mothers have already been visited by an anaesthetist and undergone various tests. The neonatologists and the staff of the delivery unit have been warned. Mothers have been instructed what to do in case of an emergency and have been told to have their suitcase ready. The well-being of the twins is closely monitored by frequent scans and Doppler blood flows. Apart from the close supervision of maternal and fetal health, all this planning also serves to ensure that an appropriate team will be present during the delivery.

Mothers

By the end of pregnancy many mothers are stretched to their limits of physical and mental endurance. A few even seem past caring about their children and just beg to get it all over and done with. Their abdomens are enormous, rendering even the simple tasks of bending or sitting up an ordeal. Sleeping, eating, even breathing may become an affliction. Their legs are often enormously swollen. They suffer from backache. 'Frequency' is the norm. Haemorrhoids cause them embarrassment and their overworked livers and over-stretched skins may provoke a constant itchiness. Even the most resilient or robust, and those who have had fairly uncomplicated pregnancies, are inevitably and understandably exhausted. Several, however – most frequently mothers of monozygotic twins – may have had to spend days, weeks or even months in hospital. Whilst this may be reassuring on the one hand, as the health of mother and twins is carefully monitored, most find hospitalisation quite unpleasant. Lack of privacy, loneliness, the need for emotional support, concern for any young children left at home, dismay about their appearance, and so on, all contribute to make their stay a depressing experience. In addition, although the hospital is a huge structure, it is a comparatively small community. Rumours, especially of tragedies, travel fast. All pregnant women, but particularly those expecting twins, seem to attract a host of those people who enjoy going into every possible minute detail of all the complications of their personal obstetric horror stories. Often these chronicles extend to the histories of friends, neighbours and ancestors. Being submitted to these accounts of frightful events, as well as to the grim reports coming from the NICU itself, greatly increases the anxiety which already assails these women.

When the great day finally arrives mothers are both relieved and terrified. Some women choose to have general anaesthesia and to be unconscious throughout the entire event. More and more, however, now ask to have an epidural. An epidural is also often administered to those who are attempting a natural delivery (Rolbin and Hew 1991). Muscular relaxation favours the expulsion of the second twin. Furthermore, pre-existent anaesthesia can speed up the process in the event of an emergency Caesarean having to be performed.

A public event

No matter how the twins are finally delivered all mothers (and fathers) are quite shocked by the sheer number of personnel attending birth. In an operating theatre at least two surgeons, two anaesthetists, two neonatologists and several assistants and attendants will be present. Mothers may be quite disoriented by all the commotion around them. Even those lucky few that have a natural delivery can hardly be said to be alone. If they had anticipated birth as an idyllic event infused with poetry, soft music and dim lights, they are immediately thrown into the tumultuous reality of noisy monitoring equipment, frequent internal inspections, repeated palpations and vociferous orders and comments.

Mrs C was one of the lucky few in the sample who did not have to undergo a Caesarean. However, she had been hospitalised before term and an induced delivery had been carefully planned. She was not a fan of light music. At her young age Death Metal Music (a world in which Marilyn Manson is considered pop) was more to her liking. Her general philosophy of life was suffused with a mixture of Zen, holistic medicine and New Age. Being a strong believer in the influence of maternal emotions and experiences upon the fetus, she spent her time whilst hospitalised dancing up and down the ward to the tune of the heaviest music possible on her Walkman. If her twins could learn anything from her before birth this, she thought, would be the way. The great day arrived and she was taken to the delivery room with her Walkman still going full blast. To begin with, notwithstanding the music, everything was peaceful in the room. Her equally young husband sat next to her alternating between holding her hand firmly and massaging her huge belly with Ayurvedic oils. Despite all warnings, they both looked confident and determined to make theirs a very natural delivery. Mr C had even brought some exotic incense with him that was meant to imprint the first olfactory experiences of the twins. As soon as the first contractions started a large crowd began to gather. First two midwives, then two obstetricians and an anaesthetist and finally neonatologists, a resuscitator and various specialist nurses appeared. In the end there were fifteen hospital staff in attendance. Mr C tried to remonstrate, but he was soon brushed aside and left mumbling angrily 'Twenty people all looking inside my wife's vagina!' By now Mrs C was wincing with pain. She soon forgot her resolution to imprint the twins with modern music and good smells. She threw her Walkman aside and began to swear like a trooper. Each member of staff was the butt of insults like 'You rapist! You filthy swine! You must be dirty minded and depraved! Keep your sordid hands off me!', and many much worse. Mrs C was later to recollect the whole experience as a very shocking one. When her twins turned out to be pretty riotous, she often mentioned their delivery as a possible determinant of their unruly behavior. More to the point, however, she swore never to give birth to a child again.

It is also true that few mothers get a chance to have a proper look at their twins on the day they are born; even fewer can experience the pleasure of attaching one or both infants to their breast. The twins are mostly whisked away and handed over to the neonatologists as soon as the delivery is over. After initial post-delivery care, most twins are transferred directly to the NICU. Some will only undergo a short 24-hour period of observation before being moved to the nursery. Others may spend months there (Papiernick 1991). Therefore, once the ordeal of delivery is over, most mothers are left to worry about the health of their twins. No amount of reassurance seems adequate until they have actually seen and preferably touched and carefully inspected them. The first contact with the twins can therefore be delayed by one or more days as the children are in the NICU and the mothers are still recovering from their Caesareans. When the moment finally arrives, most mothers show a very physical reaction to the sight and handling of their twins. They touch them, carefully explore the minutest details of their bodies. They kiss and smell them. Most are very moved and tearful. Many, however, look worried about the apparent fragility of the twins.

Fathers

Fathers are frequently left out from the entire commotion. If the mother has to undergo a Caesarean, they have to wait outside the operating theatre. The number of personnel coming and going from the theatre usually alarms them. Most fathers look worried, awkward and pale. Only a few seem elated and make repeated phone calls announcing the news to all and sundry.

Generally, the majority of those whose partners deliver spontaneously are present at childbirth. These, too, look awkward and ashen, overwhelmed by the magnitude of the event. They all seem totally unprepared for the mother's cries and moans or the sight of amniotic fluid, blood and other organic substances flooding out of their widespread legs. A few exceptions have the opposite reaction and try to act as if they were in charge, often nagging doctors and nurses with frequent questions and occasional unkind remarks. Some even seem to enter into competition with their companions. They lament sudden pains and try (without success) to divert all the attention onto themselves.

Most fathers get to see the twins before the mother does as she is usually still unconscious or being stitched up or suffering further contractions in order to expel the placental mass.

Resuscitation of the twins is usually over by the time their fathers are admitted into the room where the babies are first taken care of. To begin with most of them stand in a corner quite inhibited by all the commotion around the twins. The mere appearance of the infants seems to disconcert them. The twins do not resemble the traditional image of chubby, rosy, soft, clean and powdered tender miniature cherubs. Many look more like miniature old men with their frail, bony aspect, wrinkled faces and translucent skin. Several, given their prematurity, are still covered by fine dark hair, making them look like small primates. They are also covered by a fairly heavy coat of blood-streaked *vernix caseosa*[1] and their umbilical cords, although clamped, may still be hanging from their tummies. It is only once the twins have been cleaned, bathed and massaged with oil that fathers generally dare look at them. Many comment on the remarkable differences in their aspect. Even simple crowding and slight weight discrepancies usually render most 'identical' twins quite dissimilar at birth (see Figure 5.1). The attention of most fathers then shifts to birthweight. When asked the names of the children most take a crumpled piece of paper out of their pocket on which their companion has carefully written the names of each twin, identifying them by presentation, side, size and so on. When the twins are finally wrapped up and handed over to the father, all but a few comment, 'I am afraid of dropping them.' Some break into tears. Most are clearly intensely moved, but at the same time fearful to touch their twins. All look back and forth between the two.

Twins

Some twins look as if they are suffering at birth (see Figure 5.2). Prematurity, growth retardation, and various intrauterine problems can all contribute to make the transition to the post-natal environment an arduous one. Some may be cyanotic and gasping weakly for air. Others may just be limp and unresponsive. Still others may appear squashed by intrauterine crowding. Most seem to be too overwhelmed by gravity to attempt even the feeblest of movements. Dizygotic[2] twins are usually better off than monozygotic twins.

Despite appearances, however, many twins are born without any serious problems and have only a few minor complications or none at all. In these fortunate circumstances it is, in fact, the twins themselves who seem to take birth most naturally, and for the most part they do not look in the least perturbed. When laid down in their cots their eyes are often open and only a few cry. Bathing, gentle massaging and being tightly wrapped up in warm blankets seem to have a soothing effect on most. Being put next to each other does not evoke any apparent reaction, while physical contact may actually provoke loud screaming (see Figure 5.3).

In addition, behavioral differences are noticeable from the very beginning. One

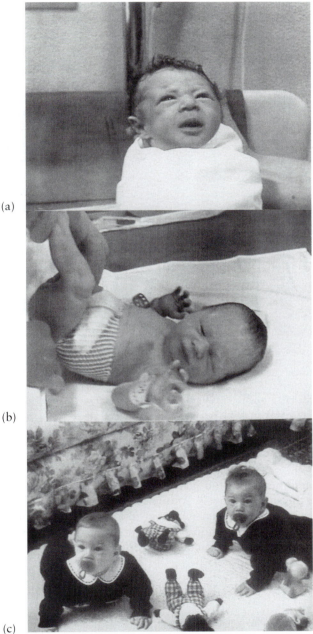

Figure 5.1 Differences in appearance at birth can be striking – monozygotic twin boys at birth, 37 weeks gestation

(a) Twin 1 weighs 300 g less than his co-twin. He is much more wrinkled and fetal crowding has left him crushed. He also has a striking dark lock of hair on the top of his head.

(b) Twin 2 has a much fuller face and is less wrinkled. The twins look very dissimilar.

(c) The same twins seven months later begin to look more alike. However, Twin 1 still looks more wrinkled and his lock of hair continues to distinguish him from his brother.

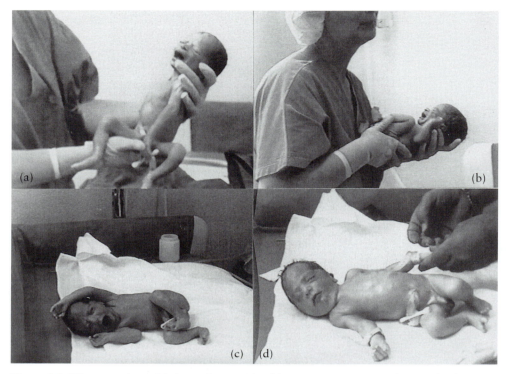

Figure 5.2 Discrepancies at birth can be considerable – monozygotic twin boys at birth, 35 weeks gestation
(a–b) Twin 2 weighs 850 g less than his co-twin and appears to be suffering. This twin had to have a fairly long stay in the NICU (twenty-one days).
(c–d) Twin 1 is clearly bigger than his brother. Except for an initial mild reaction of distress (c), he looks much more placid and unperturbed (d). Twin 1 only stayed in the NICU for two days.

may be irritable, another quiet and alert. One may be sluggish, another may show sharp reactions to the slightest touch. Another may start to suck the small aspirator-tube inserted in its windpipe avidly, while yet another may show no reaction when injected a dose of vitamin K. Obviously such initial differences could be due to the process of birth itself, which has usually been different for each and generally more difficult for one of them.

Special attention

Whilst mothers are still hospitalised they almost inevitably receive special attention and extra care. From the two rosettes on the door of their room (which reveals their status to all passers-by), to the crowd of parents and friends flocking in to see the babies during visiting hours loaded down with gifts and flowers, everything contributes to make mothers of twins feel special. In addition, whilst the mothers of singletons are generally fairly anonymous figures within the ward, the mothers of

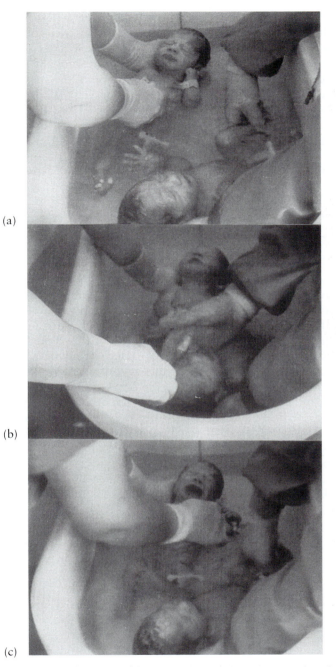

(a)

(b)

(c)

Figure 5.3 Contact is not always soothing – monoamniotic–monozygotic twin girls, 35 weeks gestation
Only minutes after birth they are being bathed together.
(a) Bathing seems to have a soothing effect on them.
(b) The nurses bring them into physical contact.
(c) This immediately produces a negative reaction and both start screaming.

twins usually know the staff well thanks to their frequent prenatal check-ups or periods of hospitalisation. Doctors, nurses and midwives often pop in to say hello, treating them like old friends. This constant flow of people gives an aura of exceptionality to the event. Furthermore, those twins who are brought to their mother's bedside to be breast-fed inevitably rivet the attention of all the visitors and relatives in the ward. Twins are already being treated like marvels. Whilst still in hospital most mothers seem to bask in this glory. Some sit up in bed like ancient fertility deities exposing their breasts with a twin hanging from each.

However, not all are so fortunate as to have their children brought to their bedside.

THE NEONATAL INTENSIVE CARE UNIT

Prematurity and discordance

Several twins have to face a more or less lengthy stay in the Neonatal Intensive Care Unit (NICU) (Botting *et al.* 1987). Given their more troubled intrauterine existence, prematurity, and growth retardation monozygotic twins are dominant in the NICU (Rydstrom 1990). The possible complications and hazards linked to an untimely birth need not be discussed here as they are not exclusive to twins.

In many cases twins are discordant in respect to potential risks. The complications affecting one do not necessarily affect the other (Ghai and Vidyasagar 1988). One twin may be full of tubes and needles, while the other may already move freely in its cot. One may be held and breast-fed whilst the other may continue to be tube-fed for a long time. One may be discharged much earlier than the other.

Within the NICU comparison between twins is the rule. Besides truly clinical parameters, nurses, paediatricians and parents all comment on the different behavior and temperament of the twins. Some may be considered sluggish and dopey, others irritable, still others quiet, but alert. Temperamental differences seem to be noticed and reported by all (Riese 1990, 1998).

Separation

In the NICU twins experience their first separation after birth. For some this will be the only separation for months or even years to come. No noticeable signs of longing or loss seem to accompany this experience. However, some simple experiment should possibly be devised to demonstrate this. It could involve, for instance, presenting vests, one worn by the co-twin the other by a control, or by contrasting the reaction to the co-twin's crying to that of the cries of a third baby. Similar experiments performed in singleton babies have shown that they are very sensitive to the voice, taste, smell and touch of their mothers (MacFarlane 1977; DeCasper and Fifer 1980). Although there is as yet no definitive proof, twins would seem to begin missing each other only later.

PARENTAL ANXIETIES AND BEHAVIOR[3]

Mothers

Within the NICU anxieties are very real. It is not easy for parents to bear the constant worries they have to contend with. In addition, they are confronted with the sight of other distressed parents with perhaps severely damaged or even terminally ill babies. Most mothers look terribly edgy and strained.

Some mothers try to obviate the anonymity of this environment by creating a personalised microhabitat within the cots. They bring coloured ribbons, small soft toys, pictures of saints and photographs of themselves from home, and hang them on the sides of the incubator.

Several mothers, particularly those living quite far away, make the hospital their temporary home and spend all day there. Many close links with other mothers in a similar condition are thus established. This seems to provide some form of mutual support for all. However, many mothers spend this time with their peers complaining about the hospital: the supposed lack of hygiene, the noisiness of the monitors, the unkindness of the staff, and so on. Major anxieties seem to be displaced onto the 'uncaring' organisation. Mothers also endlessly compare the progress and failures of their respective children. This frequently increases dissatisfaction, anxiety and uncertainty. Particularly in the room where they sit round a table pumping out milk from their breasts, all one can hear is complaints, the most frequent remark being 'We are not just cows!' Once the children are brought in, however, most group dynamics seem to vanish and mothers concentrate on their own babies. Most are excruciatingly sensitive to any, no matter how tiny, modification in the bodies of their children. They notice minute signs of punctures, microscopic scratches, insignificant rashes or irritations, substituted plasters, and worry endlessly – often reading hidden ominous signs into these details. No amount of reassurance dispels their doubts. The personnel are often suspected of keeping secrets and carrying out clandestine activities behind their backs.

In addition mothers of twins find it particularly hard being granted only the same amount of time as mothers of singletons. They feel they have to rush between the babies without having the time to enjoy a bit of peace and quiet with them. Several demand (and get) extra attention. Some want to be given special status as mothers of twins and complain twice as much. Despite their frequent complaints, most of these mothers also feel that the responsibility for the care and survival of their children has been usurped by other, more expert hands. Many, in fact, seem quite relieved by this.

Once within the NICU, no matter what the anxieties for the survival and wellbeing of their infants, the sheer state of emergency in the air somehow helps most mothers to keep going. All have to grit their teeth and bear it.

Fathers

Fathers enter the NICU less. The majority go back to work after one or two days. Therefore most come to the NICU only once a day in the evening. In this way they combine their visit with picking up a fairly exhausted partner who is more than ready to go home. Though fathers are encouraged to touch and handle the babies, only a few do so while they are still in the incubator. They look at the twins, study their charts and clinical reports carefully, speak with the personnel, but otherwise generally avoid direct physical contact. Only when the twins can be moved out of the incubator does proper handling usually begin. Most are still tentative and almost fearful in their approach.

BREAST-FEEDING

Of the group studied the majority of mothers made some attempt at breast-feeding. However, for most of them this did not last for long. Only three quite robust women continued breast-feeding for several months. Most were too drained and tired. Burdensome pregnancies, Caesareans, anxieties and lurking depression all took their toll. Mothers of monozygotic twins, due to pressure from the NICU, tried harder on the whole. Mothers of dizygotic twins had less reason for concern with their generally healthier, bigger and more mature twins. If they were unable to breast-feed their infants it was not considered a tragedy. Most mothers of monozygotic twins, on the other hand, had problems feeding their babies directly from the breast. Their nipples were too big for the tiny mouths of their premature twins and, besides, the babies tended to be dopey and had too little vigour to suck from the breast. These mothers usually tried to continue pumping out their own milk as in hospital. Generally this did not last for long either. Despite all their efforts they soon lost all milk. In a few cases not being able to breast-feed caused intense distress. The underweight infants were felt to be in special need of the protective antibodies human milk gives. Feelings of inadequacy, guilt and apprehension were frequently reinforced by their paediatricians, and by the general assumption that 'breast is best' and the 'now or never' mystique surrounding early 'bonding' (Eyer 1992). Mothers believed they were not doing all they could to help their frail children thrive both physically and emotionally.

MATERNAL CHOICE

Whilst in hospital the first encounters between parents and their twins were video-taped. In retrospect, an element of choice could already be detected in these initial contacts. These first signs of preference were often seen to continue for months and indeed years after birth. Looking back at the videos one could see a mother smiling more at one twin, another mother stroking or kissing the 'chosen' one more frequently, another deciding, contrary to all common sense, to breast-feed the dopey twin first instead of the one who was yelling. The apparent elements involved in the original choice seemed to be many and varied. The smaller or less-favoured twin could be chosen for compensatory reasons (Minde *et al.* 1982, 1990; Rowland 1991). Mothers understandably tended to feel more protective towards the twins who had suffered the most, but also the bigger, or the more attractive, or the less alert one could become the preferred twin.

However, there were differences between monozygotic and dizygotic twins. Several monozygotic pairs were markedly growth discordant at birth and weight discrepancy made them quite easy to distinguish. One twin often seemed like a smaller version of the other (see Figure 5.4). A few even looked totally dissimilar. Mothers of such twins quickly displayed a preference (Rowland 1991).

Not all monozygotic twins had a distinct appearance at birth. Some looked very similar to each other (see Figure 5.5), and it took their mothers a few days of acquaintance before bending towards one or the other. These mothers had to become familiar with the differences in the behavioral/temperamental traits of the twins in order to express a choice. Lethargic and more apathetic twins were in fact the most favoured category. Already anticipating, perhaps, the enormous pressure and incredible fatigue to come, the 'quiet' twin was probably regarded as being less demanding and easier to handle.

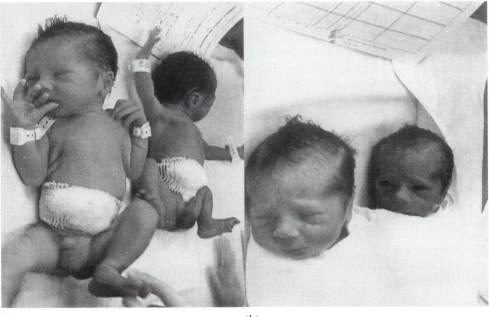

(a)   (b)

Figure 5.4 Size and weight discrepancies – monozygotic twin boys at birth, 38 weeks gestation
(a) Size disparity is evident. The small twin weighs 1,900 g and the big one 2,500 g.
(b) When wrapped after being bathed, similar facial features can be noted. However, the small twin looks only half the size of his co-twin. He also looks quite alert. This twin never recovered from his initial growth discrepancy, which was already evident at ten weeks (see Figure 3.1a).

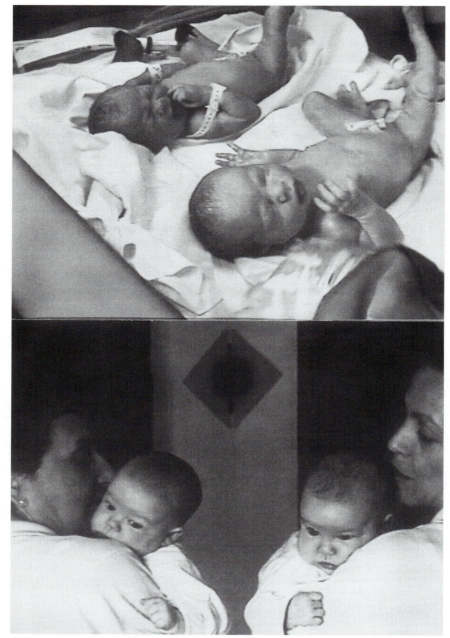

(a)

(b)

Figure 5.5 Dichorionic–monozygotic twin girls, 37 weeks gestation
(a) Weight discrepancy is minimal (60 g). Similarities in appearance and behavior are evident. Both twins hold their right leg up. This position is made possible by the scarcity of antigravity mechanisms and postures, which continues for the first 8–10 weeks after birth.
(b) The same twins, now one month old, held by their mother and grandmother. They continue to look and behave very similarly. Both have positioned their heads and hands in the same way.

For mothers of dizygotic twins, on the other hand, choice was almost immediate. In opposite-sex pairs choice was frequently and quite blatantly dictated by gender. Mothers adored their little boy. In same-sex pairs the different appearance generally also made preferences more clear-cut. Appearance played a relevant role in the choice between dizygotic twins.

> Mrs Q had just given spontaneous birth to two strikingly attractive boys. They were, however, very dissimilar. One was the 'classical' Latin type with dark hair, olive complexion and big black eyes. The other had a clearly Nordic phenotype. He was blond, with a fair and delicate complexion and unbelievably blue eyes. Their mother hesitated a second between the two. She smiled, seeming deservedly proud. When the nurse asked her if she wanted to try breast-feeding one she said, 'How can I choose? They both look so gorgeous. Well give me Bruce, he is more common.' Bruce was the one with the typically Mediterranean phenotype.

Mrs Q was quite candid in expressing her choice and some other mothers were equally open in voicing a certain degree of preference for one twin. Many, however, found it impossible to admit inegalitarian treatment. Nevertheless, preference was revealed by the way in which the children were treated differently. Choice was seldom inflexible. The other twin, particularly if in some kind of need, could temporarily become the focus of all attention and affection. However, a longitudinal reading of the tapes showed that the initial favourite often continued to be so (see Figure 5.6).

Amongst mothers of monozygotic twins choice was extreme only in a few cases. Though clearly these twins could also be the subject of preferences, on the whole they were treated more equitably within the home environment. The same gender and less clear-cut differences in appearance and behavior encouraged a more impartial treatment by mothers of monozygotic twins.

> Mrs O was one of the very few mothers of monozygotic twins who expressed a strong and enduring choice. She had just given birth to twin boys. As she had wanted to be conscious during the event the Caesarean had been performed with an epidural. The twins were very similar, but Henry was big while Nick was literally only half his weight and size. Nevertheless, Mother Nature seemed to have compensated for this injustice by endowing Nick, the smaller one, with a bright and alert disposition. Whilst this tiny little fellow scanned his new environment with an attentive inquisitive gaze, big Henry looked fairly lethargic and utterly disinterested.
>   When the twins were brought to their mother she looked at them both. The big one was asleep, whilst Nick stared her straight in the eyes. Perhaps Mrs O found his alert gaze too demanding. She chose the big dopey twin saying, 'Why is he looking at me? Give me the sleepy one.' Due to excessive weight loss and intervening intestinal complications Nick had to be detained in the NICU for nearly a month. Mrs O went home with Henry and Nick was left behind. She never visited him. As she said, 'Looking after one is quite enough. There are plenty of staff there. He certainly does not need me.' When Nick was finally discharged Mrs O complained constantly and reminisced about the blissful time when she had been alone with just one child. Nick, in fact, continued to be neglected later on.

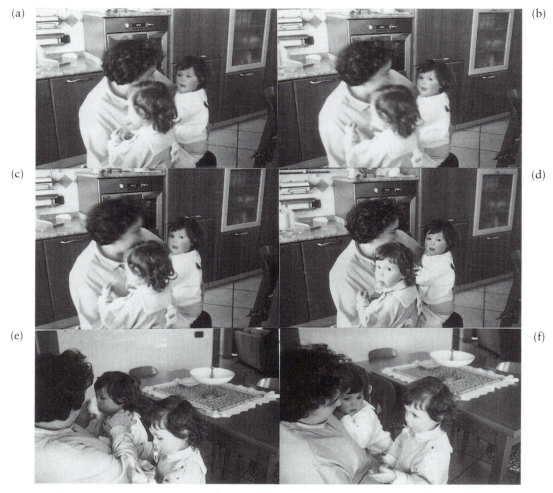

Figure 5.6 Choice can be long lasting – monozygotic twin girls, 30 months
At birth their mother immediately chose the bigger twin. Her preference can be seen to continue:
(a–d) The mother continues to look and smile at the favourite twin, completely ignoring the other.
(e) She is still very attentive to the favourite and wipes her nose without looking at the rejected one.
(f) She finally looks at the rejected twin, but close bodily contact with the favourite is maintained. The rejected girl is kept at a distance.

PATERNAL CHOICE

Fathers too made their choice (see Figure 5.7). However, fathers of monozygotic twins were generally even more equitable than their wives. Several just picked up the twin their companions had rejected. This 'one child each' distribution seemed to elicit little guilt and was frequently and easily voiced.

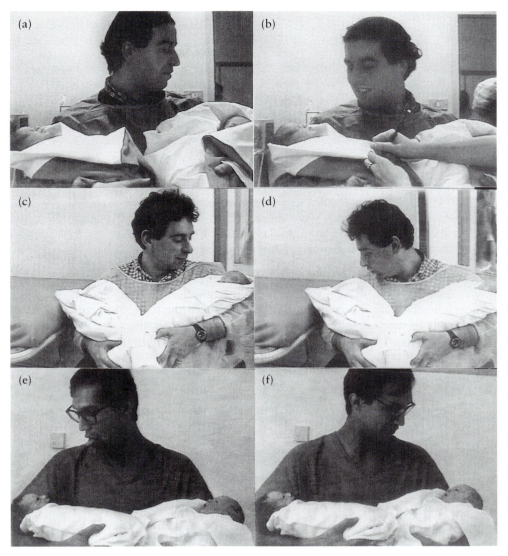

Figure 5.7 Fathers' first encounters: reacting differently to each twin – paternal choice

(a–b) This father is clearly moved when holding his dizygotic twins for the first time. However, he looks at each quite differently. When glancing at Twin 1 his expression is very serious. When staring at Twin 2 he smiles openly and looks delighted.

(c–d) This father of monozygotic twins is certainly deeply stirred. He had to sit down before holding them. When looking at Twin 1 he smiles, when looking at Twin 2 he seems perplexed.

(e–f) This father adopts an unruffled, 'manly' attitude when holding his monozygotic twins. The twins look very dissimilar. He sticks his tongue out when staring at Twin 2, whereas he smiles at Twin 1.

Mr F was one of the exceptions. His monozygotic twin boys did not have very marked weight discrepancy at birth, but by some twist of fate fetal crowding had only affected Jack. Not only did his 'squeezed' head look peculiar, almost triangular in shape, but also a single forelock of dark hair had remained on his head. He had not lost all the hirsutism or hairiness often marking prematurity. In contrast his attractive co-twin had a round, chubby face and was fair-haired with a smooth skin. Looking at Jack, their father grimaced and said, 'Yuck! He is ugly! Give me the other one! This one is all for you!' However, his wife also had very aesthetic inclinations. After some initial hesitation she also chose the attractive twin. The squashed one paid dearly for the harsh intrauterine treatment that made him look all out of shape. He was nobody's favourite.

Fathers of dizygotic twins were more openly biased towards one child. Again, gender made choice especially easy in the case of opposite-sex twins. Fathers, like the mothers, usually doted on their boys but also chose on the basis of apparent constitution. Besides the always popular 'quiet' and lethargic twin, choice also fell on twins who were ascribed slightly more 'mature' temperamental traits. Though few twins could sensibly be regarded as really being 'fun' or 'outgoing' at this stage, fathers who chose on this basis were perhaps anticipating better times to come when they would be able to enjoy that twin in the ways that fathers are generally supposed to: sharing manly interests, teaching them a sport and indulging in man's talk. None of the mothers in either group opted for temperamental traits relating to fun. Fun was, at the most, a distant mirage for them.

REJECTED TWINS

Quite a few twins were rejected by both parents. Sometimes both parents of monozygotic twins would favour the same twin to compensate for 'unfair' prenatal and perinatal treatment. No parents of dizygotic twins did that. Temperamental differences accounted for all other 'rejected' monozygotic twins. Three couples preferred a 'quiet' twin and two a more 'alert' and 'outgoing' one. In the dizygotic group five females belonging to opposite-sex pairs were rejected! In total eighteen twins were 'unwanted' by both their parents!

Most fathers were less strongly biased than their wives. Fathers were less involved in the care of the twins. This possibly favoured a more mechanical and rather distracted handling. When they came home from work and found themselves inundated by requests of all sorts, yells and lamentations from everyone, they tended to be fairly non-selective, picking up the first twin that came to hand.

An element of choice is present even with ordinary siblings. Not many parents may be willing to acknowledge this, but all children are only too aware of who prefers whom. Often preference is expressed in macroscopically inegalitarian treatment which is evident to everyone except the parents themselves. However, singletons are never confronted with a sibling born on exactly the same day. This should not be taken to mean inevitable disaster for one or both twins. More or less pronounced preferences and inevitable compatibilities accompany all of us throughout our lives. The preferred twin was not necessarily the one demonstrating a better social and emotional outcome later on.

> Though little Nick, the 'rejected' twin previously mentioned, never caught up the initial birth and weight difference with his brother, he overtook him in many other respects. He continued to be much brighter than big Henry. Having had to fight for attention from birth he also became very entertaining and popular with his peers who all ignored his whining, tedious and spoiled brother. All, that is, except Nick who was very forgiving and loved him dearly. As he said a few years later, 'Mummy loves him best, but I do too.'

LEAVING THE HOSPITAL

Though the mothers had all looked forward to leaving the hospital and had talked about this moment with great expectation for weeks or even months, when it finally came they were all anxious and fearful. Mothers were afraid of not being able to handle emergencies, or even apparent trivialities, without the expert support and advice of the staff of the NICU. Though many had had occasion to observe and learn a lot, they all felt that suddenly the entire responsibility had been dropped onto their shoulders with nobody to turn to for help. Most were in a panic when the time finally arrived. Fathers, too, anticipated a big change and looked very shaky.

Generally, all parents who have been followed during pregnancy in the Unit of Maternal/Fetal Medicine come in and say goodbye on their way home. All look fairly terrified and distraught. They stare at the usual crowd of pregnant women with a hint of nostalgia and often make their feelings felt. Many mothers, indeed, express their fears out loud.

The most striking thing is how often the twins are nearly dropped. Usually the father is holding both infants in one or perhaps two separate Moses baskets. Whilst showing the staff the twins, who are greeted with the usual exclamations of marvel, the father inevitably manages to upturn the basket almost dropping the babies! Everybody seems aware that it's going to happen and are ready to come to their rescue. When parents finally leave, their pallor, trembling and weariness all convey a sense of dread, insecurity and an intense need for help.

CHAPTER 6

BACK HOME

Although there are no such things as typical twins or even a typical type of twin, several attitudes and traits were common to all while others quite clearly were not. It certainly made a difference if twins were born to young parents in their early twenties or belonged to large families with other children. Changing patterns in childbearing meant that most twins were born to couples in their middle or late thirties without other children. This is the family situation which will be outlined first. The distinct characteristics of younger parents and of families with other children will be described later.

MOTHERS AND THE BREAKING DOWN OF IDEALISATION

'Baby blues', as with singleton pregnancies, usually started in the maternity ward. However, it was only upon leaving the protective environment of the hospital that mothers found themselves alone and wholly responsible for the care of their babies. The breakdown of idealisation was harsh for most (Linney 1983; Sandbank 1988, 1991; Hay *et al.* 1990; Robin *et al.* 1991).

Primiparae in particular had a fairly idealised and unrealistic view of maternity. Idealisation was at a maximum if the twins were the result of long fertility treatments. These mothers had generally been living with their partners for several years and were used to leading fairly free, unfettered lives. Both partners had been able to come and go as they pleased, dine out, go to the movies, travel for work or pleasure without having to make any special arrangements. However, passing time and advancing age had made pregnancy an issue for all. Most of these mothers felt that without a child life would be incomplete: a baby would change their existence, infusing it with completeness and bliss. All the unhappiness, failures and inevitable frustrations which are part of any life and become more prominent with approaching middle age were often redirected towards the lack of a child. Moreover, twins felt like a special bonus to mothers who had had any kind of fertility problem. They seemed to make up for all those years of barren waiting. However, the real children almost immediately shattered this blissful image of motherhood. Given their previous fairly carefree lives and the expectations placed upon the children, these mothers were in fact those who had the greatest problems adapting to the rough reality of bringing up twins.

Mrs T and her husband were both in their late thirties. They had been married for several years, but had decided to postpone having children. Their economic condition was not exceptional, but quite sufficient for two. Both smoked heavily, enjoyed holidays abroad, dining out, good wine, going to the movies, and a full social life with a host of friends. As Mrs T said, 'Our house is like a boarding house. People come and go as they wish.' However, at some point the biological clock began to tick for her too. Faced with an approaching deadline they decided to conceive a child. After many fruitless attempts and all sorts of tests and analyses, Mr T's sperm was found to be flawless, but Mrs T had total bilateral tubal block. IVF was the only solution and was tried countless times. By the time they came to the Maternal/Fetal Medicine Unit Mrs T was bloated with hormones, desperate and obsessed. Her whole life revolved around 'the problem'. As she said, 'I am prepared to die to have a child.' Her tension and unfailing determination were only too tangible. When the scan revealed twins Mr and Mrs T were clearly moved and both cried for joy. Having undergone innumerable fertility treatments of various kinds twins were not a surprise but a craving. At this confirmation of his virility, Mr T dropped hints during the scan that he could always impregnate somebody else if necessary. However, he seemed genuinely in love with his wife and never failed to accompany her for any appointment. All went well and Mrs T endured pregnancy without complaint. When the twins reached term they were both in the vertex position and a natural delivery was suggested. However, Mrs T burst out, 'You stupid pair! Turn round! I demand a Caesarean. If these two die I am dead too!' She made such a fuss that in the end the obstetricians had no choice but to agree to her wishes. The twin girls were both healthy, though one had to spend four days in the NICU due to excessive weight loss. Mrs T complained about her aches and pains and occasionally about her husband not being constantly at her bedside. During the first home visit it was striking how little the flat seemed geared to twins (or even a singleton for that matter). Ashtrays, empty bottles, and empty cans lay around, but no toys, no baby powder or lotions, or a space for changing diapers could be seen. Being a nursery school teacher Mrs T was certainly not unaware of the needs of young children, but the house still resembled that of a childless couple. The only items relating to children were idyllic Ann Geddes pictures portraying delightful twins dressed like little squirrels or sweet peas, all rosy and chubby and with beaming angelic smiles. During this first visit Mrs T spoke more about her friends than of the girls, but subsequent changes were dramatic. The Ann Geddes pictures disappeared and so did any idealisation of maternity. Both parents were overwhelmed, nervous and tense. Mutual verbal abuse became a constant in their lives. Tension never eased and actually increased in the following months. The girls, although physically well cared for, were progressively treated by both parents as unmanageable nuisances. All one heard was complaints. As Mrs T later confessed, 'These two have ruined my life.' Expectations had been too idealised and were too strong a match for a harsh reality. Mrs T never worked with children again as by then she considered the very thought intolerable. Her marriage was over by the time the twins were three.

Not all couples undergoing fertility treatment necessarily have marital problems. Nevertheless, these parents, particularly if the treatment is repeated and relentlessly pursued, are more liable to find the reality of twins in total contrast to what are often exaggerated and highly unrealistic expectations.

The breaking down of idealisation is, indeed, an important and little-considered aspect of all twin pregnancies, particularly when the mother is a primipara. A lot is invested in the few 'priceless' children that most women in developed countries decide they can afford to have. The reality of the simultaneous care of twins could be a particularly poor match to the expectations their mothers have. Women are often unprepared to meet the needs of one baby, let alone two.

MATERNAL FATIGUE

Maternal mental and physical fatigue can be really harrowing. Mothers emerged from an already draining pregnancy, often involving a Caesarean and exhausting journeys to and from the NICU, to find themselves thrown into a never-ending chaotic reality which allowed them little or no respite. Nights were especially harsh. Most twins, being born underweight, had to have frequent meals – some even nine or ten times a day. It also took them longer before giving up their night feeds. Not before they had reached a satisfactory weight and an adequate abdominal capacity could they finally be expected to sleep throughout the night. In addition, sleep patterns change with increasing maturation (Roffwarg et al. 1966; Parmelee and Stern 1972; Parmelee et al. 1968, 1969; Dreyfus-Brisac 1968, 1970, 1979; Prechtl 1974; Anders et al. 1995). Being born prematurely, many twins did not acquire 'mature' patterns of sleep for quite some time. All infants manifest so-called polyphasic sleep, a pattern of frequently interrupted sleep (Parmelee et al. 1969; Berg and Berg 1987; Lavie 1996). During the first month babies wake, however briefly, roughly every four hours. After the first few months their sleep becomes monophasic, without these interruptions. Premature twins possibly require longer to acquire sufficient maturity to sleep a good, sound, monophasic sleep. However, since so many twins do not acquire mature patterns for such a long time it may be that some unknown factors other than 'maturation' account for this nerve-racking delay. According to the mothers most twins did not acquire uninterrupted night-time sleep before they were one year old, and some not before fourteen months. On average monozygotic twins were born earlier, and consequently their mothers were particularly affected. In one case where the twins had been born severely premature (thirty weeks) their distressed mother reported sleeping difficulties until the boys were two.

Furthermore, it was a strain whether the twins were coincident in their rest cycles or not. Mothers were either confronted with two infants yelling simultaneously or had no respite. As soon as one was pacified, the other mercilessly began demanding its feed. Constant sleep deprivation was the greatest ordeal and the worst nightmare for all.

Few fathers helped at night. Most slept in another room or were anyway reluctant to wake up, as they had to go to work during the day. Even mothers who had substantial help during the day were alone at night. Only one upper-class woman had qualified nannies that slept with the twins; nevertheless, fatigue showed in the bags under her eyes too.

MATERNAL DEPRESSION

Post-partum maternal depression is more common in mothers of twins (Goshen-Gottstein 1980; Wohlreich 1986; Bennett and Slade 1991; Richman *et al.* 1991; Thorpe *et al.* 1991; Merenkov 1995). This condition is not recognised as a distinct disorder by the American Psychiatric Association (1994). However, it is regarded by many as a specific illness and, furthermore, as a multi-factorial one. Physical (including hormonal) and psychological factors, as well as a particular constitutional disposition, are all deemed conducive (Welburn 1980; Kumar and Brockington 1988; Hamilton and Harberger 1992; O'Hara 1994; Murray and Cooper 1997).

Therefore, when discussing maternal depression in twin births I will only report certain factors which are possible contributors and/or aggravators. No single one of these could be considered the sole determinant of such a condition. Though maternal depression was clearly linked to exhaustion, other factors also contributed.

Depression was especially profound in women who resorted to assisted reproduction of some kind. Four of the five cases had to seek long (over three years) psychiatric help, and the fifth was also severely depressed. As stated previously, this possibly indicated the harsh breakdown of what had been a very strong idealisation. The chaotic arrival of the twins could only cause acute, sometimes bitter, disappointment.

Mrs Y had been married to her devoted husband for many years. When Mrs Y turned 30 they decided it was time to have a child. After trying without success for a year, she underwent all the examinations possible. Nothing was found to be wrong with either parent and Mrs Y underwent several cycles of ovarian stimulation with Clomid. When told that she was expecting twins Mrs Y seemed very pleased and declared, 'Much better, I will not have to try again.' However, at twenty weeks she was already finding pregnancy too much. She complained, 'I hope it will all be over soon.' When advised that twenty weeks was far too soon she moaned, 'But how can I be asked to endure all this?' Her whining continued throughout the pregnancy, but reached a peak near term when she had to be hospitalised due to high blood pressure. When her exhausted obstetricians suggested some kind of psychiatric help, she replied, 'All I need is to get rid of these two. Then I will be fine.' When she was told that both twins were in an unfavourable position, she got angry with them. 'They are just doing it to torment me!' After childbirth, although surrounded by an enviable group of supportive grandparents, Mrs Y was extremely depressed. In her brooding she frequently referred to her twins as ghoulish vampires. She wailed, 'All I can hear are their incessant screams. They pierce my ears and go through my brain. My life is just a series of endless demands. They are sucking me dry.' However, she continued to breast-feed the twins. It was simply more convenient. As she repeatedly declared, 'I don't have to make any effort when breast-feeding. All you do is pull up your blouse. I can't be bothered to make any effort for these two.' When she finally sought psychiatric help, her condition got better, but the twins continued to be brought up almost exclusively by their grandparents.

Besides the 'breaking down of idealisation' and fatigue, other factors are also important in fostering depression in mothers of twins.

Caesareans *per se* are no cause for depression. However, it is interesting to note that all the women who had had spontaneous or induced deliveries either did not suffer from depression at all or were only mildly depressed. Starting the difficult task of taking care of twins in poor physical shape, with no time for recovery and many aches and pains, certainly did not help (Trowell 1982; Spillman 1993). However, spontaneous or induced labour also meant healthy and mature children. This in turn made for fewer anxieties and more mature sleeping and feeding patterns.

Most mothers had jobs and had had a more or less active social life before becoming pregnant. Already during pregnancy several had been cut off, sometimes even for months, from many social contacts. All were granted early maternity leave and some had to give up work altogether almost from the start. Now their paediatricians, given the frail condition of the children, often advised them not to take the twins out. No matter what their job had been, being excluded from outside human contacts and being confined to the house was very harsh on all (Broadbent 1985). In addition, sheer exhaustion often made many mothers reluctant to socialise. Collapsing in front of the television was the best most could manage. Furthermore, practical difficulties such as carrying a double pram down to the ground floor of an apartment block[1] or loading it into the car made going out very laborious; therefore it was difficult to have even brief normal contact with other adults. Many mothers kept the radio or television on all day to alleviate their feelings of isolation.

Being homebound became a habit for a few. Two mothers manifested mild, but clear signs of agoraphobia.

Most mothers were not totally alone at home. Though having other caregivers around clearly helped them from a practical point of view, it also meant a lack of privacy. Apartments, which had once been spacious and an oasis of peace, were now suddenly cramped and devoid of any private territory. The twins, with all their paraphernalia and their yells, invaded every inch of the house and few helpers were able simply to listen, comfort the mother and then discreetly retreat when the moment came. Having to depend on others, and thus losing independence, can be hard on any mother. In the case of young twins dependence has an urgent and essential quality of survival that makes it particularly hard to accept.

Most saw no end to their tribulations. Many confessed to being stretched to the limit and completely overwhelmed. Some admitted feeling close to hitting their children, unable to tolerate yet more demands and yells. Child abuse has indeed been found to be especially frequent in families of twins (George and Main 1980; Groothuis et al. 1982; Groothuis 1985). Though feelings of love and hate are the norm with all babies, negative emotions were exasperated and exacerbated in the case of twins. This obviously caused an enormous sense of guilt. Even having to resort to pacifiers made some mothers feel inadequate.

Another important element, which contributed to making mothers feel demoralised, was their physical aspect. Most had expected to get back into shape in next to no time. Only too often glossy magazines show beautiful models looking gorgeous in tiny bikinis straight after the birth of their equally radiant babies. However, most mothers of twins, given the extreme stretching of their abdomens during gestation, continued to look pregnant for quite a while. Their changed silhouettes made them fear that femininity was over for them. In addition, having no time for personal grooming, or a relaxing bath, let alone contemplating a visit to the hairdressers, really wore them out. Even those mothers who were not otherwise depressed complained about their bodies.

Mrs H was the only mother who rejoiced about her altered physical shape. She was already adipose before becoming pregnant, and pregnancy enlarged her body beyond belief. Her inflated size actually increased her charm in the eyes of her adoring husband. He commented, 'We will try again. After another pair she will be just perfect!' When the monozygotic twin girls were born they were markedly weight discordant. One was chubby and the other skinny. Interestingly, both parents preferred the fleshy twin. The father explained, 'She looks just like my wife.'

Mrs H was lucky to have such a revering husband. Among the main factors accounting for the high rate of post-partum depression among mothers of twins were the initial difficulties with and growing estrangement from their companions.

APPREHENSION AND DISAPPOINTMENT

During the first year of their lives (and beyond) physical problems were more serious for monozygotic twins. All the twins in this group who had had respiratory or intestinal complications and had been treated within the NICU continued to suffer the consequences. Furthermore, some twins who were growth retarded at birth remained so (see Figure 6.1) (Keet *et al.* 1986; Bleker *et al.* 1988, 1995; Koziel 1998; Buckler 1999). Interestingly, monozygotic twins generally show greater birthweight differences than dizygotic ones (Wilson 1986). If growth retardation is already noticeable during the early stages of pregnancy (as it was in all these children) long-term poor growth may follow. Twins who display growth retardation only during the second half of pregnancy are more likely to recover. The more favourable extrauterine environment generally enables these twins to catch up.

Not surprisingly, feelings of apprehension were a major source of misery especially for mothers of monozygotic twins. Anxieties were especially acute for those parents whose twins had had particular problems. Two families had to take an apnea monitor home with them when they left the hospital. In both cases there was the risk, particularly at night, that one twin might stop breathing and therefore need immediate resuscitation. Understandably, they continued to be apprehensive for a long time after.

Anything, from runny noses to mild constipation, was interpreted as an impending catastrophe. All developmental milestones were eagerly awaited and scrutinised with concern. Most stopped worrying excessively only after the children began to talk and walk.

In several cases the twins themselves were also an initial source of disappointment. Besides the clear difficulties of bonding simultaneously with two young babies, many parents had expected chubby little angels, cuddles and beaming smiles. Pictures portraying twins as delightful and immaculate cherubs were to be found in each household. As was noted earlier, most twins looked wrinkled, tiny and fragile. In addition they were often hypotonic and scarcely responsive. Social cues and interchanges were indeed very limited. Intentional smiling did not start for several weeks, fixation could be unsteady and some could not track their mothers' faces. Relating to them was often hard (Field *et al.* 1980; Tronick and Field 1987; Anastasiow and

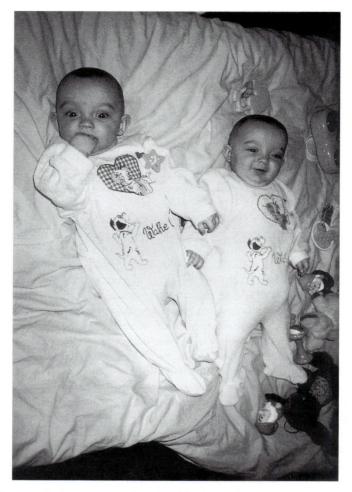

Figure 6.1 Monoamniotic–monozygotic twin girls, 6 months
The twin on the right has not recovered from initial growth discrepancy. Facial features are
very similar, but body size is quite different.

Harel 1993; Minde 1993). In addition, if a baby had been in the NICU, bonding
with it could be delayed.

Many households were now full of manuals and magazines about immature
babies. It seemed fairly common in a more or less subtle manner to place the blame
on the mother. Mothers had to bond quickly, intensely and at all costs. One insane,
supposedly scientific, book that was all the vogue at the time went as far as to
suggest doing gaze-catching exercises for hours! The natural scarcity of social and
visual interchanges of prematurely born babies was diagnosed as an ominous sign.
As a mother said, bursting into tears, 'All I seem to be able to offer them is survival.
I know this is not enough, but what else can I do?'

Anxiety, not pleasure, was prominent during the early months.

FATHERS AND CHILDCARE

As opposed to fathers of singletons, most fathers of twins were involved in their care right from the beginning. An unusual level of involvement had already started during the turbulent days of pregnancy. However, once the twins were born, most felt that they were thrown more into 'motherhood' than the 'fatherhood' they had expected (Bryan 1977; Lytton 1980; Pedersen 1980; Bronstein 1984; White and Wollett 1987; Hay *et al.* 1990; Coltrane 1996; Parke 1996; Lamb 1997). Feeding, rocking, changing diapers, cleaning floors and preparing what looked like a production line of feeding bottles, combined to form a picture far removed from the traditional one of fathers enjoying a rough and tumble with their children. For most it came as a burden and a considerable shock. Though fathers were usually spared many of the ordeals the mothers had to put up with during the day (and night), as soon as they came home from work they were immediately assigned some task or other. From sterilising bottles and pacifiers, to feeding the babies and burping them, to various and often mucky chores, their homecoming was regularly transformed into what was perceived as a torment. Many tried to escape this ordeal by finding some 'urgent' odd job to do around the house. Most preferred going shopping or taking out the trash rather than being actively engaged in the care of the twins whose relentless biological rhythms seemed to leave them drained and disconcerted. Most wives insisted they come back from work as soon as possible in the evening. Many, as soon as they entered the house, put their slippers on and quickly changed into old and tatty tracksuits. None of them could stand the idea of those whitish and smelly stains ending up on their working clothes.

A few simply fled the home and resorted to any excuse to keep away. This fleeing was always seen in a bad light by their companions, who commented acrimoniously on their absence. The majority of these absent fathers had monozygotic twins. (Possibly monozygotic twins, who are more often premature, are on the whole more tiring.) However, since fleeing fathers also had minimal contact with the observer, the potentially complex motives of their disappearance remain pure speculation.

> Mrs L was one of the very few who accepted an 'absent husband'. A woman in her early thirties, she already had three children. She and her husband had planned to stop there. When she found out that she was pregnant again she resigned herself to the fact that one more was not going to make a big difference. When she was told that she was expecting twins she started to cry. During the second scan she commented, 'God doesn't seem very helpful, but I will do my best to bring these two up.' Her husband was never by her side. However, Mrs L was used to her unco-operative husband and took life quite philosophically. Commenting on his absence during the Caesarean, she remarked, 'He is not here, but I'd better stick to him. Nobody would fancy taking on a woman with five children!'

When they were present during the observations all of the fathers poured out their bewilderment and sorrows. None had anticipated anything like this. Most felt oppressed by the sudden change from couple to large family. Even those who were obviously very caring and attentive found the turmoil just a bit too much.

In addition, most mothers frequently complained about their companions. Being homebound all day made them not only exhausted and exasperated but also often very resentful and embittered. Husbands were accused of not understanding them, whilst having the good fortune of being out at work all day. On the other hand the men too often bore resentment towards their companions. They pictured their wives taking it easy all day enjoying themselves looking after the babies. Some felt that they were missing out on a lot of things.

Trying to face the substantial added economic pressures due to the arrival of twins made many fathers complain about the exponential rise in the cost of living. Expensive medicines for premature babies, huge heaps of diapers, new washing machines, pacifiers, playpens and many other indispensable purchases were all quoted. However, though bringing up twins is clearly doubly expensive, several fathers took on extra work mainly to be away from home longer. Most admitted, 'When I am at work I can have some rest.' Several were quite bitter as they felt that their efforts both at home and at work were unappreciated. Though most began to enjoy fatherhood once the twins became toddlers, at first only three fathers seemed to take special pride and joy in the care of their baby twins.

MARITAL DIFFICULTIES

Not surprisingly marital difficulties were frequent (Robin *et al.* 1991; Hay *et al.* 1990; Spillman 1992). Most families suffered more or less transient, even fairly severe problems. Quarrels over trifles were the rule. General exhaustion played a major role in making any conflict more acute. However, simply being unable to sit down and enjoy a peaceful meal or an uninterrupted conversation were also important factors. In addition most fathers, as they had to go to work the next morning, moved out of the marital bed pretty early on, leaving the mother to look after the night shift. This clearly did not help intimacy and embittered their companions even more. The changed attitude and appearance of the women, albeit temporary, also caused a lot of friction. Mothers still looked big and out of shape. They did not smell of nice perfume, their hair was often a mess, their breasts were leaking and imposing, their clothes far from immaculate. Though this did not apply to all, many women in the first few months complained of feeling – and sometimes, indeed, looked – slightly 'brutish' and mildly 'animalised'. Most mothers were immediately put on some form of contraception, but the added lurking fear of getting pregnant again certainly did not favour the resumption of a satisfactory sex life.

OTHER CAREGIVERS

Other caregivers figure much more prominently in the lives of most twins than they normally do for singleton children. Only a very few mothers were able and willing to look after the twins with little or no help. In the best of circumstances various family members took part in the daily care of the children. A task force was created, and grandmothers, grandfathers, older sisters and retired aunts would all be recruited. They were generally felt to be a great help. Any mother whose own mother did not offer to help, however temporarily, felt very bitter and let down.

Two actually broke up with their families. Mothers-in-law were less popular, but their help was never refused. Nevertheless, since nuclear families are increasingly the rule, outsiders often had to be employed. These were the least appreciated of all. Occasionally one twin was more or less handed over completely to a helper. All these alternative caregivers had their preferences too and responded differently to each twin.

No matter what form help took most mothers tended to be rather egalitarian in trying to take turns feeding the twins. Nevertheless, the initial chaos was such that they all had to put up a noticeboard on the wall of the kitchen so that they could note who had been fed last and by whom. Confusion was rendered more acute in the case of monozygotic twins by problems of identification.

FAMILIES WITH OTHER CHILDREN

Paradoxically, families with other children on the whole coped better with the arrival of twins. Parents were generally less shocked or affected by the inevitable changes brought about by the arrival of two babies. Their marriages had already survived the advent of other children. Though they all said that having one child was on the whole easier, the reality of parenthood with its joys, sorrows and limitations did not catch them unawares. They resented their loss of freedom less, as their independence was anyway already limited. These parents were also better organised and more capable of quickly establishing a reasonable routine. Though clearly having other children, particularly if fairly young, could be an added strain, they were also company and sometimes help. Experienced mothers also felt less anxious about the health of their twins. They knew that not all illnesses are fatal and that their babies could well survive a common cold. They also knew that the initial problems were not going to last forever and that for the most part it was just a matter of biding their time. Looking back at the early stages of their other children's lives made them aware that nostalgia would be inevitable. Most were acutely conscious of the fact that after twins they could not afford to have any more children. Three mothers had actually asked to be sterilised during the Caesarean. This was therefore their last chance of enjoying having babies around. Older children also meant some previously developed contact with neighbours, other mothers, nursery school teachers and childminders. In addition, these parents did not have that superior almost scornful attitude of 'we are special and unique' which frequently isolates parents of twins from ordinary parents. They too had been normal other times around. Mothers felt and acted more like 'ordinary mums'. Besides favouring social contact, this attitude also favoured a more down-to-earth treatment of the twins. Though all parents occasionally had fun and took pride in showing off their twins, it was less of a way of life. The twins were part of the family and not its fulcrum. Those who had initially desired twins the least turned out to be the most capable and strong.

Mrs X, a woman in her late thirties, was far from wealthy. Yet she had so enjoyed the birth of her older son that she decided 'To treat myself to the luxury of having another child before it is all too late.' When she and her husband came for the initial scan aimed at determining gestational age, they both looked confident and pleased. However, when they were told they were going to have twins Mrs X broke into a desperate cry: 'We can't afford twins. One was already a luxury, but two!' Her husband was also clearly shaken, but took a more down-to-earth attitude saying, 'We will discuss this at home.' When Mrs X came back for her second scan she said, 'We are stretched to the limit, but we will try to fit these two in.' Mr X never came with her again as, to prepare for their future expenses, he took on all the extra work he could. Mrs X never complained about her husband's absence. She just concentrated on the twins, their health and their growth. She also bought a few newspapers that advertised second-hand baby clothes and articles, called upon her network of close neighbours and friends and avoided buying herself any new maternity clothes. Towards the end of her pregnancy she smiled and said, indicating her dress, 'My clothes are also stretched to the limit, but who cares.' Though enormous and clearly suffering as the twins themselves were big, she was by now beginning to take pleasure at the thought of having twins, especially as they were a boy and a girl. Her main worry was how her three-year-old son might react. Mrs X underwent her labour pains bravely and when the twins were finally delivered both she and her husband were overjoyed. Mrs X coped with everything very well. Talking about the twins she commented, 'They are such a bonus to us, but now I had better forget any longing I may have for more children.'

JEALOUSY AND DISRUPTION

In confirmation of previous studies, almost all siblings were greatly disrupted initially by the arrival of the twins and showed more or less clear signs of jealousy towards them (see Figure 6.2) (Bernstein 1980; Lytton 1980; Philips and Watkinson 1981; Dunn 1983, 1995; Dunn and Kendrick 1982; Hay *et al.* 1988). Most complained openly and bitterly about the chaos in their lives caused by the arrival 'of those two'. Young children were generally the most affected. Some showed clear signs of hostility. As soon as their mothers turned their heads, they engaged in suspicious embraces, dubious and aggressive stroking and, sometimes, clear strangling. They clung even more to their already exasperated mothers. Most also showed some form of regressive behavior. Lapses of bed-wetting and thumb-sucking were almost the rule. Although this was an extra burden on already overwhelmed mothers, nevertheless the majority of parents were very protective towards their older children. Fathers took them out alone. Mothers tried to devote some special time to them. Both parents would feel sorry and guilty for having to inflict a new and fairly chaotic routine upon them. All of these children seemed to long for the good old days. However, the real problems were still to come. As long as the twins couldn't get about, the precious possessions of siblings were at least left untouched. Their rooms were tidy and their toys were unspoiled. It was more the chaos, and the decreased availability of their parents, which affected them at first. Many also resented the special attention usually devoted to the twins, not only by their parents but also by relatives, friends and indeed even simple passers-by in the street. Twins were, if anything, more a cause of problems for their siblings than vice versa.

Slightly older children could also be somewhat overwhelmed by the arrival of the twins. Nevertheless, school-age children in particular already had other interests and friends and well-established identities within the larger community. Some were

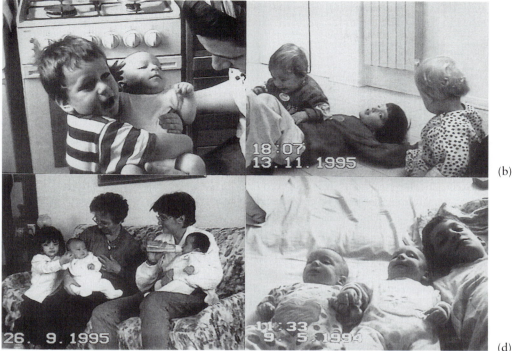

Figure 6.2 Brothers and sisters – jealousy
(a) This two-and-a-half-year-old boy tries to grab one twin from his mother's arms. This looks more like strangling than cuddling!
(b) This four-year-old boy complains bitterly to his mother, asking her to take away his monozygotic twin sisters who seem very interested in him. One is actually all over him.
(c) This two-year-old sister looks very distraught by the presence of the two-month-old dizygotic twins. The mother and grandmother are holding them. She gives a fairly vicious twist to the ear of the twin her grandmother is holding.
(d) This eight-year-old boy lies down on the bed next to three-month-old monozygotic twins, pretending to be a baby too!

actually quite proud of their new siblings and all the fascination surrounding them. They stuck pictures of the twins on their exercise books and got their mothers to bring them along when they picked them up after school.

SMALL HELPERS

A few siblings, not necessarily girls, showed a clear maternal attitude towards the twins from the beginning and took special pride and delight in helping their mothers and in playing with the babies. They were actually very helpful and understanding towards the twins. They did not even recoil, other than a grimace or two, from changing diapers or cleaning up those ever-present milky regurgitations. They were also very good at soothing the children and entertaining them – sometimes even more so than their fathers.

CHOICE

Siblings also often showed marked preferences for one twin or another. Differences in sex and temperament both played a part in this. These preferences became more evident, however, as the twins reached the toddler stage by which time they were more fun to play and interact with. At this stage it was not uncommon to see an older child taking sides with one twin against the other. This taking of sides and showing preferences was less marked in the case of monozygotic twins. Siblings showed a greater tendency to consider monozygotic twins as a pair.

YOUNG PARENTS

Only a few parents were in their early to mid-twenties. Whilst about thirty years ago this would have been the usual age for childbearing, things have now changed radically. Many reasons account for this and only a few will be mentioned here. Women nowadays generally want to progress in their chosen career before considering maternity. Couples decide to experience some freedom before settling down to a less carefree, more mature lifestyle. Economic reasons too often make it necessary to postpone parenthood. In addition, medical advances such as amniocentesis and generally improved care now allow what would have once been considered 'elderly' women to have perfectly satisfactory gestations. Very young couples have become more of a rarity. However, it does make a difference having a child at twenty rather than when you are in your early forties. Physically young mothers (and fathers) were less prone to extreme fatigue. Maternal bodies got back into shape more quickly. Mothers (and fathers) also had a more playful, joyful attitude towards the twins. Fathers participated more willingly in their care. In addition, younger parents still had a close network of friends; therefore mothers were less lonely and isolated. Taking the twins out for dinner or lunch was fun for the entire group. The great divide with childless couples was usually less acute.

In addition, life still lay ahead of these parents and so the twins were less likely to become the receptacle of all their frustrations. Most of the inevitable disappointments inherent to any life had yet to come. When indeed these finally affected them, frustrations were mostly ascribed to their marital life. All young parents had some marital problems when the children began nursery school. One couple actually split up as the still very young father sought comfort elsewhere.

PRIDE AND DELIGHT

A few mothers took special pride and delight in bringing up their twins from the very beginning. These women had a special disposition, being exceptionally giving and mature. They doted on children and would invite neighbours and friends with young babies to their homes. Occasionally they would even look after these babies as well. Two actually gave up work in order to be with their twins until they reached school age. Another two had very supportive environments, both from their families and particularly from their husbands. Another did not have such an entourage, but felt that the twins gave her strength. As she said, 'I cannot let myself go when I have to care for these two.' These were the exceptions rather than the rule. The joys of having twins usually began later for most, when they had at least reached some degree of independence as well as some form of verbal communication.

CHAPTER 7

THE INITIAL STAGES OF TWINSHIP

RESISTING TWINNING

At birth twins behave just like ordinary babies would. When a social dimension was introduced to their lives, together with demands for food, and other urgent bodily needs, they also made requests of a different kind (Stern 1974, 1977, 1985; Trevarthen 1976, 1979; Schaffer 1977; DeCasper and Fifer 1980; DeCasper and Prescott 1984; Schore 1994). They responded to being cuddled, talked to, stroked, and to being rocked and sung lullabies. They were also acutely sensitive to any individual attention aimed directly at them (see Figure 7.1). Their gaze tended to focus on the face of the caregiver (Johnson and Morton 1991). They cooed, or brightened up only if someone looked, talked, gestured, or smiled at them in particular. The only individuals they seemed to be utterly disinterested in were other babies and, specifically, their co-twin. Twins seemed very 'Darwinian' and 'selfish': their interest and attention was solely directed towards those who could offer help. Newborn babies are particularly attracted to faces (Morton and Johnson 1991; Johnson 1994). It may well be that being small, or for some other distinctive factor, the faces of other babies do not possess those characteristics which normally attract their attention (Dubowitz *et al.* 1980; Banks and Salapatek 1983; Atkinson 1984; Boothe 1988; Johnson 1990; Tyschen 1994; Daw 1995; Eliot 1999).

From the very beginning parents found themselves thrown into a baffling situation. Whilst it may be possible to breast-feed, hold or cuddle two babies at the same time, it is clearly impossible to stare and smile at them both simultaneously. Except for those occasional moments of peace when one twin was asleep, mothers (and fathers) were engaged in a constant to and fro between one twin and the other. Even in the best of circumstances individual attention and direct contact were necessarily scanty. Extreme fatigue, marital tensions and lurking depression all contributed to make concentrating on one twin as an individual a rare event (Goshen-Gottstein 1980). Most twins initially tried to resist this. Both seemed determined to get what they needed most. As soon as their mother gave undivided attention to one, the other yelled. Long before twins began to show signs of social recognition towards each other, they seemed acutely aware if a caregiver's attention was diverted towards their co-twin (see Figure 7.2). This caused frequent howls of pain and later on overt signs of jealousy. Focus on a sibling, even if only slightly older, was not accompanied by the same amount of protests. Twins seemed able to distin-

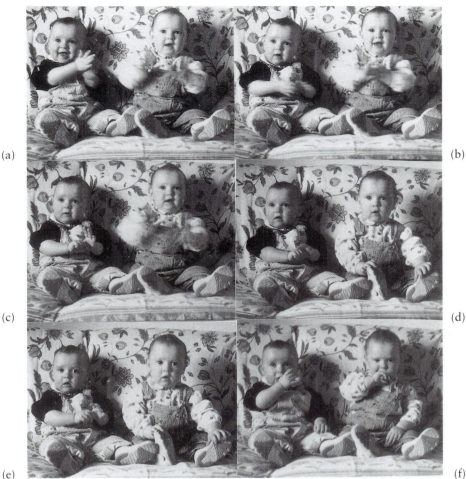

Figure 7.1 Interest in the main caregiver and other adults

(a) Both mother and grandmother are looking at these six-month-old monozygotic twin girls.
     They are clapping their hands. The twins clap their hands too and stare back. They smile.
(b) The mother has stopped looking at Twin 1, who stops smiling. The grandmother is still
     looking at Twin 2 and clapping her hands. Twin 2 continues to smile and clap her hands.
     Twin 1 still claps her hands, but only hesitantly.
(c) Twin 1 has stopped clapping her hands. She is still looking at her mother, but her gaze is
     clearly more sombre. Their grandmother has now stopped clapping and looking at Twin
     2. This twin's gaze is also less bright. She has stopped smiling, but continues to clap her
     hands tentatively.
(d) Both twins continue to look at their mother and grandmother, who are now talking to
     each other. Their gaze is rather sombre. Twin 1 holds her hands together; Twin 2 holds
     her feet.
(e) The two women continue talking to each other. The gaze of the twins is now completely
     unfocused.
(f) As their mother and grandmother continue to ignore them, the twins now start sucking
     their thumbs. Twin 1 looks tentatively towards her mother; Twin 2's gaze is now averted.
During all this time the twins have never looked at each other.

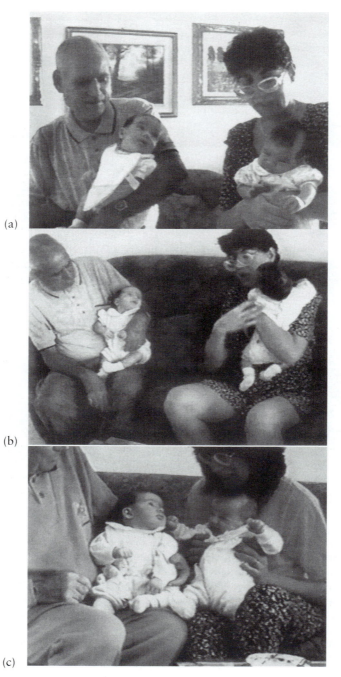

(a)

(b)

(c)

Figure 7.2 Attention is directed towards the main caregiver – opposite-sex pair, 3 months
(a–b) This mother is holding the boy and the paternal grandfather the girl. The girl continues
to gaze at her mother, who seems quite oblivious.
(c) A month later the mother is still holding the boy and the paternal grandfather the girl.
The girl continues to focus only on her mother, who looks back at her on this occasion.

guish the level of handling and communication most suited to their age. Therefore, they objected less before even only slightly more 'mature' signals or age-adequate manifestations of attention were directed towards older siblings. Infant auditory threshold and speech perception change with age (Aslin *et al.* 1983; Trehub and Schneider 1985; Ehret 1988; Peck 1995). Possibly these more 'mature' visual and auditory signals were scarcely perceived. Certainly, however, baby twins seemed particularly determined to be treated as individuals.

Their pressing demands to be handled as 'lone twins' were almost inevitably met with resistance and mounting exasperation. Many twins merely increased the volume and piercing tone of their protests, which provoked further feelings of annoyance in caregivers. Hearing is far from mature at birth and infants are insensitive to low sounds (Eliot 1999). Twins were not, however, insensitive to their co-twins' loud yells (Simner 1971). Even to an outsider their cries seemed particularly acute. One could well understand why many distressed mothers expressed the need for some peace and quiet. Twins' voices remained particularly loud. They continued to try to make themselves heard above the voice of their co-twin well past the initial stages of verbal communication. Sooner or later though, no matter how strong their early attempts at obtaining undivided attention were, all twins complied and adapted to the circumstances. Those who conformed first were often awarded the label of 'the good one' and received extra cuddles and smiles. Individuality was clearly discouraged.

ATTACHMENT TO TWO

Attachment is particularly intricate and, in some respects, different in twins.

After observing mothers with their infants for many years, John Bowlby put forward the Attachment Theory (Bowlby 1969, 1973, 1980). He regarded attachment, the emotional bond to a caregiver, as an essential and instinctive behavior guaranteeing the survival of the child. Attachment being a two-way process, both the child and the caregiver derive great pleasure from their mutual bond. A 'safely' attached infant not only receives protection and care but from this 'secure base' can proceed to explore the world. A secure attachment is seen as the foundation for future healthy mental development. Bowlby has had many followers (Ainsworth *et al.* 1978; Main *et al.* 1985; Greenberg *et al.* 1990; Murray Parkes *et al.* 1991), yet, even though the Attachment Theory has been tested in the most diverse situations, its predictive value is currently being seriously questioned (Kagan 1998).

Strangely, this aspect has been studied very little in twins despite the fact that in their case the vicissitudes of attachment are quite particular. Some aspects are shared with singletons, others are not (Dickerson 1981; Gromada 1981; Vandell *et al.* 1988; Anderson and Anderson 1990).

Several of the twins were kept in the NICU for a more or less prolonged period. Others (Richards 1979; Affleck *et al.* 1991; Minde 1993) have described how such a harsh environment favours the handing over of the babies to the staff. In particular, mothers often feel inadequate and intimidated by all the sophisticated equipment and constant monitoring of their children. They also cower at the thought of interfering in any way with the relentless routine of such fairly grim settings.

Prematurity itself does not make matters any easier for many mothers. Attachment to tiny, fragile and unresponsive babies can be quite hard.

When the twins were finally discharged from hospital, the problems linked to prematurity tended to persist at least for a while. Furthermore, it was not until both twins were home that parents were fully confronted with the task of simultaneously looking after two babies. Relating to two is quite different from relating to one (Lytton *et al.* 1977; Schaffer and Liddell 1984; Josse and Robin 1986; Robin *et al.* 1988). Absolute concomitance was simply not possible. To try to be impartial, mothers often held one twin whilst looking at the other (see Figure 7.3). Gazing,

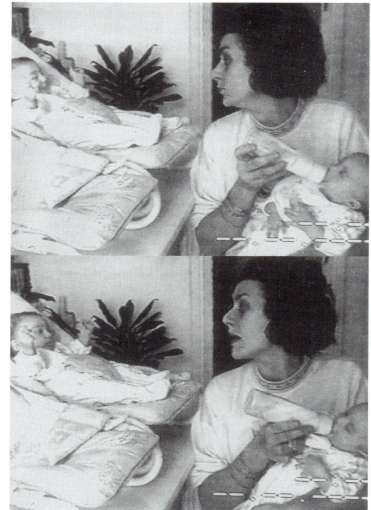

(a)

(b)

Figure 7.3 Trying to relate simultaneously with two – dizygotic twin girls, 3 months
(a) This mother is bottle-feeding one twin. The twin is looking at her mother. However, her
    mother is devoting her attention to the other twin who smiles back and flaps her arms.
(b) The girl being fed has fallen asleep, while her mother continues to look and talk to the
    other who responds.

facial expression, hand movements, talking, breast-feeding, rocking, cuddling and stroking were all frequently dissociated. Out of sheer necessity mothers also tended to engage in any of these activities for fairly short intervals. Individual attention was characterised by its brevity and the continuous oscillation from one baby to the other. Two mothers resorted to an extreme 'choice' in order to try to deal with these frustrating circumstances. Even then, however, the other twin could never be completely blotted out (see Figure 7.4)! Furthermore, practical aspects necessarily

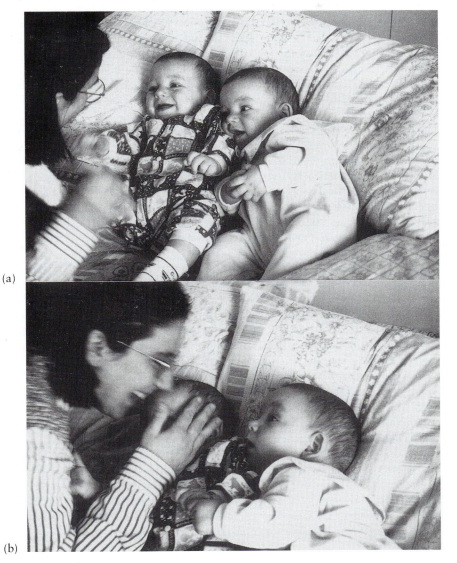

(a)

(b)

Figure 7.4 Attachment to two
(a) These four-month-old monozygotic twin boys focus all their attention on their mother. From the expression in their eyes it is clear that their mother is looking at the one on her left, who immediately 'brightens up'. The other twin is only half-smiling.
(b) In order to relate to the other, the mother has to 'blot out' the co-twin.

dominated the daily routine of the lives of young twins. By the time the twins had been changed, cleaned, fed eight to ten times a day, burped and rocked to sleep, there was very little space left for individual emotional interchanges or anything else.

Attachment also tended to be more 'promiscuous' and scattered over several people. To begin with, twins were in the unique condition of having simultaneously to share their main attachment figures with another baby. Though the main focus was generally directed towards the principal caregiver, fathers and other caregivers (including brothers and sisters) were especially prominent in the lives of the twins. They picked up attention whenever and wherever it was available. This did not mean disaster. Children can be very resilient and can do a lot with what they are given, no matter how little it may be (Rutter 1971, 1988; Kagan 1998).

Furthermore, the importance of other family members (including fathers, other siblings and co-twins), and of the social network around families, is often underestimated. All children, but doubly so twins, have lots of important contacts outside the mother–infant dyad (Lewis 1987; Parke and Tinsley 1987).

In addition, twins – especially monozygotic ones – have each other to rely upon. This unique link gave many of them a lot of support. The most constant and steady presence in the life of any twin is its co-twin. In many cases, sooner or later, each necessarily became the major figure of attachment for the other. Twins began to rely on each other for comfort, company and support (see Figure 7.5). Unlike singletons, who have a vertical pattern of attachment, contemporarily, a strong horizontal one was established with an uncommon intensity and at an unusually early age. This horizontal attachment was particularly solid and secure in the case of monozygotic twins.

The twins' attachment to each other and to the main caregiver was tested by the psychologist using the Strange Situation Test in a specific session between the ages of twelve and fifteen months. This procedure is described in detail in the original study (Ainsworth *et al.* 1978). Briefly: in a twenty-minute session a child is left alone with a stranger and reunited with its mother in various combinations. The reactions to separation and reunion are classified according to four standard categories indicative of the quality of attachment. This procedure is normally carried out in a laboratory setting. However, this proved to be impossible. Therefore all the twins were tested less formally within their home environment. A laboratory setting clearly would have offered a situation more conducive to a finer assessment, and this domestic version is obviously open to criticism and should only be taken for what it is worth. Hopefully, it may stimulate further more rigorous and appropriate research.

It is often not realised how mothers of twins very rarely go out without the twins, unless for work. Waving hands and apparently happily saying goodbye, therefore, while considered fairly usual for singletons, can be regarded as quite exceptional and hence potentially 'stressful' for twins. Besides separation and reunion with the mother, various forms of separation of the twins were tested (alone; mother only present; co-twin only present; both mother and co-twin present).

All monozygotic twins, except for two pairs, only cried and rejoiced when separated from or reunited with each other. When their mother went out most just carried on with their shared activities. By this age a strong and prevailing horizontal attachment had already formed in most monozygotic twins. Matters were quite different for dizygotic twins. Only three pairs displayed prevailing horizontal attachment. Two of these came from very severely emotionally deprived backgrounds.

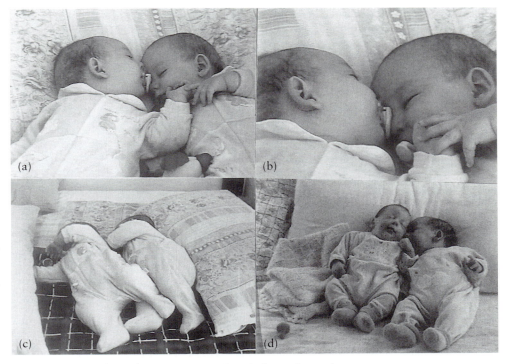

Figure 7.5 Mutual comfort – monozygotic twin boys, 3 months

These twins seem to find a special comfort in close contact with each other. Both are asleep on their parents' bed. The mother has put them next to each other spontaneously. She justifies this, saying that they cannot sleep alone in their cots.

(a) Both twins keep their heads in close contact. Twin 1 sucks a comforter and keeps his hand on his brother's face. Twin 2 holds his right arm behind his brother's body. With his left index finger he gently touches his brother's hand.

(b) Twin 2 is also sucking a comforter. His mother gave him one when he woke briefly. The heads of both twins have returned to the same position as before. Twin 2 now holds his brother's hand, which is again on his face.

(c) Their mother has moved the twins further down the bed. She has also put two pillows on one side of each twin, as if to protect them from falling; she explains, however, that the pillows give them extra comfort. Both twins sleep on the same side and keep their left arm high up, slightly bent, covering their faces. Their bodies are touching. Twin 1 keeps his left leg over his brother's right leg.

(d) A fortnight later the same twin boys are asleep on their parents' bed again. Twin 2 keeps his head in close contact with that of his brother. Twin 1 holds his hand on his brother's face.

'CUTENESS'

Initially one of the greatest joys parents derived from having twins was putting them together and seeing them next to each other. Identical clothes added an essential touch of overwhelming charm. Two little babies dressed alike in the same crib look enchantingly 'cute' (see Figure 7.6). This seems to have a universal and irresistible

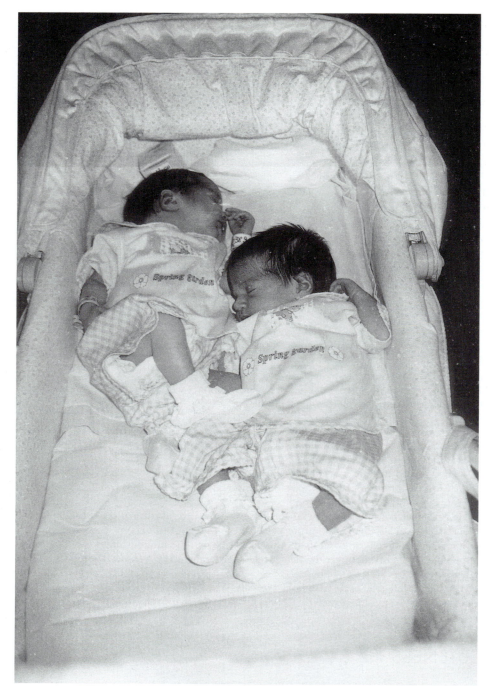

Figure 7.6 Cuteness – monozygotic twin girls leaving the hospital
The girls dressed in identical, frilly outfits, and sleeping next to each other in the same carry-cot look enchantingly cute. Indeed, these two displayed an incredibly high quota of social glamour when brought to the unit of Maternal/Fetal Medicine to say goodbye.

appeal. 'Cuteness' often implies that romanticised conventions about childhood are taken to such a degree as to make a baby or infant look funny (Higonnet 1998). What better candidates than monozygotic twins? Doubly cute. Smiles and cries of wonder were inevitable. Understandably, no parent could resist this temptation. Proximity and identical clothes also made a statement of twinship in the case of very unlike twins. Even a group of unrelated infants wearing the same garments is strongly engaging. Advertising agencies are well aware of this attraction. However, obvious physical differences soon made most dizygotic twins cease to be so appealing. After the first few months most onlookers assumed that they were just ordinary siblings born very close in time.

Contrary to dizygotic twins, time often mitigated the initial, frequently striking differences in appearance of monozygotic twins. Most of them looked more similar as they grew up. Although some monozygotic twins never recovered from their original differences in weight and size, forced proximity and identical clothes often overcame even quite macroscopic inequalities. The 'cuteness' did not run out for these twins. It was merely replaced by sheer glamorous 'amazement' or a different kind of 'funniness' in later years.

THE MAGIC BOND

To begin with (and sometimes from then on) certain twins did not react well to mutual physical proximity. Being put next to each other seemed to have little or no significance at this point. Often parents were actually surprised and disappointed by the scarcity or even total absence of interactions between their newborn twins. Many, in order to try and re-create their union within the womb and to offer them some form of comfort, put them in the same cot only to have them cry in protest over the apparent lack of space (see Figure 7.7). When placed together, most twins lay in distant corners of their cradle and showed signs of irritation at any stimulation originating from the other twin. Dizygotic twins in particular seemed quite disturbed by the vicinity of another baby. Parents of dizygotic twins were on the whole less tenacious in their attempts at reunion, and dizygotic twins were more persistent in their rebellion. With one exception, all dizygotic twins slept separately by the age of one.

Most monozygotic twins, however, quickly adapted to their parents' insistence on putting them next to each other and began to find comfort in the proximity of their co-twin. Within a month or two almost all monozygotic twins found close physical propinquity soothing. Monozygotic twins seemed especially 'compatible'. However, explanations other than a 'magic bond' uniting monozygotic twins from prenatal life may have accounted for this increased sharing. The thin septum dividing most of them *in utero* could possibly have favoured greater habituation to each other's motions and blows. After birth their howls may be more akin and hence less disruptive for each other. In addition, smell certainly figures prominently in the lives of young babies (MacFarlane 1975; Blass and Teicher 1980; Schaall *et al.* 1980; Balogh and Porter 1986; Pedersen *et al.* 1986; Schaall 1988). Babies recognise maternal breast and axillary odours, and singletons find comfort in the smell of their older siblings (Porter and Moore 1981; Chernoch and Porter 1985; Makin and

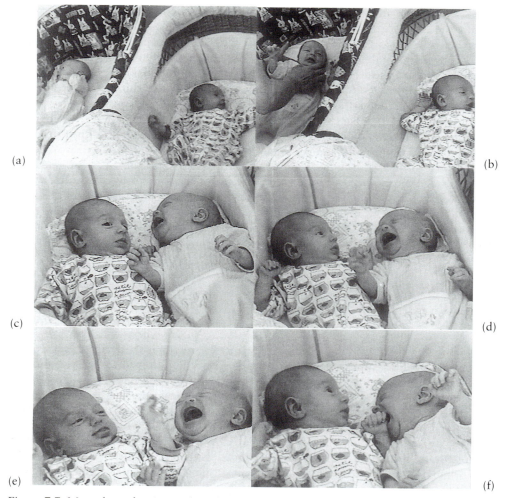

Figure 7.7 Mutual comfort is not the rule – monozygotic twin girls, 3 months
(a) Both twins are in separate cots.
(b) The mother picks one up in order to put her into her sister's cot.
(c–f) Twin 2 immediately starts crying and continues to do so. Eventually she ends up with
      her sister's hand in her mouth! Twin 1 seems unperturbed by her screaming co-twin.

Porter 1989). One could postulate that monozygotic twins may give out more similar and therefore more 'compatible' and comforting odours. Of the innumerable studies centring on twins, one ingenious piece of research uses specially trained search-and-rescue dogs. The dogs were presented with piles of dirty socks belonging to various individuals, including several dizygotic and monozygotic twins. Whilst dizygotic twins were easily distinguished, these highly trained canines could not tell monozygotic twins apart, basing their judgement on olfactory senses alone (Gedda *et al.* 1980). However, other studies have found that the distinctive olfactory 'signature' of monozygotic twins can be more easily recognised when twins are given different diets (Wallace 1977; Porter and Moore 1981; Porter *et al.* 1985, 1986, 1989;

Hepper 1988b; Halpin 1991). Save for extreme cases with consequential differential dietary requirements, the twins always ate the same food.

Besides odours, mutual licking and sucking promptly began and therefore taste became another element of sharing. Taste, though not fully developed, also figures prominently in the lives of infants (Mistretta and Bradley 1986; Crook 1987; Bartoshuk and Beauchamp 1994). Though nobody seems to have done any research on this, monozygotic twins may also 'taste' more similarly. Furthermore, the texture of their skin may be more alike.

Modes of reacting to physical proximity did not necessarily anticipate more complex patterns of social relating. Affection or mutual antipathy became manifest when proper social intrapair relationships gradually grew more elaborate and evolved. Though mutual comfort often heralded later affection, the two were not to be confused.

FIRST CONTACTS

The first contacts between the twins initially took the form of mutual sucking, licking and stroking. Placed face to face, they readily sucked each other's nose or chin and licked each other's cheeks. They also sucked each other's fingers, fists or wrist if one's hand happened to fall into the mouth of the other. Each part of the co-twin's body could be used as a kind of pacifier. Parents revelled in these initial contacts. Smiles, cuddles, kisses and laughter immediately reinforced any joint activities. Some caregivers found these actions such fun that they themselves inserted the nose or the fingers of one twin in the other's open mouth. Mutual licking and sucking was often interpreted, and not solely by parents, as a lack of awareness of each other's boundaries. Frequently people would exclaim 'How funny! She thinks it's her hand!' or 'He thinks it's his thumb!' Possibly no twin had such elaborate thoughts: at this early stage whatever part of the co-twin could be used would be used as a more or less 'compatible' pacifier. The twins also sucked their caregivers' nose and in most instances showed some sign of surprise and even distaste when sucking some bodily part of their co-twin. Equally the other twin usually tried to turn its face round, thus removing its nose, chin or cheeks from the mouth of the co-twin.

SOCIAL SIGNALLING

Usually 'social' mutual signalling involving visual contact and some form of facial expression and vocalisation between the two only started at around 3–4 months after birth. Before then twins directed their attention almost exclusively towards adults, or even towards slightly older children. They seemed attracted solely by more 'mature' facial features and expressions. However, this did not mean they were oblivious to the presence of another baby. Their yells when competing for attention testified to this. At this stage kin recognition may not take truly 'social' and 'adult' forms and as such should not be confused with social recognition. Auditory, tactile and olfactory senses, as well as familiarity with each other, are more important sources of information (Bekoff 1981; Porter 1987; Hepper 1990, 1991). Only when their vision began to mature (Dubowitz *et al.* 1980; Johnson 1990; Daw 1995) and when placed face to face in the same cot did the twins begin to show the earliest signs of visual social signalling. Even then the focus on the other twin was usually only fleeting. Monozygotic twins on average smiled and brightened up at seeing their co-twin slightly earlier than dizygotic twins did. However, they were also made to face each other more frequently. All parents of monozygotic twins eagerly awaited mutual smiles, and since monozygotic twins normally shared the same cot the possibilities of mutual direct ocular contact were greater (see Figures 7.8, 7.9).

Most parents were overjoyed as soon as they realised that their twins had begun to exchange unintentional and very transitory looks. Most tried to transform this into a daily exercise. As soon as another adult was available to pick up a twin, the babies were made to face each other. Often nothing happened and the twins just stared at the adult facing them. But when mutual gazing was sustained even for a fleeting second many reinforcing comments and smiles accompanied this happy event.

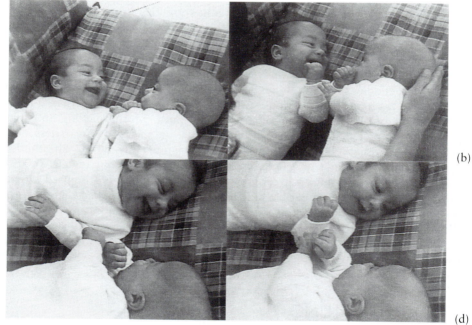

(a) (b) (c) (d)

Figure 7.8 Initial social signalling – monozygotic twin boys, 4 months
(a–b) The boys are in the same cot. Twin 1 is looking and smiling at Twin 2. Twin 2 does not respond.
(c) Twin 2 now responds and Twin 1 seems to brighten up.
(d) Twin 2 now smiles back at Twin 1, who is looking intently at his co-twin.

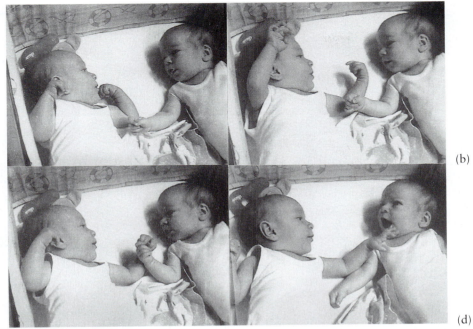

(a)

(b)

(c)

(d)

Figure 7.9 Initial social signalling – opposite-sex twins, 4 months
The twins are placed face to face in the same cot.
(a) They start looking at each other.
(b) They continue to look at each other. The boy raises his arms.
(c) They continue to look at each other. The boy touches his sister's hand.
(d) The boy touches his sister's face. She makes a grimace and looks away. Eye contact has been very brief.

BEHAVIORAL DIFFERENCES

From birth, mothers in particular could tell even very similar twins apart basing their judgement on behavioral traits alone.

Behavioral differences tended to be more clear-cut in the case of dizygotic twins. Genetic explanations apart, differences in appearance – and even more so differences in gender – generally favoured a distinct intrapair differentiation.

Remarkably, most monozygotic twins were generally as behaviorally dissimilar as dizygotic ones at the beginning of their post-natal lives. Cuddliness, fearfulness, jerkiness, tranquillity, particular sucking and sleeping rhythms were all mentioned and noted as characteristic and dissimilar traits (see Figures 7.10, 7.11). Innumerable examples could be quoted.

The mother of one set of monozygotic twin girls showed their teats, one quite smooth and the other nearly torn, to illustrate their different ways of sucking. Another mother when breast-feeding her monozygotic twin boys showed how one always clung to her body, whilst the other always kept at a distance. As she

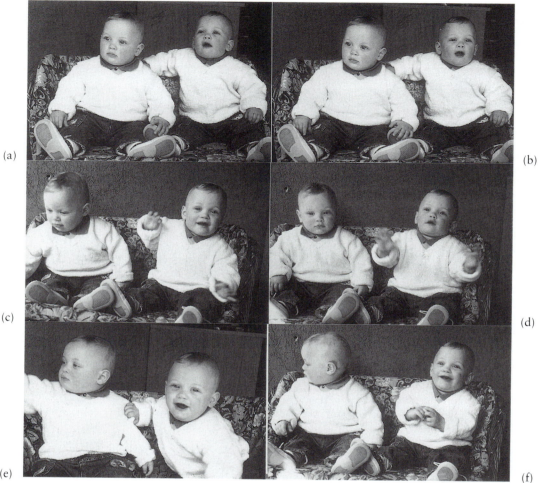

Figure 7.10 Behavioral differences – monozygotic twin boys, 1 year
The twins look very alike. However, behavioral differences are evident.
(a–f) Twin 1 looks dull, moves very little and seems scarcely interested in social interactions.
When he looks down or looks sideways (d–e) he is staring at an inanimate object, a
lamp (not visible in the picture), which he briefly tries to touch (f). Twin 2 appears
demonstrative and outgoing, shows a variety of expressions and accompanies them with
gesticulations. He is also interested in social contact and looks, smiles and gurgles at his
mother (also not visible in the picture).

said, 'He buries his head in my breast whilst his brother just sucks from the tip of
my nipple.'

Very soon mothers were also able to distinguish various noises and cries: 'This
must be Tom waking up', or 'This is clearly Dick making a fuss.' Only two
very exhausted mothers ever confessed to having got their babies mixed up once at
night.

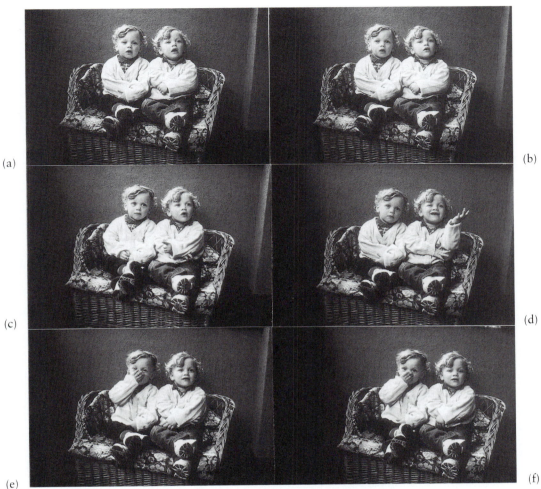

(a)

(b)

(c)

(d)

(e)

(f)

Figure 7.11 Behavioral differences – the same monozygotic twin boys, 3 years

(a–b) The boys are sitting on a settee next to each other. Arms and legs are all kept in the same position. However, the extrovert keeps his head turned slightly upward in a less rigid pose. His left hand is more relaxed. He does not hold his jumper with it as his co-twin does.

(c) The extrovert begins to open his mouth ready to utter some words and to move his hands preparing to gesticulate. The introvert closes his mouth and brings both hands together between his legs.

(d) The extrovert is now talking and gesticulating. The introvert's lips are closed tightly and his arms protect his body as before.

(e) The extrovert continues smiling and the introvert smiles too, but covering his mouth with his hand.

(f) The extrovert keeps smiling. His arms and hands are almost back in the initial position. The introvert has stopped smiling, still covers his face with one hand, and holds his sweater tightly with the other.

MOST DIFFERENT, MOST SIMILAR

One pair of dichorionic twin girls was found to be monozygotic at birth. These twins were the most similar of the entire group (see Figure 7.12). When the girls were tiny fetuses they moved and rested for almost exactly the same number of seconds. Activity and reactivity levels were virtually the same. Their rest–activity cycles were also strikingly simultaneous and coincidental. As soon as one began to move, the other also moved. When movements ceased, they ceased for both. Though many fetuses sometimes engage in rocking motions, these did so frequently and in synchrony (see Figure 7.13). When watching the scans their mother often commented, 'I hope they will look different because they move the same.' Legs up was the favourite position of both; however, a few days before term they simultaneously turned into the podalic version thus rendering a natural delivery impossible. When she finally saw them after the Caesarean their mother exclaimed, 'They are identical! Give me one, it doesn't matter which. They look the same.' While she was talking the girls were crying in correspondence. To begin with a tiny mole on the wrist of one was the only distinguishing mark to help their mother tell them apart. Besides appearance other features were confusingly similar. The tone of their voices was very alike and their behavioral manifestations were disquieting in their similarity and almost perfect synchrony. Long before imitation could be postulated the girls acted in perfect accord. However, some minute temperamental differences were noted and these guided their parents in telling them apart. One was slightly more outgoing and the other more withdrawn. One was slightly more cuddly, the other more rigid. One sucked rather voraciously and the other was fairly slow. No open preference was ever shown in their case and fairly interchangeable handling continued to characterise the lives of these girls.

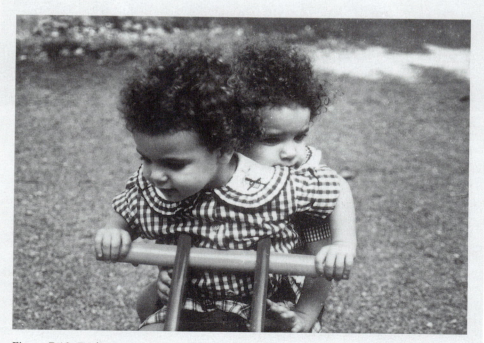

Figure 7.12 Dichorionic–monozygotic twin girls – similarity in aspect and behavior is evident, 3 years

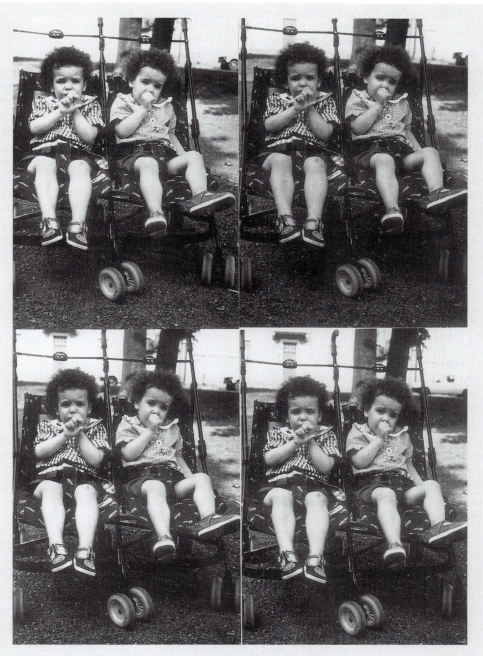

Figure 7.13 Dichorionic–monozygotic twin girls, 3 years
The similarity in aspect and behavior are even more evident in this sequence. Behavioral differences are minimal. Both twins are sucking their fingers and have similar, rather sad expressions. However, Twin 1 is sucking her index finger and Twin 2 her thumb. Twin 1 has her legs slightly more closed. Both move very little.

As mentioned before these twins were dichorionic. Having thickly divided amniotic sacs and totally separate placentas this sub-type of monozygotic twins should theoretically experience the most different of intrauterine environments. Theoretically this in turn would lead to greater differences between the twins. Some researchers have indeed found this to be the case in a retrospective study comparing monozygotic twins according to their shared or non-shared placentas (Karras Sokol *et al.* 1995). Unquestionably one cannot reach a general conclusion from one case alone. However, this example does raise several questions. Since their placentas were separate the split of the zygote had to have been a very early one. Could this earlier division have entailed a greater possibility of an equitable distribution? Could divisions taking place later, at multicellular stages, possibly favour a less even allotment? The intrauterine environments of these girls were as separate as those of all dizygotic twins. No vascular placental communications existed between them. Dizygotic twins are usually favoured by this relative intrauterine independence. Could a less-troubled environment have had a lesser impact upon them? Does the turbulence experienced by monozygotic twins during intrauterine life, especially when monochorionic, foster differences in them?

DIFFERENT OUTCOME OF AN APPARENTLY IDENTICAL CONDITION

Two very rare pairs of monoamniotic twin girls were included in the sample. They are contained within the same amniotic sac, with no partition in between – the closest twins can get apart from conjoined ones.

Both pairs were badly affected by their uncommon degree of sharing. Both were premature deliveries. All four babies had low birthweights and underwent prolonged stays in the NICU. One pair also suffered from extremely severe and distressing complications. However, there were also profound differences between the two pairs which led to quite different outcomes. At birth, weight difference was fairly minimal in one case (70g) and pronounced in the other (330g). The growth-discordant twin never regained the weight to make up the size discrepancy.

Besides this, behavioral discrepancies were also marked from the start.

One set of twins screamed when put together minutes after birth and this pattern of mutual irritability continued at least for the first few months. The other pair showed an almost opposite response. Mutual closeness immediately calmed them down. In addition, one girl of this pair, the substantially smaller one, showed an interesting phenomenon for the first six months. Her more intrusive sister often flapped her arms, thus unintentionally hitting her in the eyes. However, the less-favoured twin appeared to get used to her sister's blows. The blink reflex is absent at birth, but can first be observed at around two months (Peiper 1963; Berg and Berg 1987). When hit on the eyes by her sister, the smaller twin continued not to blink well beyond the second month (see Figure 7.14). In other circumstances, such as her mother moving her hands towards her eyes, she blinked. Mrs N, having realised this, frequently tried to make her blink.

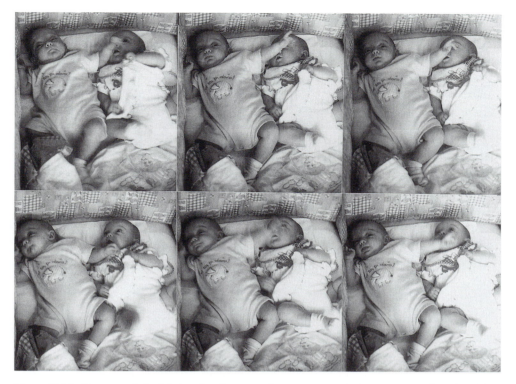

Figure 7.14 Absence of the blink reflex in one twin – monoamniotic–monozygotic twin girls, 4 months
Both twins are in the same cot. Twin 1 continuously, though inadvertently, strikes Twin 2 on the face. Twin 2 does not react to the blows. The blink reflex seems absent in her.

Irritability was later replaced by indifference in the girls with similar birthweights. Both twins seemed somewhat disinterested and indifferent to human faces, including that of their co-twin. Though by no means autistic these girls did display some very mild autistic traits. Physical contact with hard surfaces, bright colours and music all gave them greater pleasure than looking at each other (see Figure 7.15). Despite this apparent detachment the girls were in fact very strongly attached.

On the other hand, the growth-discordant girls were both lively and cheerful (see Figure 7.16). They enjoyed each other's company and as soon as they were old enough they began to share some good laughs together.

An apparently very similar and unusually close intrauterine condition had prompted quite divergent outcomes in these two fairly exceptional sets of twins. Whatever the reason, maximum prenatal propinquity had not automatically favoured later closeness.

Again, some purely speculative hypotheses come to mind. The greatly enhanced intrauterine mutual stimulation could have been too disruptive for the 'avoidant' pair. Their reaction to mutual contact after birth was very strong, even when barely touching each other. This constant disruption could have fostered the growth of what may be inherent traits of aversion towards bodily stimulation. On the other

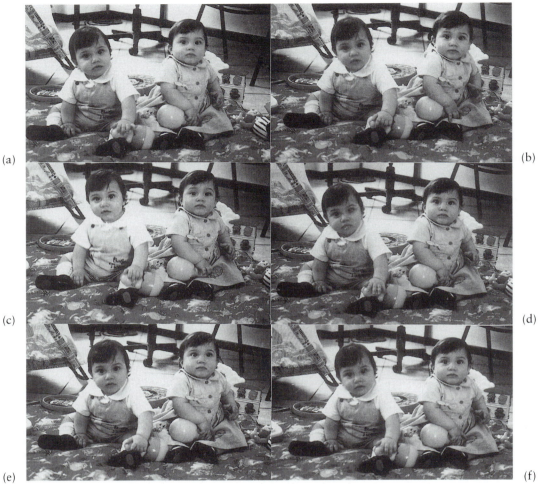

Figure 7.15 Different outcome of an apparently identical situation –
monoamniotic–monozygotic twin girls, 11 months
(a–d) Both girls, although physically close, seem quite disinterested in each other. They look
       at the camera.
(e) Twin 2 briefly looks up at her mother.
(f) Twin 2 has stopped looking at her mother and looks at the camera again.

hand, the cheerful pair displayed an unusual degree of tolerance to mutual blows
soon after birth. A higher threshold to tactile and proprioceptive stimuli could have
had a protective effect on these girls. This in turn could have favoured greater
tolerance.

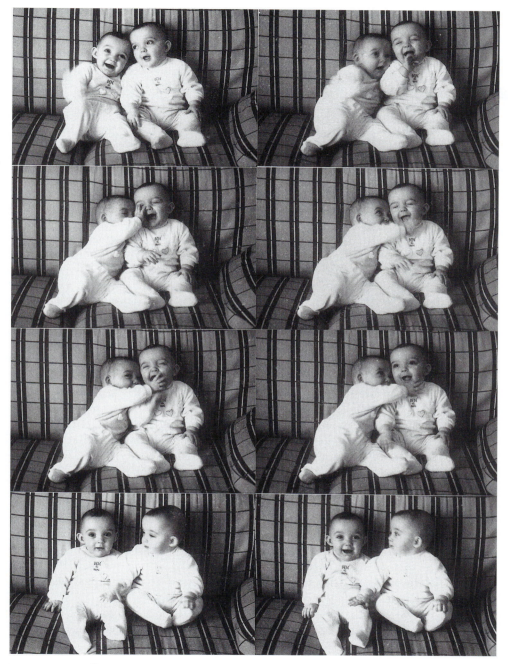

Figure 7.16 Different outcome of an apparently identical situation –
monoamniotic–monozygotic twin girls, 1 year
The contrast with the behavior of the pair in Figure 7.15 is evident. Both twins touch each
other's body and face, they laugh and vocalise and look at each other.

CHAPTER 8

'TWINNING'

PRACTICAL CONSIDERATIONS

'Twinning' refers to various environmental manoeuvres, some intentional and some completely involuntary, which contribute to the social and emotional post-natal making of twins as uniquely related individuals.

Most parents were initially driven by eminently practical considerations in forcibly 'twinning' their children. As mentioned before, many twins initially slept in the same cradle. Being so tiny there was certainly room for both. Parents understandably preferred to reserve their already strained economic outlays for the subsequent purchase of two long-lasting bar beds. Many parents actually slept with the twins. This arrangement made their restless nights somewhat less arduous. Even those who lived in large houses understandably opted for one bedroom for both twins as this made night feeds and various daytime tasks more manageable. After all, many ordinary siblings often share the same room. When bottle-feeding began, mothers often sat the twins in their baby-bouncers and fed them both at the same time. This speeded-up yet another chore and avoided unnecessary crying. As soon as the twins were able to sit unsupported most families bought playpens. The twins were often a bit cramped inside these narrow cells, but at least basic security was assured if a mother had to go out of the room for a bit. When the twins began to crawl, and even more so when they reached the toddler stage, they inevitably had to be kept under constant control; this was only achieved by keeping them both in the same room. One could add a long list of the many other occasions on which parents were forced, out of sheer necessity, for questions of safety, to keep the twins together or close to each other. Unavoidable practical considerations necessarily meant that the twins lived an uncommonly communal life.

While to begin with the twins themselves had little or no say in the type or degree of any twinning, they were not passive either. Twins had an impact on their caregivers as well (Brazelton 1974).

Mrs F, a woman in her early thirties, had read all the manuals available on twins from the moment she had been given the news. She dismissed most of them as nonsensical and full of platitudes. However, as an architect, she assimilated the notion that the house had to be 'twin-proofed'. She, therefore, proceeded to redecorate and reorganise her fairly spacious apartment. Her immaculate and sparkling white walls were covered with brightly coloured floral wallpaper. She explained that, 'It looks too cosy and English countryside for my taste, but at least their fingermarks will blend in with the flowers.' Walls were knocked down to make her bathroom and the children's bedroom more spacious. 'This room would have been plenty for one, but was definitely too cramped for two. I am sure they will spread out into the sitting room, but at least in principle they should be able to use this as their playroom as well.' In fact, any potentially dangerous furniture had been removed from every room, plugs had been covered, fragile objects had been moved out of reach, and the windows had been protected with wire-net frames. Everything had been carefully thought out in the minutest detail. Mrs F said, 'The only extravagance is keeping our hi-fi in view. But we love opera and I hope these two will too. Children like arias, don't they?' Mrs F never for a moment imagined what her monozygotic twins' musical tastes and their particular temperamental dispositions were really going to be. As soon as her boys heard *Rigoletto* or *La Traviata* they started to scream at the top of their lungs. When their maternal grandmother played them pop songs the twins loved it. Mrs F commented, 'We have really hit rock bottom.' Furthermore, both boys displayed a particular intolerance and irritability towards physical contact and proximity of any kind. This aversion included their mother and co-twin. Mrs F complained, 'I can't hug them or else they cry.' When the moment came Mrs F bought a huge playpen which occupied almost all of her spacious sitting room. The twins, however, objected loudly to being 'confined' together. Mrs F commented, 'They are very territorial. Nothing wrong with it. The trouble is they would need at least one country each!' Separate cots and beds were never put in doubt, but soon the twins even objected to sleeping in the same room together. When they were two years old Mrs F moved to an even bigger flat in order to have plenty of separate space for each twin. Though less 'twinned' than all other pairs as far as territory and proximity were concerned, these twins were deeply attached to each other – but from a distance! Their emotional link was strong but not 'banal', and lay outside the conventions generally associated with twins. Mrs F commented, 'They love each other dearly, but they both need their vital space.'

After the initial stages most other monozygotic twins, on the other hand, displayed a more or less strong inclination towards mutual physical proximity.

IDENTICAL CLOTHES, IDENTICAL HAIRSTYLE, SAME TOYS

Appearance certainly plays the largest part in the special charisma of monozygotic twins. Parents could not resist the lure of dressing their twins alike. After so much effort, the worries and sometimes incredible suffering, a little compensation was quite understandable.

Parents of growth-discordant twins were, of course, at a disadvantage. It was more difficult to find identical clothes of different sizes. This didn't mean, however, that they all gave up.

The mother of severely growth-discordant monoamniotic girls, for instance, often could not find the same clothes in such different sizes. One of the twins was about half the size of the other. When she couldn't find identical clothes this mother resorted to dressing the girls in matching, strikingly bright colours. This perceptual strategy often paid off. The girls were frequently identified as twins.

All dizygotic twins, except for one pair, looked very different at birth. They simply looked like ordinary and often quite dissimilar siblings. Besides gender, hair colour and general facial features strongly distinguished them. Even in the initial stages of their post-natal existence their parents had to resort to much more elaborate stratagems to try and hide their differences in appearance. To render monozygotic twins discernible, as such, it was often enough to give them an identical ribbon or hat.

Gender difference generally discouraged even initial attempts in opposite-sex pairs.

> The only exceptions were Antonia and Agustin. These twins had already been the targets of many sexual innuendoes while still *in utero*. Once they were born their parents enjoyed dressing them up the same. They often shared jokes about breaking the twins' sexual roles. However, after the first six months the twins hardly looked like twins at all. Furthermore, different gender was now a pressing issue even in this case. Fostering transvestism at this time fell into disgrace. Sexual jokes about heterosexual games between the twins replaced former 'deviance'. Any activities alluded to were now rigorously 'straight'.

Apart from this couple, the parents of dizygotic twins simply gave up after the first six months. Even when wearing identical clothes most of these twins merely looked like ordinary siblings who were nearly the same age.

Most parents of monozygotic twins did not give up until they were confronted with day care placement of some kind. The same applied to hairstyles.

Faces are generally the most distinctive constituents of our bodily appearance. Though buttocks, breasts, shoulders, legs and general demeanour may all give out clues to our identity, it is only when looking at someone's face that we can be sure about his or her identity (Goffman 1959, 1967; Morris 1977). Parents of monozygotic twins, and progressively even the twins themselves, were prepared to make concessions on clothes, but were reluctant to alter anything to do with their facial appearance. Although some differentiation in clothing had already started due to pressure from the external environment of day care, hairstyles remained the same for the majority of monozygotic twin pairs at two and three years of age.

Hairstyle was never an issue for dizygotic twins. Most of them had quite distinct looks and frequently the colour of their hair was different as well. Same hairstyles were simply the result of their mothers finding it more convenient to get their hair cut the same: when taking reluctant twins to the hairdresser it was easier and faster to say, 'Give them the same haircut.'

Toys varied among the two groups. Parents and friends frequently brought identical toys when visiting monozygotic twins. This rarely happened with dizygotic ones. Furthermore, opposite-sex pairs were generally bought traditionally gender-related toys.

> After the first six months even the parents of Antonia and Agustin (mentioned previously) gave them gender-specific toys. Antonia was, somewhat precociously, given a Barbie doll with 'sexy' underwear, a make-up set and a small coquettish dressing-table so that she could learn 'the arts of seduction'. Agustin was regaled with a collection of bright-red toy Ferraris, gymnasium equipment and a heap of fake gold credit cards.

Besides identical presents from their friends, parents of monozygotic twins often bought identical toys themselves purely as a matter of convenience. The twins them-selves, attentive as they were to any material possession of the other, reinforced equal distribution of tangible properties (see Figures 8.1, 8.2). Parents felt guilty if one twin yelled because the other was holding a big cuddly teddy bear. Buying another identical teddy bear avoided many unnecessary battles and screams. 'Twin' dolls, 'twin' cars and generally 'twin' toys abounded so that the twins could be given one each. As one mother said, 'Everything has been duplicated in the house. I only buy identical things. Nevertheless, they even object to that. When they have identical toys, they each want the one the other is holding!'

Constant mutual monitoring was a feature of monozygotic twins. Of course, from the very early days they were much more frequently placed next to each other. Reciprocal monitoring was certainly made easier by these environmental factors. Ini-tially they grabbed anything the other was holding fairly indiscriminately, while their later tendency to demand the same toys possibly reflected the twins' general inclination to prefer similar kinds of play activities.

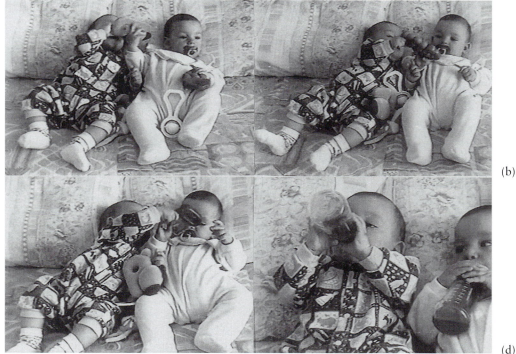

(a)

(b)

(c)

(d)

Figure 8.1 Mutual monitoring (1)
These five-month-old monozygotic twin boys do not look at each other. However, each is very aware of what the other is holding.
(a) Twin 1 takes a toy off Twin 2.
(b) Twin 1 takes another toy.
(c) Twin 1 takes yet another toy.
(d) To stop all this, their mother has given them each a bottle. Twin 1 is sucking from it. Twin 2 keeps the teat in his mouth. However, he is not sucking, but is looking intently at his brother's bottle.

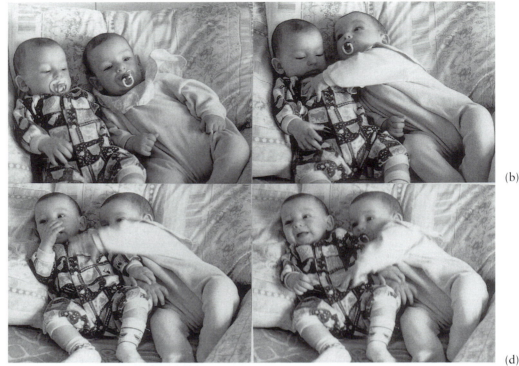

(a)

(b)

(c)

(d)

Figure 8.2 Mutual monitoring (2)

(a) The monozygotic twin boys in Figure 8.1 are now next to each other on the bed sucking their comforters.

(b) Twin 2 tries to grab his brother's comforter. The comforter falls down. Twin 1 looks at his brother's hand, which is still near his mouth.

(c) The mother talks to Twin 1 who 'brightens up' and brings his hand to his mouth. Twin 2 tries to grab his brother's right hand with his own left hand. Twin 1's left hand is resting on Twin 2's right hand.

All these activities have been carried out without looking at each other.

(d) Twin 1 smiles at his mother. Twin 2 now also looks at his mother, apparently no longer focused on his brother's activities.

In the end many monozygotic twins, besides matching clothes and hairstyles, also had duplicate toys.

Mrs D, a woman in her early thirties, worked in the fashion business. When she and her husband were told that they were expecting monozygotic twins they were overjoyed, 'Fancy that! This is so unique! None of our friends will be able to copy that! It's wonderful!', and so on. From then on Mrs D carried out an extensive study of all the books she could find relating to children's clothes. She turned up to each scan with a pile of pictures which she showed to everyone. Fortunately she discarded twins dressed like little squirrels, bunnies, sweet peas or bumblebees. She concentrated instead on the traditional romantic image of children as innocent angelic creatures wearing ornate costumes (Higonnet 1998). Once she knew that the twins were boys Little Lord Fauntleroy and Gainsborough's

'Blue Boy' became her models. These were then dutifully reproduced in various versions to match the passing seasons and growing size. When Mrs D finally delivered her twin boys they matched her dreams perfectly, with big blue eyes, curly Titian hair, and peaches-and-cream complexion. Both parents were radiant, 'Just as we had imagined them.' Once back home the twins were always dressed identically and quite fancily. To begin with they were a bit encumbered in their movements, but soon adapted. Enchanting pictures of the boys promptly appeared on every available surface in the house. A few were even published in a glossy fashion magazine. When the twins were one year old Mrs D decided to give a big birthday party for them. An extra observation was arranged to coincide with this event. All was lavishly prepared and the twins looked like clones of Little Lord Fauntleroy. All the adults beamed, uttered exclamations of wonder, applauded and took lots of pictures. The twins didn't seem to mind. They were used to this kind of attention. However, many other children of different ages were there now. A few older ones began to come up to the twins. 'Take your mask off, you look ridiculous with the same mask', said one and, not convinced, he pulled the twins' cheeks trying to take their faces off! Increasingly perplexed he mumbled, 'Ridiculous! Why did their mummy want to have two the same? I am a boy and I have a sister. Why two the same?' However, the worst comments were still to come, and all revolved around the costumes and the matching appearance of the twins. 'Can you play football in that?' and 'Which is you and which is your brother?' were the least harsh. In the end a menacing crowd surrounded the twins. The exact meaning of the remarks was possibly beyond their comprehension, but the threatening tones were not. They clung to each other and cried. In the end Mrs D was tearful too. Her image of childhood as 'innocent' and 'angelic' was shattered by all these cruel remarks. From that day the costumes were discarded, the children were made to wear modern clothes with different colours and, as soon as their hair was long enough, different hairstyles. Mrs D never tried twinning again.

All other parents of monozygotic twins, however, persisted with matching clothes and hairstyles.

MODE OF ADDRESSING: COLLECTIVE DENOMINATIONS

Many twins were frequently referred to as 'the twins' – just as one would say 'the Smiths' or 'the Joneses'. Plurals were also frequently used instead of singular forms. 'You two' often replaced individual names. More often than not this was done totally unconsciously just to speed up communication with frequently boisterous twins. Mothers had to shout 'you two' in order to prevent impending catastrophes without wasting any time. A collective denomination was simply more synthetic. However, this especially applied in the case of monozygotic twins. Similar appearance made collective names almost natural. Furthermore, monozygotic twins, as soon as they were able to, generally acted in unison. Opposite-sex or physically dissimilar twins always had quite distinct names. Dizygotic twins were called 'the twins' mainly in particularly busy moments. In any large family mothers will call out things like, 'Children! Dinner is ready. Please go and wash your hands.' Busy mothers of singletons and of twins would not dream of specifying each single name in such circumstances. Dizygotic twins were much closer to ordinary siblings in this respect.

PRAISE OF JOINT ACTIVITIES: PAIRING

Having overcome any initial dismay, everybody had great fun in watching monozygotic twins together. Pairing was particularly strong and reinforced in them. Though 'pairing' also stemmed from practical considerations, a strong element of pleasure and pride contributed to it as well. Actions done together were not only 'cute', but were also felt to be an intrinsic element of being a pair. Therefore from the very beginning twins were often 'paired', encouraged or even pushed to perform mutual and joint actions. Twins responded to any smile by intensifying what had been acclaimed. Dancing together, playing ring-a-ring-a-roses, or waving goodbye and blowing kisses in perfect unison were especially popular joint acts. Two little monozygotic girls delighted everybody when dressed up to stage a rudimentary French can-can whilst singing, 'We are the little twins.'

TRYING TO BE EGALITARIAN

All parents with more than one child are faced with the problem of trying to be impartial. No parent gives each individual child exactly 'equal rights'. Preferences, opposite gender, unlike talents, asymmetric weaknesses, changed life circumstances and many other causes all contribute to make the upbringing of any single son or daughter different and distinct from that of another (Dunn and Kendrick 1982; Dunn 1985). In the case of singletons inequalities can be rationalised with factors such as different age, gender and disposition. Mothers and fathers of singletons are clearly favoured by the age gap and obvious differences in their children in justifying sometimes even very macroscopic inegalitarian treatment. Parents of twins find themselves in a very peculiar situation. Since the children are the same age, unequal treatment is somewhat more difficult to justify.

Inegalitarian treatment was especially pronounced in dizygotic pairs. Different appearance, highly distinct temperamental inclinations and, in particular, different gender facilitated often marked preferences for one or the other twin. However, parents of opposite-sex pairs, though often blatantly more biased towards one, were adamant in denying any preference. Possibly marked partiality aroused increased guilt and concomitant denial.

Parents of monozygotic twins found themselves in an even more puzzling condition. The twins were the same age, the same gender, had similar behavioral inclinations, and often a very similar appearance. Preferences were more difficult to put into practice. Inequalities were clearly there from the very beginning in the lives of all 'identical' twins. Often, so was a quite pronounced parental choice. However, the inequalities were less marked than in dizygotic twins and possibly any preference was also more difficult to justify. Same toys, same food, equal turns and joint outings were examples of this. Even identical clothes were sometimes justified as impartiality.

Parents of monozygotic twins were on the whole much more candid and open about admitting any, albeit mild, preference for one or the other. Being generally much more egalitarian they possibly had less remorse about their inclinations. Growing independence, parallel to increased strength in the link between the twins, also seemed to buffer preferences. Parents seemed to perceive that the effects of inequalities were anyway mitigated by the progressive mutual pleasure, support and sometimes even 'self-sufficiency' of the twins as a pair. The twins, being more involved with each other, were less inclined to notice or resent mild external disparities affecting one of them.

COMPARISONS

Comparison was the rule for both monozygotic and dizygotic twins. Most frequently it centred on developmental milestones. One twin cut his first tooth several weeks earlier, the other crawled or walked or said 'Mama' first, and all these disparities were inevitably evidenced and often discussed at length.

However, this recurrent contrasting often had upsetting consequences on both the parents and the children. Parents worried unduly that some undetected prenatal or perinatal damage might be responsible for any delayed development. The twins, on the other hand, seemed to find such comparisons humiliating. When everybody applauded the first step of one, the still insecure twin looked pathetically miserable. In the long run comparison accentuated competition and fostered imitation. If one had achieved something, no matter what, the other wanted to attain the same. Twins were often driven by mere comparisons to follow in each other's footsteps.

LABELLING

From their early prenatal days twins were often given contrasting labels. Though at birth most of the old classifications seemed to vanish, for a few they did not. These twins were already codified from before birth.

Alex and Phil were one such case. When their mother was told that she was expecting twins she was furious and remonstrated with the obstetrician in charge until, in the end, this latter had to point out, 'But look, this is not my fault!' Mrs E irritated everybody in the unit. From around week 20 marked growth discrepancy became clearly evident. Alex was big and Phil was not. From then on Mrs E became enraged with Alex. It was impossible to convince her he was not deliberately stealing the vital juices of his brother. She nicknamed Alex 'the Vampire', immediately ascribing him bloodsucker qualities. His brother became 'the Victim'. Weight discrepancy at birth was considerable. Mrs E was outraged with 'the Vampire'. Needless to say post-natal 'choice' immediately fell upon the so-called victim. Although Phil soon gained weight, and after one year had caught up with his brother in all overt physical respects, their mother continued with very open favouritism. Only when both twins reached verbal communication did 'the Vampire' begin to speak up for himself and whine. His nickname was changed into 'Mosquito', another bloodsucking creature, but less overtly sinister. However, the unequal conditions of intrauterine life had long-lasting effects on Alex, who continued to be treated and reprimanded as a predator of some kind. Roles were reversed in post-natal life and 'the Victim' became the acclaimed tyrant.

Mrs E was a fairly extreme example of prenatal psychological maternal elements reverberating on post-natal life. These also affected a few other parents, albeit to a less irrational degree.

At birth, contrasting was more accentuated and clear-cut in all cases of dizygotic twins. The qualification 'less so' was used for more than half the cases, but for none of the monozygotic ones. Possibly their parents did not have the same cogent necessity of differentiating temperamental and physical traits.

REINFORCEMENT FROM SOCIETY: REFLECTED GLORY AND DIRECT GLAMOUR

From the early days of pregnancy many mothers began to feel 'special' and most fathers quite proud. Women already tended to consider themselves as 'super-moms', and their companions often experienced being the father of twins as proof of superior virility.

However, once the pregnancy was over the limelight inevitably shifted from the parents to the twins. Without both children present nobody paid special attention to either the mother or the father. On the other hand, when both twins were there their parents basked in reflected glory. Few could resist the temptation of achieving, albeit indirectly, this special status. In order to attract the maximum attention the twinning had to be maximised (see Figure 8.3). This applied almost exclusively to monozygotic twins. However, some dizygotic twins may look similar or even very similar.[1]

At birth Eric and Michel's facial features were fairly similar but, above all, their bright red hair made them stick out as twins. They were the result of IVF. After endless attempts to have a child the father was found to have a very low sperm count and IVF was tried repeatedly. The father seemed very wounded by this. Although it is no longer considered the case by science, for him his dizygotic twins were the proof to the outside world that conception had been spontaneous. Both parents tried to reinforce any existing similarities between the twins for as long as they could. Identical clothes in matching bright colours and identical hairstyles were the rule. Needless to say, as soon as they were taken out the twins received a special amount of attention. Their father in particular was delighted. He made a point of coming back early from work to take the twins out in their double stroller. This rarely happened with other twins. However, 'cliché' twinning manoeuvres also continued within the house. The same cot, the same toys, praising of joint activities, plural denominations, and so on, were all used. The twins had very different temperamental dispositions, Eric being

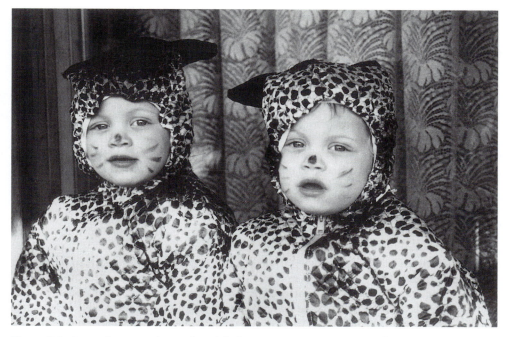

Figure 8.3 Attracting attention and social glamour – monozygotic twin boys, 2 years
The twins are dressed up in identical leopard costumes. This outing produced maximum glamour.

quiet and rather withdrawn whilst Michel was extremely expressive and outgoing. Compared to other dizygotic twins they also had areas of greater affinity and seemed to be particularly cognate. Interestingly, when the children were two years old a younger sister was spontaneously and quite unexpectedly conceived. The father was overjoyed and possibly no longer felt the need to demonstrate his virility. Identical clothes disappeared altogether and the boys were immediately given different haircuts. However, it was now the twins themselves who objected loudly when asked to give up other 'markers' of twinning. For instance, they were still sharing the same bed even beyond the age of three.

Matters were quite different for monozygotic twins. As with their pregnant mothers, their public appearances broke down one of the rules dominating our daily social contacts. Even perfect strangers felt entitled to come up and look, touch and talk to them and to their parents (Goffman 1959, 1961, 1967). Twins rarely went unnoticed during the early years of their lives.

Though several parents protested about the amount of attention their twins received, they all seemed quite pleased actually. The fact that none of them avoided using any of the elementary Gestalt stratagems which loudly announced that their children were twins clearly attested to this. If two people want to pass unnoticed, wearing different, plain clothes is unquestionably a good start. Film stars and prima donnas who base their fame on being special and unique can become quite enraged if their stylist sells an identical dress to someone else. They know quite well that the special attention they crave for inevitably shifts to the matching clothes, clouding and diminishing their individual prestige. Parents of twins acted in exactly the opposite direction by dressing their children alike. Confusing the individual identities of the twins was precisely what attracted all the attention.

Even close relatives and regular caregivers made no effort to distinguish monozygotic twins when they were dressed alike. They only pointed out in an amused tone that they could no longer tell who was who.

Only when urged to do so by nursery school teachers did some parents start to dress their children differently. Even then, once home most were changed back into matching clothes.

From the beginning direct 'glamour' accompanied most monozygotic twins. Passers-by turned round to stare at them and cried out 'Oh, look! How cute!' Long before the twins were aware that they looked alike, they seemed to discern the fact that each time they were together their joint spectacle caused a lot of excitement, compliments and smiles. On the few occasions they were alone, none of this commotion was aroused. They simply merged into the crowd.

To begin with most young twins looked quite frightened and began to yell when perfect strangers came up to them making a lot of fuss, with loud and excited exclamations, pinching their cheeks, patting their heads and stroking their faces. Nevertheless, sooner or later monozygotic twins got used to all this attention. Frequently by the age of two they were already unwilling to relinquish a celebrity which they themselves had not chosen in the first place. For several of the twins, feeling 'special' and being constantly in the limelight became a kind of habit.

The little girls who were frequently asked to dance a can-can together were one such case. Up to the age of three they always wore identical flowery pinafores and matching Victorian style clothes. However, at nursery school the teachers were adamant, 'No identical clothes!' Mrs K, their mother, tried hard to comply, but the twins themselves were inflexible. They screamed when dressed in different outfits. Different colours made them yell. Different shoes were kicked off. Different socks were rejected. Small, different ribbons were torn to shreds. Their mother was desperate. Finally she resorted to embroidered names on the back of the girls' clothes. As she said, 'This will only last until they can read. Then, God help me!' At a later stage the girls confessed candidly, 'Nobody looks at us otherwise and we have no fun.'

Glamour may be one of the many and complex reasons accounting for the fact that 'divorce' can later become much more costly for monozygotic twins.

One could well imagine this problem becoming more acute during the insecure and tumultuous age of adolescence. However, not even middle age seems immune to the temptations of rekindling glamour. Recently, the newspapers (*Marie Claire*: October 1998) wrote of a plastic surgeon based in New York who specialises in 're-twinning' monozygotic twins. He operates on those whose unshared existential vicissitudes and the unequal wear and tear of life have made fairly dissimilar in appearance. Once their former allure as a pair is re-established, thanks to the miracles of modern cosmetic surgery, these twins apparently feel 'reborn', ready once more to take up all the glitter that accompanied the beginnings of their lives. Though these are clearly extreme cases, they do nevertheless indicate that this apparently superficial aspect of twins' lives may be more than skin deep.

CHAPTER 9

BECOMING 'TWINNED' – THE COUPLE EFFECT

FROM PAIR TO COUPLE

Save for those rare twins who are adopted by two separate families and, therefore, reared apart (Bouchard and McCue 1981; Bouchard 1984; Pedersen *et al.* 1988; Plomin *et al.* 1980; Bouchard Jr. *et al.* 1990; Bouchard Jr. 1994), each twin inevitably continues to be an essential part of the environment of the other after they are born. However, their link progressively takes on psychological/emotional dimensions. A 'couple effect' begins to be operative as well.

The French psychologist René Zazzo was the first to describe and investigate the 'couple effect' in twins (Zazzo 1960, 1984). He maintained that the additional element of specific inner dynamics in all pairs of twins removes the rigid dichotomy between nature and nurture *per se*. According to Zazzo the uncanny similarities noted in twins reared apart (Lykken *et al.* 1992; Wright 1997; Segal 1999) are due to the fact that some genetic traits could only be expressed when the twins are not living together. When they are the 'couple effect' has the power to mask, attenuate and counterbalance the powers of heredity.

Twins are neither moulded by their genes alone nor can they be regarded as helpless receptacles of the home environment. Intrapair forces are an essential constituent of their lives.

However, one should be very clear about the meaning of the word 'couple' in this particular context. Whilst studying twins Zazzo had in mind, amongst other things, that the relationship between them might prove to be yet another 'experiment in nature' which could clarify aspects belonging to other couples, especially those united by wedlock or any form of mature love. Traditional couples and twins are profoundly and inherently different and therefore hardly comparable. Adult love, of whatever nature, generally stems from mutual choice.

From the moment they are taken home, twins live together and are seldom alone or apart. They share their bedroom and often their bed, their meals, their recreation, their means of transportation and are taken out together. The most constant presence in each twin's life is its co-twin. To begin with all twins are forced into being a couple. Only later does a growing independence permit them to express their will.

Adult love is also based on various affinities, including sexual attraction. Though love often suggests different gender, this is far from being the rule. However, adult partnership certainly implies sexual and reproductive maturity.

In adult love the age group of the partners displays all sorts of variations. They can be peers, but there can also be a huge difference in age. Furthermore, no close biological contiguity normally links any companion. The incest taboo is a fairly universal and very strong prohibition. Although some superficial semblance of the lives of young twins may be identified in adult couples, twins can hardly be used to illuminate any aspects of mature partnerships. When referring to apparently shared phenomena such as cohabitation or mutual masturbation, a profound distinction in age, grade of maturity, volition, quality of intercourse and many other factors have to be considered.

MUTUAL COMFORT AND UNDERSTANDING

Twins were made to rely upon each other for comfort and help from a very early age. Sometimes this happened quite spontaneously. When some twins were put close together in their cots they showed clear signs of solace. More often physical proximity was simply forced upon them for purely pragmatic reasons. Initial enforced propinquity in many cases developed into reciprocal support.

Ordinary siblings too can rely on each other a lot for support (Dunn 1983, 1988; Dunn and Kendrick 1982; Foot *et al.* 1990). However, twins live an incommensurably more communal life. Monozygotic twins on the whole experienced an even more shared life. Furthermore, their genetic similarity may have been an additional factor in rendering their general behavior and its physical manifestations more alike and therefore more understandable to each other. They were indeed even more prone than dizygotic twins to display extreme manifestations of mutual comfort and understanding (see Figure 9.1). If a twin needed physical comfort, was in a playful mood or was beginning to practice verbal communication, there was often nobody available save the co-twin. When starting to exercise for independent locomotion it was not uncommon to see one twin use the body of the other as a kind of walking stick. Twins often seemed to 'know' better than anyone else the moods, rhythms and needs of the other. Often all they needed was a glance. At times this heightened awareness increased closeness and tolerance. On other occasions it provoked flight: better to keep away from a companion in a bad mood!

> As a toddler Henry, a monozygotic twin boy, went through a phase of frequently being in a temper. Nick, his co-twin, was able to anticipate these changes of mood. Consequently, at these times, he would keep well clear of his brother even before Henry had manifested any apparent signs of temper. Their mother commented, 'Nick works just like a barometer for Henry. He can predict the sun or rain, and by looking at him I know exactly what to expect next from Henry.'

Silent understanding frequently develops in old couples, this usually being preceded by long years of verbal entente. Twins, on the other hand, engage in preverbal and non-verbal forms of mutual comprehension and perception which precede, and sometimes possibly even delay, language.

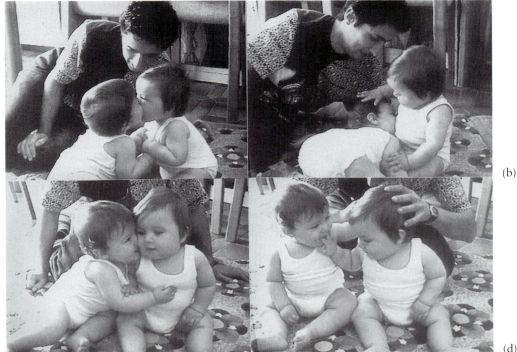

Figure 9.1 Intrapair relationships attachment to each other – monozygotic twin boys, 10 months

Their father is with them. Proximity seeking behavior is very evident.

(a) They kiss each other and hold hands.

(b) Twin 1 is all over Twin 2's body. Twin 2 holds his brother's arm and touches his head.

(c) Twin 1 approaches, touches and kisses Twin 2, who seems slightly more distant.
      However, Twin 2 does not protest or move away and touches his brother's arm.

(d) Twin 1 puts his arm around his brother's shoulder while looking directly at him. Twin 2
      puts his hand inside his brother's mouth while looking down. Their father strokes Twin
      2's head.

In none of the pictures do the twins turn round to look at their father.

The step from what was initially purely physical comfort to mutual awareness and cognisance was very short for all twins. In several cases dependence became very strong.

For three pairs of twins from emotionally very deprived backgrounds, mutual reliance was almost all they were left with. Except for their most basic needs, nobody took any care of them at all.

Greg and Victor were the first-born children of two university lecturers whose ideal of the maximum lifestyle was successful careers combined with a large family. When told that they were going to have monozygotic twins, both parents were elated – another symbol of excellence! The mother said, 'Our friends will die of envy', and her husband added, 'Nature is unparalleled.' Curiously, while saying this he had the prestigious magazine *Nature* in his hands. Pregnancy was rather laborious, especially as Mrs A began to suffer from severe hypertension towards the end of week 28. She was hospitalised for twenty days. At thirty weeks maternal and fetal conditions suddenly worsened and an emergency Caesarean had to be performed. The twins were tiny and quite immature. They were immediately transferred to the NICU and had to spend two months there; they both survived. Whilst they were in the NICU their parents rarely visited them. 'We are too busy,' Mrs A said. They continued to be busy even when the twins were finally discharged. Both parents were absolutely determined not to have their lives disrupted by the arrival of the children. Feeding times had to be met on the dot, naps had to be very long, toilet training was planned to start at six months, and when the twins cried their parents simply shut all the doors. The twins practically lived confined to the cot they shared within the cramped space of their tiny bedroom. Mrs A reiterated, 'We are too busy. They have to get used to it.' Except for when they were being fed and the odd occasions when they were cleaned, the twins were always alone and only had each other's company. Mrs A justified this, 'They will learn from each other.' As they grew older Greg and Victor lagged behind in every possible developmental respect. Of course, during pregnancy they had given worrying signs of fetal suffering, they were born premature and had suffered from severe respiratory complications. However, post-natal environmental neglect was also striking. Only when the children were placed in nursery school did they utter their first words. Greg said 'Victor', and Victor said 'Greg'. Nobody had taught them to speak. Soon the teachers also began to point out the developmental delay. Finally the evidence became too strong and the contrast with other children too marked to be denied any longer. At long last the twins got remedial help. As a teacher's report says, 'These twins have been relying on each other for too long. But at least they had each other! This has probably saved them from even worse consequences. Against all the odds they are now responding to treatment.'

THE TELEPATHIC LINK

Unusually early and intense mutual comprehension, including a particular capacity to decipher each other's body language (Hall 1959; Morris 1985), could perhaps explain some of the paranormal qualities often attributed to twins (Sommer *et al.* 1961; Playfair 1999).

When they reached independent locomotion, and even more so when verbal communication began, it was not uncommon to see one twin indicating, by gestures or words, that the other was in some kind of need.

This phenomenon started even earlier in three cases of particular proximity-seeking monozygotic twin pairs. Sometimes one twin would cry to signal that the other was experiencing some kind of discomfort. Eileen cried when Frances had to be fed. Their mother immediately warmed a bottle when she heard Eileen's distinctive cry.

When starting to crawl, Jan frequently bumped his head. He just looked surprised, while his co-twin cried. Their mother often laughed saying, 'But why are you crying? Jan hurt himself, not you!'

However, there was probably nothing eerie or paranormal about all this. It would not be unreasonable to hypothesise that an uncommonly early and constant exposure to each other's rhythms, bodily substances, behavioral patterns, and body language may foster a heightened reciprocal sensitivity in some twins. Some kind of familiarity with each other's rhythms may already start before birth. This would not imply esoteric 'telepathic understanding'. It may only suggest that twins, being constantly exposed to the manifestations of their co-twins, could sense from an unusually early age, and hence later perceive in an uncommon way, the signals of the other twin. Monozygotic twins, given their doubly unique genetic and prenatal sharing, could be particularly liable to experience especially intense mutual sensitivities. After all, heightened understanding is 'the' most often reported joy of sharing one's life with a monozygotic twin.

Interestingly, all twins that displayed some form of 'telepathic phenomena'[1] had shared their cot up to at least six months. This can in no way be made into a general rule, nor can other explanations be ruled out. Although it is difficult to make anything of these phenomena, the coincidence is puzzling.

IMITATION

That old couples end up resembling each other in many ways, sometimes even physically, is a fairly common notion. Though certain similarities may have been there from the beginning, thus prompting the initial choice to form a couple (Segal 1999), time often emphasises them.

Monozygotic twins are already an uncommonly alike pair right from the very beginning. Nevertheless, no twins are immune to the developmental steps which concern any child. Imitation plays a major role in the lives of young children as a means of learning (Meltzoff and Moore 1977, 1983a, 1983b; Uzgiris 1981, 1984, 1990, 1993). The so-called 'proto-conversations' (Wollf 1963, 1969) babies entertain with their mothers are a clear example of the importance of mimicry (Stern et al. 1983; Trevarthen and Marwick 1986; Papousek and Papousek 1993; Schore 1994).

Twins, albeit naturally inclined to learn from older human beings, are constantly confronted with their co-twin. Long before they give any reciprocal sign of social communication, almost subliminal monitoring of the behavior of the other invariably and inevitably takes place. No matter how hard they apparently try to ignore their co-twin, he or she is always there next to them. Monozygotic twins are on the whole made to share life together more than others. Their genetic similarity may be an additional factor in finding mutual facial expressions and general behavioral displays more in tune with their natural inclinations.

As time evolves twins not only continue to constantly 'study' each other, but also begin to imitate the activities and 'solutions' of the other. Imitation soon becomes routine practice. However, while most monozygotic twins can be regarded as strong imitators (see Figure 9.2) the majority of dizygotic twins imitate their co-twin only minimally.

Other children, too, imitate their peers (Eisenberg and Mussen 1989). However, imitation of another peer has distinctive features in twins. Twins start imitating and 'learning' from each other at an uncommonly precocious age. In a like manner to attachment, a horizontal 'learning' takes place parallel to the prevalent vertical one.

Though starting earlier, imitation became particularly evident around the toddler stage. Twins immediately notice if their co-twin has been successful in performing any task. They are also particularly sensitive to any praise this elicited from those

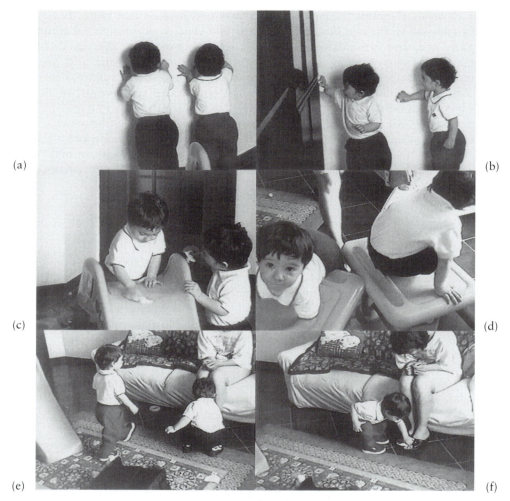

Figure 9.2 Imitation – monozygotic twin boys, 2 years
(a) Twin 1 is cleaning the wall and so is Twin 2.
(b) Twin 1 moves to clean another surface and Twin 2 follows him.
(c) Twin 2 cleans their plastic slide and so does Twin 1.
(d) Twin 1 has now climbed onto a small table and Twin 2 is climbing onto an identical one.
(e) Twin 1 cleans his mother's shoes and Twin 2 approaches him.
(f) Twin 1 has left, but Twin 2 imitates what his co-twin has just done. He cleans his mother's shoes.

around them. Through imitation they try to perform the same task, thereby obtaining their share of acclaim. Monozygotic twins almost constantly find reinforcement in the delighted response elicited by any joint performance. This is often extended to simple mannerisms. Therefore they sometimes clearly imitate each other simply in order to receive applause.

Those watching twins performing similar actions frequently confused mimicry with total genetic alikeness. 'Incredible! They act just the same!' was a frequent comment.

The human eye can be deceived, but videotapes played back at slow motion and 'micro-analysed' clearly showed how twins had not acted simultaneously. One twin had glanced at the other and then copied the other's behavior (see Figures 9.3, 9.4).

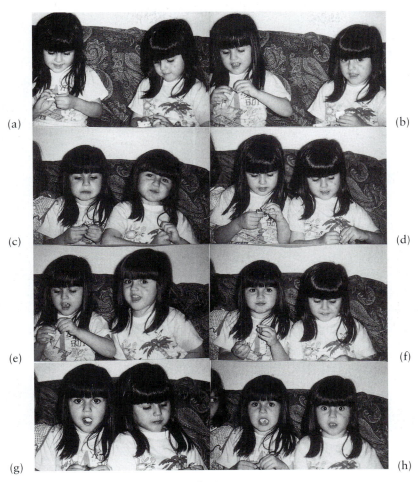

(a)   (b)   (c)   (d)   (e)   (f)   (g)   (h)

Figure 9.3   Imitation – monozygotic twin girls, 3 years
Twin 1 is the dominant twin. Twin 2 copies everything she does, but without ever looking directly at her.
(a) Both are sitting on the settee and are unwrapping a sweet. Twin 1 smiles. Twin 2 looks serious.
(b) Twin 1 smiles happily. Twin 2 also smiles happily and looks up at the observer.
(c) Twin 1 makes a grimace and Twin 2 also makes a similar grimace. She again looks up at the observer.
(d) Twin 1 and Twin 2 look down at their sweets simultaneously.
(e) Twin 1 opens her mouth wide. Twin 2 does the same and looks up at the observer.
(f) Twin 1 now prepares to put her sweet in her mouth and looks up at the observer. Twin 2 is still unwrapping hers.
(g) Twin 1 opens her mouth wide showing the sweet inside. She looks at the observer rather provocatively. Twin 2 leans against her.
(h) Twin 2 also opens her mouth and looks at the observer, imitating her sister.

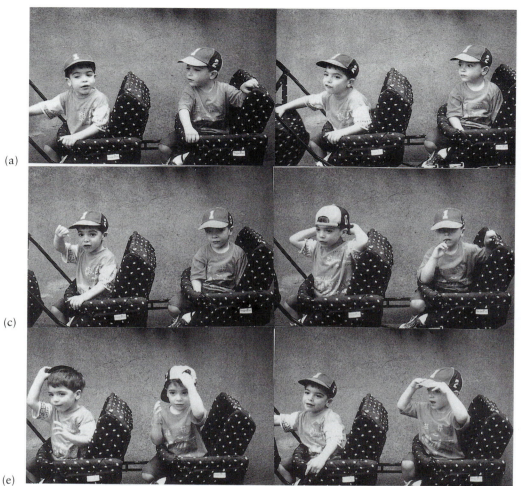

Figure 9.4 Imitation – monozygotic twin boys, 3 years
Both twins are sitting in their pushchair.
(a) Twin 1 glances sideways at Twin 2, while Twin 2 looks straight at him.
(b) Twin 1 makes a grimace. Twin 2 continues to monitor his brother as if waiting for his
     next move.
(c) Twin 1 moves his hand towards his sun hat. Twin 2 has turned his head round and
     appears not to be looking at his brother any more.
(d) Twin 1 has turned his hat round. Twin 2 does not seem to notice this, but looks
     perplexed. He keeps his index finger in his mouth.
(e) Twin 1 turns his hat back again. Simultaneously Twin 2 turns his hat round as his brother
     had done just a second ago.
(f) Twin 2 quickly corrects his move and turns his hat back again. Now both twins have their
     hats turned in the same direction. Twin 1 appears relaxed, whilst Twin 2 clearly continues
     to monitor him.

SECRET LANGUAGE

The idea of some twins sharing a secret language (also called autonomous language, cryptophasia and idioglossia) to the exclusion of outside communication often kindles popular imagination. Exceedingly few twins develop this form of language barrier (Luria and Yudovitch 1959; Mittler 1971). These very rare cases usually come from extremely deprived backgrounds (Koluchova 1972, 1976). Secret language seems to belong to the mystique of twins communicating in strange, paranormal ways. However, several of the twins, when practising for verbal communication, exchanged some verbal babble, nodded or acted in accordance to what had been 'said' and often laughed. Other workers have reported transitory forms of 'secret language' in twins (Mittler 1970; Dodd and McEvey 1994; Mogford-Bevan 1999) and some have found it to be more common in monozygotic twins (Alm 1953; Zazzo 1979a, 1979b).

Though monozygotic twins were better 'interpreters' of each other's utterances, many dizygotic twins were also good at deciphering. Though other forms of familiarity between the twins were not strong, mutual 'language' comprehension came easily to them. Nevertheless these fairly cryptic mutual utterances did have the resonance, pitch and tone of a normal conversation. Only their content was obscure (Bakker 1987). Nor did the twins seem unable or unwilling to communicate with other people. Usually they made their needs and feelings very clear to anyone willing to listen to them. Their shared 'secret language' had the quality of a fairly primitive sort of signalling, reminiscent of that amongst animals of the same species. Communication is incomprehensible only for the uninitiated and, indeed, nobody else could understand the alleged 'secrets' the twins were trying to share. Other children outside the family, although at the same level of maturation, did not have the same familiarity with their long-established forms of communication. Adults and older children within the household were at a different degree of evolution.

Interestingly those twins who manifested some kind of 'secret language' were at the same levels of verbal communication. Cases with marked discrepancies did not show the same degree of mutual idiomatic understanding. Once the step towards communicating with others in mature, prevalent language had been taken, the jabbering of the less advanced co-twin seemed unworthy of attention or even perhaps unintelligible. Verbal maturity had to be the same.

Mrs X had previously lived in Venezuela for several years and she had travelled around quite a lot while residing there. Her already colourful use of language was interspersed with metaphors referring to that country's luxuriant countryside. During a visit her opposite-sex twins started calling each other and communicating with high-pitched incomprehensible utterances from one room to another. Mrs X smiled and said, 'Many books on twins say that I should worry about this sort of communication. But to me their cries sound more like the call of parrots in the jungle. Birds signalling their whereabouts in and above the lush vegetation. What else could they do at this early stage? Have erudite disquisitions in an elaborate idiom? I actually love to hear them calling each other in the morning. They will soon move up in the evolutionary scale, but I will miss their cries.'

As soon as they were able to utter proper words all twins just dropped their transitory idiom and seemed only too glad to have finally achieved more sophisticated, comprehensible and widespread forms of communication.

LIVING AS A COUPLE

In conformity to the stereotype of monozygotic twins united by boundless love, they were frequently asked to kiss and hug each other.

In 1905 Sigmund Freud first pointed out that all children have natural 'sexual' curiosities and derive some pleasure from masturbatory fondling of their genitals (Freud 1905). This caused an uproar at the time, but is now widely accepted. As every mother knows, little boys have erections. Most people, however, are unaware that even tiny fetuses intermittently display erect penises too.

Occasional self-stimulation has been observed to begin at between seven and ten months of age in boys. Girls are slightly behind in this respect and their self-fondling is less focused and less frequent as well as apparently less intentional (Galenson and Rophie 1971, 1974; Kleeman 1975; Rophie and Galenson 1981). Most people simply regard infantile sexual curiosity, masturbatory activities in children and periodic erections in young boys as perfectly physiological phenomena.

Young twins were no different from other children in this respect. They too were naturally curious and occasionally engaged in masturbatory practices.

However, the treatment of monozygotic twins as 'couples' went far beyond being asked to perform fairly superficial demonstrations of fondness. Certain taboos which normally apply to all siblings, including most dizygotic twins, did not count in their case. Adults looking after monozygotic twins considered behavior that would not have been tolerated in ordinary brothers and sisters as normal and natural, if not downright fun. Many were allowed to sleep together and to hop into each other's bed at night or at any time during the day. Only one pair of particularly similar dizygotic twins was allowed to do the same. Even mutual masturbation[2] was not considered a forbidden activity for many monozygotic twins. These manifestations were usually carried out quite openly, and when twins were caught in the act everybody smiled or even laughed. Several parents gave their own videos of the children to the observer. A favourite was to film them unawares, as they awoke, in the act of embracing and fondling each other's genitals.

At this stage monozygotic twins possibly derived only a certain comfort and gratification from these activities. Fondness, softness, skin-to-skin contact, body odours, pleasure and natural curiosity all played their part. Furthermore, mutual explorations were probably much easier to perform with a life-long companion sleeping in the same bed. Monozygotic twins had no need to play at doctors and nurses if they wanted to explore each other's secret parts (see Figure 9.5).

Whether, and to what degree, these early activities have an impact on the development of the future sexuality of twins one cannot say. This facet of the lives of twins has hardly been considered and seems to be a taboo subject.

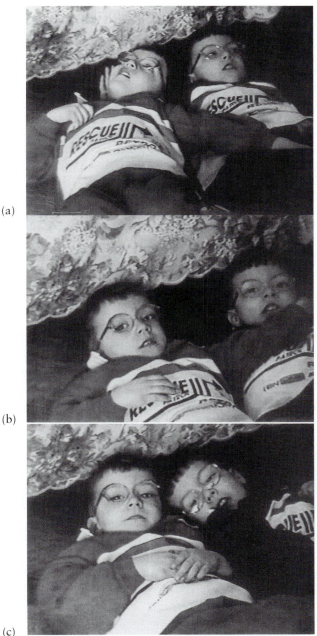

Figure 9.5 Mutual masturbation – monozygotic twin boys, 4 years
(a) The twins are unaware of the observer's presence. Twin 1 is fondling Twin 2's covered genitals.
(b) Both twins have realised that the observer is there. Twin 1 moves his hand to Twin 2's face.
(c) Twin 1 keeps his hand in an 'innocent' pose. Somewhat defiantly, Twin 2 is beginning to put his own hand inside his trousers.

DOMINANCE

'Dominance' also excites a lot of popular interest and is one of the favourite and most talked-about issues regarding the psychology of twins (Moilanen 1987; Goshen-Gottstein 1980; Lytton 1980). Even during an early ultrasounds visit it is not uncommon to be asked, 'Which is the dominant one?' At this stage 'dominance' can only possibly refer to a more active twin.

After birth other, necessarily more complex, intrapair dynamics were very strong. Each pair had its own equilibrium which was not based solely on boundless love and equality. A psychophysical imbalance frequently led one to predominate and in some cases even oppress the other.

It may sound paradoxical that more monozygotic twins were strongly domineering towards their co-twins. Monozygotic twins might be expected to be less divergent in their behavioral manifestations. However, most monozygotic twins shared an incomparably more complex relationship.

In both monozygotic and dizygotic twins dominance most frequently seemed to originate from truly different physical characteristics and 'temperamental' traits (see Figure 9.6). One twin could be more passive and 'lazy' and found it convenient to allow the other to take the lead. Another twin could be 'dominant' in the sense of

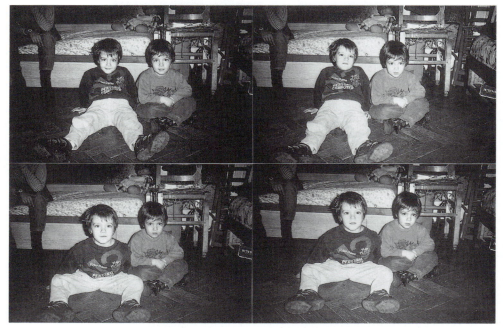

(a)

(b)

(c)

(d)

Figure 9.6 Dominance – monozygotic twin boys, 3 years 6 months
Twin 1 was always domineering, but dominance in this case seemed to stem from differential temperamental traits.
(a–b) Twin 1 is keeping his legs rather defiantly open. Twin 2 sits properly.
(c–d) Twin 1 is now even more defiant towards his mother and the observer. Twin 2 continues to sit in the background.

being more independent, enterprising, and more open towards novelties or less fearful or shy. Supremacy did not necessarily coincide with physical strength or with parental choice (see Figure 9.7). Sometimes the smaller and apparently frailer twin seemed to have an inborn tendency to be the leader, and the sturdier co-twin recognised this

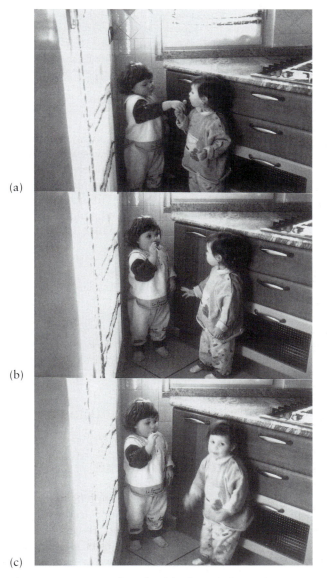

(a)

(b)

(c)

Figure 9.7 Dominance – monozygotic twin girls, 2 years 6 months
Dominance in this case was fostered by maternal preference.
(a) The non-favoured twin is sucking a lollipop. The dominant one grabs it.
(b) The lollipop is now in the mouth of the dominant sister. The other does not rebel or protest.
(c) The dominant twin continues to suck the lollipop. Her sister turns away without protesting.

'supremacy' and acted accordingly. The less favoured could also be less whiny and timid and hence endowed with an inherent disposition to be domineering.

> Ian and Damien, monozygotic twin boys, were one such case. Already during pregnancy Ian tossed and turned and kicked incessantly, whilst Damien hardly moved – to the extent that Ian was labelled a 'hooligan' and Damien 'quiet'. At birth the twins were very similar physically, but their behavior was not. Both parents chose 'quiet and cuddly' Damien without any hesitation and Ian was 'rejected'. Maternal prenatal perceptions seemed quite correct in this case. As time passed Ian became a real hooligan and a pest. Despite being preferred by everyone, 'quiet and cuddly' Damien was clearly dominated by his unruly co-twin.

Most parents felt that dominance was simply part of the general pattern of twin-ship. Therefore a fairly innocuous initial dominance was often allowed to become true assertion. In a few cases dominance eventually bordered on torment. One twin would be the perpetrator of torture, the other a somewhat passive recipient. Tyranny had its limits and when it went too far the subordinate twin rebelled even physically. However, the underlying pattern of dominance did not seem readily liable to inversion. Compared to other roles, dominance seemed more steady and fixed.

> One mother expressed this well, saying: 'Henry is definitely the leader and Nick the fol-lower. But Nick will not comply if Henry goes too far. They have a kind of equilibrium. Just like in communicating vessels one is not allowed to go too high or the other too low.' This was the same mother, particularly cognisant of the laws of physics, who had compared Nick to a barometer of Henry's moods. In order to receive some of their mother's scanty attention Nick complied with most of his bigger brother's requests. In this way he occasion-ally received his mother's praise for being so good. Furthermore, his much stronger co-twin did not hit him. Little Nick knew he would always lose on purely physical grounds.

SHIFTING ROLES

Not infrequently twins unexpectedly switched the complementary and binding roles assigned them. Since this sudden exchange is more frequently encountered in monozygotic twins, the shift is generally interpreted as genetics taking their toll: identical genes expressing identical temperamental traits at slightly different times (Lytton 1980).

One mother of monozygotic twin boys said, 'It's incredible. He has become the other one!' Another remarked, 'Extraordinary! They are perfectly interchangeable!' Monozygotic twins more often than not reached many developmental milestones at different times. One started walking, began to use the potty or teethed and the other followed within a few days or weeks. Exchanged roles could not just be confusing delayed manifestations of equal physical characteristics, but seemed to originate from more subtle intrapair dynamics.

Genetic similarity certainly played a part in facilitating such switches. Nevertheless, other reasons may also have contributed to these sudden shifts. All twins, sometimes even from prenatal life, were attributed different labels and roles. As explained earlier, dichotomies and role attribution were much more clear-cut, rigid and oversimplified in the case of monozygotic twins. As in many classifications, labels were generally based on fairly inflexible standardisations. Subtle tones and half-measures were inevitably absent. Differences were taken to their extremes without taking into account any of their nuances, including undoubted similarities, which went to make up the distinct personalities of each twin. One twin was good, the other bad; one cuddly, the other independent; one sociable, the other shy; one always on the move, the other a thinker.

Often both twins seemed to find it difficult to accept the rigid roles they had been assigned. Putting themselves into the other's shoes allowed them to express different aspects of their temperament. The other members of their family finally had to acknowledge these different needs, though they would re-create the original division with the roles switched. This recreation of the original division, albeit with roles reversed, did not alter environmental or intrapair equilibrium. Though parents were frequently taken slightly aback, a balance was soon re-established. Labels were simply exchanged.

Later swapping of roles sometimes took on different meanings as well. Switches often occurred around some major change. At these vulnerable moments, when confronted with new or unusual situations, twins reacted to these potentially disturbing events by adopting and imitating the solution used so far by the other twin.

In a pair of monozygotic twin boys Fred had always been adventurous, apparently not in the least fearful or shy, and extremely independent. His mother remarked, 'He is very independent. Paul is just the opposite. He is very cuddly, affectionate and not at all daring.' However, Paul, the shy one, by being fearful and withdrawn, received a lot of extra attention and affectionate care from all the adults. When the children were about three years old their parents decided to place them in a day-care group. Suddenly their roles were switched. Fred became shy and Paul bold. Their mother remarked on their genetic identity. The twins themselves, however, were of a different opinion. Fred said, 'When I cry, teachers look at me', and Paul explained, 'They call me naughty, but I have fun and they leave me alone.' Both had probably found the former role of their co-twin more congenial for facing this new situation. Fred needed reassurance once outside the safe boundaries of his home. Paul enjoyed some of the freedom which only Fred had savoured up until then.

The exchanging of roles seemed to take on an additional significance later. When twins became aware of their similarities in appearance, both seemed to enjoy fooling others. A 'Comedy of Errors' had by then begun.

POSSESSION, JEALOUSY AND RIVALRY

Before twins showed any apparent interest in each other they were intensely aware of reciprocal possessions. If one had a pacifier, in a matter of seconds the precious possession would end up in the other's mouth. Rattles, bibs, bottles and toys were all grabbed with great speed. Although their distraught parents immediately tried to substitute the stolen prize with something else, twins seemed determined to want the same thing at the same time. As described before, most toys were soon duplicated. Even the slightest difference was quickly noted and objected to with loud signs of distress.

Beyond material possessions, twins were acutely aware of any sign of undivided attention. As with ordinary siblings, in due time jealousy and rivalry appeared (Eisenberg and Mussen 1989; Dunn 1993). Both sat on their mother's lap, both wanted to be held by their father and both simultaneously tried to attract any older sibling's attention. Though experience soon taught them that they couldn't both have everything at the same time, varying degrees of jealousy continued to be a permanent feature of their relationship.

To start with, jealousy principally revolved around objects and third persons. However, mutual jealousy soon appeared. If one smiled at a caregiver instead of paying attention to its co-twin, this latter yelled. If one showed an interest in a guest, the other objected. Older siblings, who often had a marked preference for one twin, were an endless cause of misery for the second.

> The lives of Linda and Mary, the fat and thin monozygotic girls, had always been charac-terised by their parents' marked preference for Linda. From birth poor skinny Mary did not suit the taste of either parent. Mary put up with this blatant unfairness for quite some time and with incredible stoicism. Both parents basked in Linda's chubbiness and Mary did not protest. However, they also had an elder brother, Ricky. When the girls were born he apparently ignored them, though he regressed to fairly babyish behavior for a while. Nevertheless, when he turned twelve Ricky suddenly began to take a keen and rather carnal interest in Linda's curves. Possibly some steroids heralding puberty had begun to stir his blood. He kissed and hugged and fondled her all the time. This proved too much for poor neglected Mary who was fairly advanced for her age in verbal communication. One day she just exploded shouting, 'Whore!' Everybody was stupefied. Where could she have learned such language? Mary went even further than that. Shaking Linda by the shoulders she continued, 'You slut! You harlot! You tart!' She seemed to know the whole gamut of similar expressions. Mary could clearly endure her parents' partiality, but could not tolerate a rival in her life with her sister, no matter how clumsy and inept he might be. Perhaps a young admirer was felt to be a much bigger threat than unequal parental love.
>
> Differential achievement at nursery school also brought further conflicts into view. Given the overt preference everyone in the family demonstrated towards Linda, the abundant twin, she always expected to get her way. Mary tried to beat her on other, less 'fleshy' grounds. By the age of three 'thin' Mary was becoming the intellectual of the family. She was extremely advanced at nursery school. Her sister was greatly annoyed and endless family disputes ensued, but the teachers were adamant. They favoured intellect and, as a con-sequence, Mary.

All twins could be up one moment and down the next, as they were so frequently being compared to each other. However, antagonism appeared more overtly in dizy-gotic twins, as they were less frequently paired and more openly appraised on their differences. Those dizygotic twins that did not show signs of strong rivalry either simply ignored each other or were less frequently submitted to comparison by those around them.

CANNIBALISTIC FIGHTS

Even the best couples fight occasionally. All twins, monozygotic or otherwise, were no exception. Just as in ordinary life some unions worked, others clearly did not.

Given the widespread mystique which often surrounds twins, not all parents had considered the possibility of fights. Mutual bites began when the twins were still toothless. Hair pulling, eye poking, scratching and the use of any object at hand to deal blows to the other's head were soon added to their repertoire. To begin with, given their lack of force, twins could cause each other little harm. For most of them their impromptu fights appeared to be age-appropriate ways of obtaining something they wanted. Sometimes what appeared like hostile moves, such as biting or hair pulling, also seemed simply to represent age-related ways of approaching the other. When the twins were young, though parents usually intervened, they themselves took such conflicts in their stride. To begin with parents were not unduly worried. After all babies and young children do not play with each other much at first (Lewis *et al.* 1975; Rubenstein and Howes 1976; Mueller and Brenner 1977; Vandell 1980). Almost all they do is to pull each other's hair or scratch each other's faces (Maudry and Nekula 1939; Hay and Ross 1981, 1982). Twins fell within the normality.

Beyond these early stages, fights increasingly became a cause of concern for parents. Twins as toddlers could and often really did hurt each other. Distraught parents began to be afraid that their little cherubs had changed into fierce monsters. 'Savageness' protracted well beyond the stage in which it can occasionally still be observed in singleton children. Twins continued to be fairly 'primitive' and 'barbarian' in their fights. As they grew older their skirmishes resembled those of cavemen, dragging the other by the scalp and the widespread use of any handy tool as a bludgeon.

As in many primitive groups 'territorialism' clearly played a part in this. The narrow playpens that were meant to protect them from outside dangers caged them together in a very close space, which soon became a perilous battlefield. Parents quickly put these playpens aside and substituted them with the wider confines of a totally 'twin-proofed' room. Despite having more space, fights continued to occur. This seemed their most 'natural' and familiar way of dealing with their disputes. Nascent verbalisation did not substitute physical savageness, but only added another component to it.

There were differences between monozygotic and dizygotic twins. Though dizygotic twins could be fairly ferocious with each other, they applied appropriate social rules to others. Violence only continued within the couple and very seldom spilled over this boundary. Fights were also kept within the walls of the home. Most monozygotic twins did not apply such social rules. To their parents' dismay, their private fights often took place under the critical eyes of perfect strangers. As other studies have found, monozygotic twins seemed to act as 'reinforcing agents' for each other (Charlesworth and Hartup 1967; Hartup 1974; Hartup and deWitt 1974). Things became even worse when their savage fights burst out at nursery school.

However, once their initial temper had subsided, monozygotic twins tended not to bear a grudge. Their battles simply erupted and then vanished as quickly as they had come. Often it was quite impossible to discern the internal dynamics that set these struggles off. The twins themselves seemed fairly unruffled by their unrestrained attacks. Most tore at each other savagely one moment, and ignored or even hugged each other the next. Only a few pairs were constantly at each other's throats.

Dizygotic twins frequently continued with rancour and needed to call an adult in to solve their dispute. In opposite-sex pairs the environment tended to protect 'weaker' females from their male co-twins. Nevertheless, neither opposite nor same gender guaranteed peace.

> Martha and Bella, dizygotic twin girls, were possibly the most combative pair. Their parents had eagerly awaited their birth after repeated use of fertility drugs. They were elated when told the news that they were expecting twins. They were also elated when a few weeks later they were informed that the twins were both girls. Mrs Z said, 'That's marvellous! They will be able to play together and keep each other company!' Some inkling of doubt started during ultrasounds. The girls reacted to each other's unintentional blows with mounting force. Mrs Z commented, 'My tummy looks like a battlefield!' When 'quickening' started Mrs Z noted, 'Now my tummy even feels like a battleground!' After birth Martha was labelled 'an angel'; Bella was classified as 'a nervy type'. Long before the girls could get about they transformed the house into a battleground. They both just screamed and yelled all day and all night as if enraged. They were also extremely sensitive to any special attention given to the other and would immediately howl furiously. Mrs Z simply hoped that time would heal. However, with growing independence matters became even worse. Any attempt to sit the girls next to each other immediately set off a paroxysm of kicks, bites, scratches, pulled hair and punches. With increasing strength matters got worse and worse. One day 'angelic' Martha even managed to break her sister's front teeth with an accurately placed kick. Needless to say, as soon as the girls were able to utter their first words, verbal abuse followed. Bella's first words were 'Silly cow!'; Martha's first word was 'Witch'. Mrs Z commented, 'Their first words are insults. I am afraid these two are a very poor match.'

Martha and Bella are an extreme example, but mixed feelings were present even in the fondest of pairs.

CHAPTER 10

CHANGES IN THE TWINS

THE TODDLER STAGE: THE TERRIBLE TWINS

In the early days most parents had looked forward to the time when the twins would start acquiring some independence. Apart from anything else, carrying two babies around was an arduous task. The mother of one pair of especially robust twin boys noted, 'Thank goodness that Nature occasionally thinks about mothers of twins too! They get heavier, but luckily this does not happen all of a sudden. Our arms have time to adapt to their weight. By now my biceps are as big as Popeye's!' All mothers complained of terrible backache and various muscular aches and pains. Most envisaged the acquisition of some independence, especially independent loco-motion, as a huge relief for them. The first doubts assailed them when the twins started to crawl. At that point, it was difficult – but not impossible – to keep the twins under control.

Not even the most experienced mothers had even remotely guessed at what having two toddlers meant. By themselves even capable mothers could hardly cope with 'the terrible twins'. That same mother of the robust boys said, 'Why on earth did the Almighty decide to give twins the upright stance?' Oblivious to all danger the twins were by this time moving in every possible direction – usually the opposite one. All doors had to be closed; all windows shut. Everything possible had to be moved out of sight, let alone reach. Every possible sharp angle had to be removed, as tumbles and bumps were the rule. Fragile objects were the first things to vanish, as were any small objects. The twins were inclined to swallow anything they could, indiscriminately. Anything – even a co-twin! – could be used as a ladder for climbing to unimaginable heights. Subservient Nick often got down on his hands and knees so that Henry could climb on his back to grab what he fancied. Parents stopped using tablecloths after the crockery had finished on the floor a few times. Tables, chairs, lamps, even curtains, aquariums and hi-fi would all suddenly have to disappear. Mattresses and pillows were placed around the twins' bar beds, as they could now climb (and fall) out of these. Most parents actually bought new, very low beds. Taking the twins out became a nightmare too. Some parents decided not to go out unless they were together. It was impossible for one person to run after two children – one heading towards the road and the other towards the fishpond. Double tantrums in the middle of the street were another strong deterrent. In any case, it was impossible to go to supermarkets or shops of any kind. Twins became embarrassingly skilful shoplifters.

Already-exhausted parents were once more plunged into a seething turmoil. Of course parents of singletons also go through a stormy stage when their children begin to walk. But twins as toddlers seemed strident advocates of the relative unfitness of the human species to care for two children simultaneously. Not until the twins became a bit more cognisant of potential dangers did the strain, constant vigilance, perpetual shouting and incessant alarm that characterised this frightful period begin to recede.

PLAYING TOGETHER

Understandably all parents looked forward to the days when the twins would start entertaining each other. Parents would finally be able to enjoy one of the advantages of having twins.

Mutual interactions started quite early in most twins. These were obviously age-related. Grabbing or hitting, but also offering the other a toy, smiling at each other, and showing signs of pleasure or aversion towards mutual company were all displayed. Passing time increased the complexity of the twins' mutual interactions as others have already described (Radke-Yarrow et al. 1983; Eckerman and Didow 1988, 1996; Eisenberg and Mussen 1989; Eckerman et al. 1989; Barnett 1990).

To begin with many parents were dismayed by the fact that toys were mainly used as weapons. Anything could become a bludgeon. Also, toys broke at an alarming rate. When they played the twins only seemed capable of making an unbelievable mess.

It was only at around the age of two and a half that twins began to really play constructively with each other (Hartup 1983; Garvey 1990). At that stage many parents were pleasantly surprised. There were others, however, that suffered bitter disappointment. Their twins could not stand each other.

Twins have been described as fairly poor, shallow and unimaginative players (Wilson and Harpring 1972; Wilson 1974, 1975; Clark and Dickman 1984), the same causes being called into play as those postulated to underlie language delay. However, this was not found to be the case.

By and large monozygotic twins were better playmates. Most of them were quite co-operative (Loehlin and Nichols 1976; Lytton 1980; Segal 1984) and imaginative players. Their mutual games far exceeded the play activities of their singleton peers in sophistication and duration. Their interactions were sustained and their imagination was reinforced by their long acquaintance and possibly by a greater similarity in their tastes (Howes 1985). Monozygotic twins were in fact quite 'smart'. The psychologists noted, too, that when the twins were assessed separately with tests adjusted for singletons their scores clearly did not reflect the high sophistication and ingeniousness of their shared exchanges.

Adrian and Arthur had always been a delight for their parents. They were very alert, very prone to respond to social cues and found mutual comfort greatly soothing. They were also both extremely musical. Already as tiny babies they delighted in any melody or song. Their parents noted this and indeed there was always music of some sort or other in the house.

As the twins grew older it became evident that they diverged in their musical talents. Adrian danced incredibly well, while Arthur was a born singer and musician. Needless to say, the twins became almost professional performers. Their roles were distinct, but co-operation was impeccable: one played and sang and the other danced.

Dizygotic twins were less companionable in their playing. Many tended to go fairly separate ways. Others just fought. Only a few were co-operative. Initially co-operation amongst opposite-sex pairs was as good (or as bad) as that of same-sex pairs. However, around the age of four opposite-sex pairs tended to split along the general trend of their peers – boys on one side, girls on the other (Kohlberg and Ziegler 1967; Maccoby and Jacklin 1987; Archer 1992; Maccoby 1994).

Nevertheless, even when playing together dizygotic twins, on the whole, tended to be less imaginative and duller in their play. Monozygotic twins were generally a better team and acted more as a close-knit system.

Curiously, Antonia and Agustin, the twins whose parents liked to make sexy witticisms about their gender-related roles, were very collaborative in their games. Antonia played the male and Agustin the female! Antonia was the doctor and Agustin the nurse. Antonia was the manager and Agustin the secretary who followed her round. She was the football player and he the applauding crowd. Traditional roles were blatantly reversed in their non-conflictual games. Antonia seemed endowed with a more traditionally 'masculine' disposition and Agustin with more conventionally 'feminine' temperamental traits. Their by-now-resigned mother commented, 'He will make an excellent wife for someone and she an ideal husband!' In their case these opposite tendencies made a good match and resulted in co-operative play for quite a while.

Shared entertainment implied that their caregivers were no longer the main or even sole focus of the twins' attention. Most parents were pleased and relieved. However, a few mothers resented the special intimacy between their monozygotic twins.

The mother of Ian and Damien complained, 'I waited so eagerly for one of the big advantages of having twins: mutual companionship. But now I am no longer sure. I feel completely superfluous. The other day Ian suggested that my husband and I went out for the evening, saying that he was with Damien so they didn't need me.'

TOILET TRAINING

Another, previously ignored, aspect also seemed to indicate the deep 'biological' compatibility of monozygotic twins at this time. Very few twins were clean and dry before the age of three. However, the advent of nursery school meant toilet training was a prerequisite for all. Disgust for foul odours also emerges around this age (Schaall 1988; Schmidt and Beauchamp 1988).

Mothers of dizygotic twins barely mentioned this aspect of twins' lives. However, occasional accidents and sudden 'calls of nature' would occur during the observations. Each twin signalled the misfortune of their co-twin with strong expressions of disgust. Equally the right to privacy in the bathroom was not questioned. This was not so with monozygotic twins. Although they indicated the discomfort of their unfortunate co-twin, they showed hardly any signs of disgust. Nor did they contemplate privacy. If one went to the toilet, the other followed. At this stage the diets of most twins were still largely the same. Though this is no more than a guess, one had the impression that the odours of their bodily wastes were more similar and therefore elicited no clear aversion.

> This was partly confirmed by one mother. In order to train her twin girls she had to sit them next to each other on their potty and did not allow them to get up until both had done their 'duty'. After a while she became suspicious of their remarkable simultaneity. She decided to investigate the matter further by keeping watch on them from behind the door. As soon as one produced the desired result, both kneeled around the full potty and part of its content was transferred to the empty one without any sign of disgust. Then they cried out, 'We have finished!' and were embarrassed when they realised that their mother had spied their misdeed. Their mother commented, 'It was only the timing that made me suspicious. It may be their diet, but their faeces are in fact very much alike.'

THE MIRROR STAGE

In her classic study, Burlingham (1952) was the first to note that dizygotic twins identify their mirror images before monozygotic ones. However, only the French psychologist Zazzo systematically studied the reactions of twins when confronted with their reflected image in a mirror (Zazzo 1960, 1979b, 1993). According to Zazzo children generally recognise their mirrored image by two and a half years. Dizygotic twins do too. Things are much more complex and baffling with monozygotic twins. Zazzo pointed out that they took at least six months longer before recognising themselves in a mirror.

From one year onwards several minutes of video recording were devoted to the study of the reactions of the twins in front of a mirror. To begin with all twins just saw another child in the mirror. They tried to touch and explore it, but were soon baffled and driven back by the apparent discrepancy between the smiles and tentative approaches of the 'virtual' child and the cold, flat, two-dimensional surface of the mirror. However, by the age of two and a half all dizygotic twins had indeed realised that this was their image and not that of another child.

On the other hand, for quite a long time monozygotic twins did not see just any other child in the mirror image but rather recognised their co-twin (see Figure 10.1). This was testified by the fact that after repeated attempts to touch and stroke the assumed face of the other twin, they often turned round, seemingly quite disconcerted, until finally they spotted the real thing. Growth-discordant pairs, though very dissimilar in height and weight, had very similar facial features. These too saw their co-twin in their mirror image. This never happened with dizygotic twins. They never looked around for their co-twins.

Not until the age of three (and for some not until they were nearly four) did monozygotic twins begin to realise that what they were looking at in the mirror was indeed their own face. Until then monozygotic twins had not 'known' about their often striking similarity in appearance. Many were quite confused. Some asked

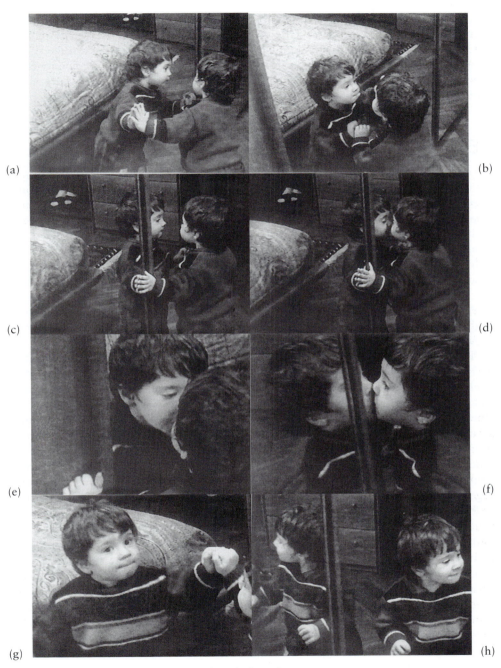

Figure 10.1 Mirror stage – monozygotic twin boy, 2 years

(a–d) This monozygotic twin boy 'sees' his brother in the mirror. He looks sideways at his
mirror image, touches it, mimics it and finally begins to kiss it.

(e–f) The boy is now kissing his own mirror image.

(g–h) Only after kissing the hard surface of the mirror does the boy look perplexed and
finally turns round to look at the 'real thing' with a baffled smile.

themselves, 'But who am I?' Deep doubts about their identities began to assail their young minds. Some even cried. One girl asked, 'But why two? Is she me or am I her?' Parents reported confusion and bafflement well beyond this initial stage.

Awareness of their own image in the mirror also brought dawning awareness of their condition to monozygotic twins. A young girl asked, 'Is this why everybody looks at us?'

VERBAL COMMUNICATION

Twins have been found to be generally delayed in language development. Although everybody agrees that twins display so-called intentional pre-linguistic communication – that is, they appear to understand what is said to them and are quite capable of indicating their needs and wishes (Camaioni 1993) – consensus on delayed language also seems to be fairly widespread (Mittler 1971; Savic 1980; Sandbank and Brown 1990; Rutter and Redshaw 1991; Lewis and Thompson 1992; McEvoy and Dodd 1992; Mogford-Bevan 1999). Language acquisition in twins is commonly considered to be about six months behind singletons.

According to many experts, twins utter their first words later, speak in shorter and structurally simpler sentences, their vocabulary is more limited, and generally they persist with immature forms of expression for longer.

This has been ascribed to a number of causes (Day 1932; Davis 1937; Mittler 1970; Myrianthopolous 1975; Hay et al. 1990; Lytton et al. 1977). Prematurity in itself may predispose to developmental delay. However, other premature infants do not show the same regularity and specificity in verbal delay as many twins do. Therefore other joint causes have been postulated. The most frequent explanation regards the quality of maternal (and paternal) communication. Undoubtedly mothers who must communicate simultaneously with two children of the same age tend to shift from one to the other and therefore engage in less prolonged interchanges with each single twin. Since maternal facial expression whilst talking is regarded as an important source of learning verbal communication (Gopnik et al. 1999), twins may also miss out on this. Mothers tend to look at each individual twin less. Furthermore, busy, tired mothers also tend to address the twins as a unit and to speak in shorter sentences and simplified language in order to speed up communication. This blame-it-all-on-the-mother explanation does not explain why singletons from truly deprived backgrounds often start speaking, albeit perhaps in rudimentary and unsophisticated ways, before twins generally do. Another reason accounting for this delay is thought to reside in the coerced proximity of all twins. Language cannot be learnt from another baby (Chomsky 1988; Bloom 1993; Pinker 1994). Possibly all of these are in part true as each explains different facets of this unusual developmental trait. There may well be other as-yet-unknown reasons which account for this delay. Nevertheless, save for a very few pathologic exceptions, all twins begin to speak in the end.

The twins in the sample varied regarding language development. Those who were born prematurely or had had major problems at birth were often late developers. Furthermore, those who came from emotionally deprived backgrounds also suffered from this developmental delay. Severe maternal depression, with consequent increased mutual reliance of the twins, seemed another aggravating factor. However, developmental linguistic delay was not ubiquitous even when more than one of these components were present. Other factors often intervened.

For instance, the monozygotic twin boys, Wes and Stephen, were born prematurely. Their mother was not depressed, but clearly very busy having to cope on her own with three older children in addition to the twins. However, having so many siblings around probably gave the twins plenty of opportunities to learn (Woollett 1986). They soon became very verbal.

The mother of Alex and Phil, the 'vampire/victim' monozygotic twin boys, was deeply depressed and went back to work even before completing maternity leave. Two very competent grandmothers took over the care of the twins. Alex and Phil were quite precocious in their verbal manifestations even by singleton standards.

Multiple caregivers and social networks around the twins helped a lot (Zimmerman and McDonald 1995).

Peer communications are hardly dialogues at the stage when verbal communication begins (Boysson-Bardies 1999). They are generally brief, superficial and fairly indiscriminate. Piaget regarded the earliest stage of peer verbal communication as essentially 'egocentric' (Piaget 1923). Subsequent research has challenged this concept of an exclusively 'egocentric' nature of the linguistic interactions of children aged from two to seven. 'Social' peer language is now postulated to start between the ages of three and five (Luria and Yudovitch 1959; Keenan 1974; Shatz 1983; Garvey 1984; Pinker 1984). However, for example, a three-year-old child may go up and say something to another child of the same age. This latter may or may not acknowledge what has been said. Frequently the first child, without waiting for or indeed expecting a response, simply dashes off to another activity or says something to a third child. Though tentative friendships and affinities begin to form, unrelated three-year-olds rarely engage in prolonged verbal interchanges (Shatz 1983).

Twins, particularly monozygotic twins, on the other hand, given their special and long familiarity, did engage in albeit simple dialogues. These included comments on their parents such as 'Mommy is angry, isn't she?' 'Yes, let's move to another room so she will leave us in peace.' Shared projects and reciprocal observations were also part of their discourse: 'You are really doing well.' 'No, I am afraid!' 'You can climb this too. It's a small table. Try!' 'All right. But then we will play with the cars.'

Again the psychologists commented on their scores when they were subjected separately to tests adapted to singletons. The generally poor performances of the twins when alone contrasted strongly to the verbal interactions observed when they were playing together.

Verbal interchanges with anyone outside the dyad were less conspicuous. It took more time and effort to engage them in conversation. If asked something a grunt was often the only reply. Furthermore, the other twin was seldom left out from any dialogue.

Von Bracken describes how one twin – whom he called the Minister of Foreign Affairs – often did all the talking. The other – the Minister of Internal Affairs – quietly supervised the interchange (Von Bracken 1934a).

During one observation only the Minister of Internal Affairs of a pair of monozygotic twin boys was present to begin with. He sat on the sofa in obstinate and passive silence, making no effort whatsoever to communicate with his mother. Only when his brother came back from a short appointment with a paediatrician did he look at her. His brother now did all the talking. Soon both went off to another room to carry on some private activity. Only then did the silent twin start to talk, albeit in a whispering, conspiratory tone. Verbal communication seemed to have introduced another element of union between monozygotic twins.

A new dimension was opened up by verbal communication even in the relationship of Toby and Jack, the monozygotic twins who had been extremely averse to each other and who displayed an indiscriminate irritation towards physical contact of any kind. Now they could, and indeed did, interact, and even play, but at a distance. Their verbal exchanges were highly sophisticated and brought them closer to each other, though not in the physical sense of the word.

Dizygotic pairs were quite different. They were generally only too willing to have one-to-one interchanges with people from outside the dyad.

Interestingly, the red-headed dizygotic boys who had always been treated like monozygotic twins were very unlike in their verbal outcome. Eric was extremely alert and vociferous. He was precocious in acquiring verbal communication, whilst his generally more withdrawn brother had a linguistic delay of about six months. Needless to say, this gap did not favour verbal exchanges between them. Even when Michel finally began to speak, their shared games continued to remain largely non-verbal.

The attainment of verbal communication, whether it was delayed or not, was a turning point in family life.

Conversations did not mean ceasefires between the twins. Fights continued unabated, but a verbal weapon was added to the arsenal (Tesla and Dunn 1992). Many parents, hearing their twins arguing cleverly with each other, commented that they would make good lawyers. A surfeit of potential students of law testified to the special quality of the twins' verbal communication.

ENTERING COMMUNITY LIFE

Impact on dizygotic twins

By the age of two the lives of monozygotic and dizygotic twins began to diverge in other important respects. Most twins were placed in some kind of day care, as all but three mothers went back to work. By the age of three all twins had made their entry into the slightly more formal environment of nursery school.

Although it was possible to observe very few twins in their day-care placement (two dizygotic and three monozygotic pairs), there were other occasions to observe the twins interact with their peers. The visits now took place just after nursery school. This usually meant picking up the twins from school and, weather permitting, spending at least some time, often the entire observation, in nearby playgrounds where both school friends and other children were present in abundance. In addition, copies of all the twins' school reports were obtained.

Although their teachers knew that dizygotic twins were twins, they always referred to them in the reports as single individuals. It is now almost standard practice in many

European countries to assign twins to separate classes or groups. Only three particularly shy twins were reported as having any difficulty separating from their co-twin.

When dizygotic twins reunited after nursery school, most pairs just seemed pleased to see their mother. As soon as they spotted her they hung to her skirt and simultaneously started to flood her with confused and fragmentary information about their activities. Quite often mothers were overwhelmed and had to say, 'Please, one at a time!' In trying to make themselves both heard at the same time, the twins' always raised their voices and could be heard from a distance.

What was very evident whilst observing dizygotic twins playing with or alongside their peers was that other children did not treat them as twins. Given their different appearance they were not singled out, but were treated just like any other ordinary member of the group (Dunn 1993). The concept of twinship clearly eluded their peers as well. Children would ask if they were brothers or sisters, but that was all. Though time spent in the home environment was still necessarily spent together, once dizygotic twins began to move their first tentative steps into the wider community they were no longer regarded socially as twins. Peer interaction was clearly eased by this and most twins seemed quite relieved to enlarge their circle of contacts (Corsaro 1985; Volling *et al.* 1997; Rich-Harris 1998).

Entering nursery school did pose problems, however, for Lenny. His twin sister, Claire, was in the same school. She was double his size and weight. Lenny had never recovered from his intrauterine growth retardation. At birth Claire weighed over a kilo more than him. This difference always bothered him. When children saw him next to Claire they often came up to him and asked, 'Are you her younger brother?' His self-esteem suffered greatly at all these remarks. So much so that later he managed to convince his parents to take him to a different school. Without Claire's overwhelming presence he proved to be very popular.

Impact on monozygotic twins

Contrary to dizygotic twins, monozygotic ones found their link further reinforced once they began to move out of the home environment. Outsiders and peers looked upon them as a single entity. Even when placed in separate groups, their peers identified them anyway. When they arrived or left nursery school together, or when their classes were united, their appearance invariably gave them away. Young children are very good at detecting any deviation from the norm and usually react by isolating anyone who is different, sometimes in quite a cruel manner (Asher and Coie 1992; Coie and Cillessen 1993; Diamond *et al.* 1993; Kindermann 1995; Volling *et al.* 1997). Monozygotic twins were regarded as a discordant oddity. One day, in a playgroup, a boy came up to an especially similar-looking pair of girls and asked, 'What are you? Photocopies?'

The debut of monozygotic twins in a peer group was thus characterised by isolation that made them cling to each other even more (Kim *et al.* 1969; Vandell *et al.* 1988). However, the twins themselves also rejected their peers. Given their close union, mutual fun and far superior ways of entertaining each other, they were generally quite oblivious of the others (Bank and Kahn 1997). Suspicion and lack of effort stemmed from both sides.

Nor was selective treatment of monozygotic twins limited to their peers alone.

When reading their teachers' reports it was striking how frequently the co-twin was mentioned and problems were analysed and anticipated. Teachers had a tendency to consider monozygotic twins 'clinical cases' and exerted frequently ungrounded therapeutic efforts on them. One report went as far as to declare that the twins did not have separate egos! Their mother was in tears when she read this. However, the twins themselves promptly dispelled her anxiety. One announced, 'I want tea!' while the other countered, 'No tea! I only like orange juice.'

Besides teachers, other adults also contributed to further isolate monozygotic twins. Invitations to birthday parties and other social events were beginning. Though three-year-olds do not interact all that much with their peers, society now puts a strong accent on the importance of early socialisation. Consequently, all mothers began to look out for potential young friends for their children at around this age. Monozygotic twins did not qualify as very suitable candidates for such early inter-changes. They probably came last on anyone's list. Few mothers were willing to invite two young children instead of just one. When they did the union between the twins inevitably resulted in their singleton child getting left out or, even worse, ganged up on. On the other hand, asking just one twin was felt to be unfair, especially in the case of monozygotic twins. Gender and other obvious differences made such selective invitations more feasible in the case of dizygotic twins. Mothers of monozygotic twins would themselves invite other children to their house, but this often ended in disaster with insults, blows and tears. The twins would quite openly create an unholy alliance against the outsider. Therefore, monozygotic twins tended to get left out of the minor network of individual non-institutional contacts with their peers.

GANGING UP AND 'ILLICIT ACTIVITIES'

Growing up brought out other more complex manifestations in pairs of monozygotic twins. By the age of three a new dimension to mutual closeness was beginning to emerge. An element of defiance, mockery and aggressive fun was added to the union of many monozygotic twins. Parents now found them difficult again (Hay and O'Brien 1984). The twins had 'ganged up'. This could be observed even more clearly in older pairs (Burlingham 1949).

The mini-gang resembled much later adolescent bands in its spirit. Triumph, obstinacy and bravado: two against the world. In most cases these manifestations were barely perceptible and quite subtle, but in a few instances they were not.

A pair of twin boys, at around the age of three, started ganging up on others. Anti-social behavior increased in the following years. The twins mocked their teachers; they deliberately tried to hurt one little girl; and certainly did hurt their grandmother's cat when they hung it up by its tail.

Ian and Damien, the other case that displayed defiant ganging up, were particularly riotous monozygotic twin boys. Up to then Damien had been slightly more subdued. At around the age of two he could no longer resist the lure of becoming the true rebel his brother had always been. Their mother believed in the principles of enlightened education. No limits, no coercion, no rules. Children had to decide what suited them best. The twins certainly always had great fun being allowed to make the most unbelievable mess: flooding the house with water; eating with their hands like savages; pasting their meals all over the walls; and belching like heavy beer drinkers well beyond the age of infantile burping. Furthermore, they gave full leash to fairly ravenous masturbatory appetites and defiantly fondled each other's genitals in front of everyone. It was only when confronted with nursery school that their parents began to question the way they were bringing them up. If anything, nursery school, by giving them boundaries to their bad behavior, had done them some good. Mrs C tried to modify her principles, but Ian and Damien behaved like little hooligans and continued to act as a fairly dangerous and well-organised gang.

A pair of very pretty and precociously 'sexy' twin girls found a more conventionally 'feminine' way of ganging up. Besides fondling each other's genitals, they formed an alliance in seducing their much older brother. They took turns in kissing and caressing him in all sorts of ways, including stroking his genitals with their feet. They literally drove their brother crazy with their constant and carefully aimed stimulation. So much so that he failed his exams at school. Without openly mentioning this pleasurable masturbatory aspect, the boy justified his failure by saying, 'I have no peace. How can I study when they are both all over me?'

This particular household was a fairly deprived environment, and nobody took any effective measures to stop the girls' behavior. Furthermore, they all lived in a few cramped rooms. All three children slept in the same room as their parents. What they were exposed to there could perhaps explain a lot.

These are worst-case scenarios. Very few twins actually turn into defiant hooligans or promiscuous 'duos' later on.

However, the often visible aspects of a small and generally much more innocuous 'gang' were never taken into account by the many 'experts' involved in the care of the twins. The accent was so much on individualisation and forced separation that teachers and school psychologists did not know what happened when the twins were re-united. Coerced separations can bring lovers closer together against all odds and quite often with tragic consequences for all. Twins are certainly not lovers, but their union is unique and sometimes very special. If professionals want to break this 'link' they have to offer twins equally special alternatives (Schwarz 1972; Gleenson *et al.* 1990; Segal and Russell 1992). Growing up probably brings with it differing interests and talents. A passion for a job can dilute exclusive love. In later life passionate love for someone can also weaken the links uniting most monozygotic twins. However, at the early age of between three and five it was difficult to envisage any other sufficiently powerful attraction (social or otherwise) capable of weakening the natural bonds and affinities which bind them.

COALITION AGAINST AN INTRUDER

Two families decided to have another child when their twins were three years old. In another case an unplanned pregnancy came as a complete surprise to overjoyed parents. All three children were girls.

None of the twins themselves seemed very enthusiastic about the new addition to the family. As with the birth of any new sibling jealousy clearly played a part in this. The twins were no longer the sole centre of attention and they resented it. Possibly seeing another child enjoy the kind of one-to-one relationships they had never experienced made them all the more envious. Probably the different gender of the new child also roused further jealousy. No inkling of this showed through their verbal interchanges. The twins were totally silent about the new arrival. Their little sister did not exist in their conversations. When asked about her, they replied with silence and a sly smile.

All three pairs (two monozygotic and one dizygotic) adopted the same strategy towards the recent addition to the family: a united front against the intruder (see Figure 10.2). The birth of a new sister brought about a clever, focalised coalition

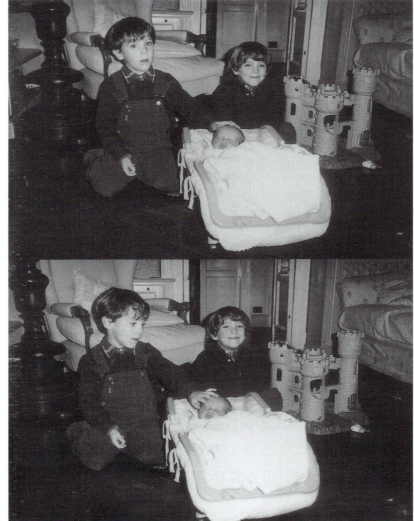

(a)

(b)

Figure 10.2 Coalition against the intruder: a little sister is born – monozygotic twin boys, 4 years
(a) Twin 1 strokes his sister's head. Twin 2 smiles, apparently angelically.
(b) Twin 2 continues to distract everybody with his smiles which now do not seem so much angelic as sly. Twin 1 pokes his finger in his sister's (closed) eye.

aimed at ignoring and tormenting her. The behavior of all three pairs betrayed no sign of either interest, affection or pride. Total disdain can be heartless in itself. However, parallel to this disregard a more or less tacit hostile conspiracy was put into action. All three mothers reported that as soon as the twins were alone with their sisters they started torturing them in all sorts of insidious ways. Scratches, twisted arms, near strangling, and overturned cradles were all reported. The parents all complained that they could not leave the twins alone with their baby sisters. Even when mothers or other attentive caregivers were there the twins acted in unison, and in one way or another managed to cause some upset. One would go up and talk to their mother, while the other pulled the girl's hair. One would smile angelically, while the other would viciously punch her on the nose. One would complain an urgent need, while the other would shake her cot violently. They would start making a din the moment their sister fell asleep. They would both demand attention when she cried out. Synergy made their combined actions very effective. It would be virtually impossible for a singleton child to cause so much chaos. Mothers seemed almost intimidated by this united front. The little girls seemed to receive scanty attention compared to their boisterous brothers. All mothers declared that their daughters had very gentle, shy, undemanding dispositions. However, the joint efforts of their twin brothers possibly helped foster an undemanding and fairly withdrawn disposition in the girls.

When twins were born into families with older siblings, all siblings on the whole were greatly disrupted by their arrival. However, these younger siblings of twins seemed to suffer even more. The twins were no longer babies and were well organised.

Indifference and oppression were soon reciprocated. Whilst young children are normally very interested in even slightly older ones, the three younger sisters seemed to completely ignore their brothers. They crawled or walked in the opposite direction as soon as they were able.

CHAPTER 11

DIFFERENT TYPES OF TWINS

THE *'FAUX JUMEAUX'*: DIZYGOTIC TWINS

The French expression *'faux jumeaux'*, meaning false twins, which is used to indicate dizygotic twins, may contain a grain of truth. Though they can be very similar, many resemble each other no more than ordinary siblings often do. However, it would be rather tactless and quite startling for them to be asked if they were 'true' or 'false' twins. Besides any other considerations the expression 'false' carries a strong moral connotation which even young children can grasp.

A pair of very bright and particularly articulate three-year-old twins cried and protested loudly when a rather insensitive visitor asked if they were true or false. They both sobbed and replied in unison, 'But we don't tell lies!'

The English expressions 'fraternal twins' and 'identical twins', which also have their equivalents in some Latin languages, equally denote certain truly distinctive features characterising these two groups of twins. However, it would also be inopportune for twins to be constantly asked if they were fraternal or identical. A dizygotic twin girl replied, 'Fraternal or identical? What do you mean? I have a sister, no brothers. Why identical? She is blonde and I am auburn.' It is especially unfitting for monozygotic twins to be defined as 'identical' when in only too many ways they clearly are not.

Nevertheless, it is undeniable that dizygotic twins are in many respects different to and less 'extreme' than monozygotic ones. Not only is their genetic similarity more like that of ordinary siblings, but many environmental factors also progressively come into play to reinforce this innate tendency.

GOING DIFFERENT WAYS

Dizygotic twins were necessarily made to share most aspects of their early existence, just like monozygotic twins. However, although this certainly did have an impact on them, they were at the same time inevitably regarded as quite distinct. Their often marked behavioral differences prompted increasingly different treatment by all those interacting with them.

The mutual involvement of dizygotic twins never reached the same intensity noted in monozygotic pairs. As they grew more independent, autonomy and differential treatment were reinforced in the dizygotic twins. After the first two years of their lives social recognition of marked differences between them had an influence on their caregivers as well. 'Twinning' was generally reserved only for special occasions such as nursery school parties and important social gatherings.

Most parents adjusted promptly to the changed circumstances. They forgot the limelight that came with twinning and concentrated on the unmistakable emergent individuality of their children. Their differences began to be the source of real joy. Having children who were progressively treated more as ordinary siblings by everyone, was, they felt, one problem less. Many now actually pitied parents of monozygotic twins.

One mother confided, 'Identical twins are delightful and fun to begin with, but I can't bear to imagine the problems at adolescence! In any case, I love variety and difference.'

This change in attitude soon also brought with it practical consequences. Three sets of twins acquired separate rooms. More and more the twins' individual needs for space, solitude and time to themselves were taken into account. Though dizygotic twins, given how young they were, did not cease to live a shared life they were no longer constantly reminded of their original union.

THE REMAINS OF TWINSHIP

Social emphasis on differences began to change the lives of dizygotic twins by fostering independence and individuality in them. However, the increasing urge to grow apart also stemmed from deeper intrinsic drives. The twins' different 'nature' also began to have its effect. Before reaching a certain independence they could do little about being treated as a unit. Baby twins could not move away from each other when placed in the same cot or made to share the same bathtub.

As their independence grew dizygotic twins started to behave according to how they felt about each other, just as ordinary siblings would (Dunn and Kendrick 1982; Dunn 1985). Some got on, others did not. Some simply kept apart and played in separate rooms or corners. One dizygotic twin declared, 'I cannot stand him. He always gets in my way.' A girl asked, 'Why don't you get rid of her? She takes up all my space.'

Until the age of two the real meaning of the word 'twins' naturally escaped the twins themselves. Even if enlightened parents tried to explain to them that they had once been in Mummy's tummy together, and that this was the reason they were referred to as 'twins', the true essence of twinship was clearly beyond their understanding. At this stage nobody ventured to introduce notions of genetics. Only one mother ever mentioned different eggs and seeds to her two-year-old twins. For a while these two refused to eat eggs, perhaps fearing cannibalistic implications. Some time later the same explanation was listened to with keen interest and laughter. No mother of monozygotic twins ever bothered to mention the splitting of an egg.

By nursery school age most dizygotic twins objected quite loudly when they were still occasionally referred to as 'the twins'. This had ceased to be just a simple nickname. As one said, 'I am not a twin, I am Mark.' Or as one little girl declared, indicating her co-twin, 'I am Jane, perhaps she is the twin.'

'Me' was the first word uttered by many dizygotic twins. They also used 'I' more frequently than 'we'. This did not occur so frequently with monozygotic twins.

However, not all the conundrums and ties of twinship were unravelled. Their forced union, which generally still continued, actually accentuated feelings of animosity in some particularly incompatible pairs. As one girl put it, 'I want to divorce from her. She gets on my nerves.'

In their early years most dizygotic twins could be considered by and large to be midway between monozygotic twins and ordinary siblings.

OPPOSITE-SEX PAIRS: GROWING UNEQUAL

From the very beginning matters were more clear-cut for opposite-sex pairs. Gender rendered them different beyond any possible doubt. Opposite-sex pairs were also what most parents had hoped for. 'Now that we have one of each sex, we don't need to try again', was a quite understandable attitude. The family could be completed with just one gestation. This seemed a special bonus to those couples who had decided to postpone pregnancy to the limit of childbearing age or who had had any kind of fertility problems.

However, there is nothing like witnessing parents being told the sex of the fetuses during ultrasound scans to make one realise how deeply rooted gender issues are. Parents still prefer males. People from different countries and different cultures frequently come to the Unit. This seems to be a fairly universal (and not just a Latin) bias.

In the case of opposite-sex twins more or less explicit preferences may be expressed long before birth. Role attribution and role radicalisation (Goshen-Gottstein 1981) are an almost irresistible temptation for all parents when told that they are expecting opposite-sex twins. Incredible as it may seem, given that we are talking about the non-social, non-verbal intrauterine environment, girls are frequently described as seductive temptresses, chatty, gossipy and over-emotional. Boys are ascribed athletic dispositions or reckless inclinations. Their level of activity can sometimes be well below that of their sister, but any motion of even the most torpid male fetus is almost invariably interpreted as a sign of greater vivacity.

Differential treatment of opposite-sex twins has been described by others in various studies (Lytton and Romney 1991; Burnham and Harris 1992).

Once the twins were born most parents doted on the boys and were fairly dismissive of the girls. Boys were cuddled, picked up, talked to and looked at for longer intervals. Girl twins, after some initial protest, generally came to accept their 'subordinate' role much earlier than singleton females (Gilligan 1982; Levy and Haaf 1994).

Maurice and Sharon were the first children of parents in their late thirties. Mrs U had seemed quite happy not to have children but, as they approached forty, her husband had convinced her that it was now or never. Somewhat reluctantly Mrs U had complied and was soon pregnant. However, when they were told that they were expecting twins, Mrs U burst into tears. She said, 'This is too much! I am too old for twins!' She continued to despair until told that one was a boy. At that point she exclaimed, 'Thank god for that! My worst nightmare was the idea of having two girls!' During prenatal life, despite the overabundance of fluid in his amniotic sac, the boy seemed definitely sluggish and passive compared to his sister. Despite this, their mother (their father was rarely present) already started attributing 'superior' and quite 'mature' qualities to the boy. Contrary to all the evidence she regarded him as more active, and even more intelligent and more imaginative than his sister. When clinical parameters began to diverge between the twins, Mrs U blamed it on the girl, saying, 'Couldn't she absorb some amniotic fluid into her sac? She should be drinking more. She cannot expect her brother to swallow it all!' The situation continued to be difficult for the girl after they were born. Mrs U was severely depressed. The twins were placed in the same cot and she looked after them very little. Any attention or demonstration of affection she did give was directed solely towards the boy. Yet favouritism was vehemently denied. She maintained that, 'For me they are exactly the same.' Up to the age of six months the girl seemed more alert, vivacious and sociable than her brother. In fact she scored better in all tests at this age. Nevertheless, sadly she could not endure such markedly unequal treatment forever. From then on she began to lag behind her brother in many respects.

Besides influencing parental preference, opposite-sex pairs highlighted many stereotypes of male/female roles (see Figure 11.1). Natural gender-related inclinations (Ruble and Martin 1998) exhibited by the twins themselves were also taken to the extreme.

Girls were often dressed with frills, ribbons and laces that made them look like pretty little dolls but also rendered many activities rather difficult to perform. Boys, on the contrary, were dressed in practical hardwearing clothes. Three different male twins were even dressed up in little pinstriped suits on special occasions! There were no equivalent *tailleurs* for the three girls, however.

To the dismay of many liberal-minded parents both girls and boys tend to be attracted by respective traditional gender-linked toys (Bjorrkqvist *et al.* 1992). Many parents declare, for example, that they will never buy their sons a gun, but sooner or later they surrender to the evidence that their little angels use anything from newspapers to plants and toilet rolls as weapons. The same applies to girls, who can make any old rag become a doll. However, opposite-sex twins invariably brought out the most extreme caricatures and stereotypes of aspects of gender in everyone around them. Girls were given kitchenettes and boys racing cars. Girls were pushed to be flirtatious and boys to be tough. Girls were appraised for their physical attributes and boys for their mental abilities. The divide that normally exists between opposite-sex peers was transformed into an even bigger gulf for these twins.

OPPOSITE-SEX PAIRS: NATURE AND NURTURE

There is no denying that gender-linked differences are not imposed solely by culture. Although *la différence*, as the French call it, may not be as extreme as parents of opposite-sex twins make out, boys and girls do have specific natures (Kelly 1991). Nature itself, indeed, often took its revenge. Up to adolescence girls are often more precocious and advanced than boys in several areas of development (Ruble and Martin 1998). This frequently brought about comparisons that clearly annoyed both boys and girls, especially when they began nursery school.

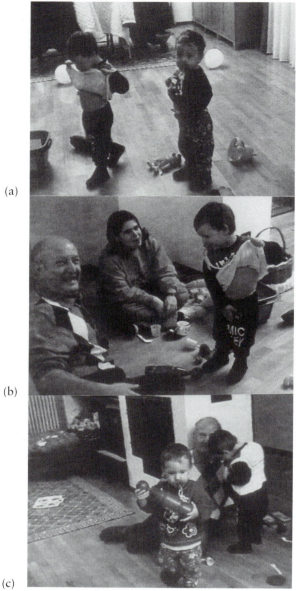

(a)

(b)

(c)

Figure 11.1 Opposite-sex pair, 20 months
All the family takes pride in the 'masculinity' of the boy, while the girl is left to one side.
(a) The boy begins his performance. He shows his tummy and moves towards his mother and maternal grandfather (not visible in this picture). His sister just touches her belly slightly and looks towards me.
(b) The boy touches his penis and shows off in front of his mother and grandfather, who both laugh and comment on this.
(c) The boy continues to show off to his grandfather. The grandfather is still smiling, but now looks away. The girl takes a huge plastic skittle and moves away. She is sucking her pacifier and nobody seems to pay any attention to her.

Furthermore, entering the community of their peers reinforced the division of roles as boys began to play with boys and girls to play with girls (Bayley *et al.* 1993; Alexander and Hines 1994; Serbin *et al.* 1994).

Paradoxically, despite all the comparisons, peer-group divisions and frankly unequal treatment, male–female pairs seemed to develop a special mutual tolerance. They fought less and supported each other more compared to same-sex dizygotic pairs. In addition, they seemed to have developed a particular understanding of each other's different needs. A girl once noted, 'He bumped his head, but Mummy told him not to cry. He is a boy. But still, it hurts.' Her sobbing brother smiled, looked up and touched his sore forehead.

This may apply to families of singletons as well. Empathy for siblings of a different gender is not exclusively displayed by twins (Radke-Yarrow *et al.* 1983; Dunn 1988). However, there seemed to exist a special empathy between opposite-sex twins. Possibly their long familiarity, as well as their distinct and generally excessively clear-cut roles, may have favoured the attitude 'we are all brothers and sisters under the skin'.

SAME-SEX PAIRS, THE LESS POPULAR TYPE OF DIZYGOTIC TWINS

When told that the twins were probably dizygotic, most parents strongly wished for a boy and a girl. Same-sex pairs were generally a disappointment. However, most parents soon got over this and commented, 'Provided they are both well, it is all right.'

Parents of same-sex twins began to diverge from those of opposite-sex pairs right from their initial choice of preferred twin. Gender, obviously, was not an issue. For these parents, apart from the favourite 'torpid' twins, appearance was important, as it can also be in favouring ordinary siblings (Burns and Farina 1992). A more attractive twin was frequently preferred by parents of same-sex pairs.

Curiously, openly ignored or uncared-for twins were more common in this category.

Intense rivalry developed quite soon between most of these twins. The two pairs who were not strongly antagonistic had both been favoured by nature. All four children were very attractive and highly intelligent. Each twin found its compensation in quite unlike, but pronounced talents. All other same-sex twins suffered greatly from antagonism.

Differential appraisal and constant contrasting were very frequent.

Stuart and Donald were very different physically. Their conception had been a surprise for parents in their late thirties. They already had one son and neither had wanted another child, let alone two. This mother, too, exclaimed, 'I am too old for twins.' However, resignation soon set in. Though the pregnancy went well and the twins had more than adequate birthweight, genetics had been far from impartial with the twins. Stuart was very attractive and Donald was not. Both parents were immediately taken by

Stuart's good looks and neither chose Donald. Donald was handed over totally to the care of his grandmother. Not even time seemed to favour Donald. He lagged behind in developmental milestones. However, Stuart could not tolerate even a very inferior rival. He soon began to bash Donald about. Donald was not inclined towards martyrdom and so he punched back. Both got heavily reprimanded, but they continued totally unperturbed by the clamour around them. Only when Donald risked ruining Stuart's good looks, nearly breaking his fine Greek nose, were drastic measures finally taken. They were made to play in separate rooms. Rivalry never ceased. On the contrary, it actually increased as the boys grew older. Even nursery school only opened up new horizons of competition between them.

MONOZYGOTIC TWINS: THE *'VRAIS JUMEAUX'*

Monozygotic twins on the whole were far more 'congenial' behaviorally, physically and psychologically (von Bracken 1934b).

Though monozygotic twins often have striking temperamental as well as physical differences, there is no denying that what they share is quite unusual and 'excessive'. It would be quite ridiculous to deny the importance of their unique genetic sharing. Nobody else shares as much as they do, from genes to prenatal and post-natal environments and the external signs of twinship. It is quite understandable, though not necessarily commendable, that they should continue to be called *'vrais jumeaux'*, the real twins.

Not that these twins were truly identical, far from it. Though popular opinion may contain some truth it often stops at very superficial qualities and has a tendency to simplify, unify and classify. Most people do not bother to look for individual differences. For most, twins are identical in all respects.

In reality monozygotic twins were neither completely different, nor totally identical.

Their well-defined identities were always beyond doubt, especially for themselves. One twin replied testily to an old aunt who remarked on his similarity to his brother, 'I am me and he is he.' Apart, perhaps, from old aunts, no one in any of the families ever doubted the fact. Twins showed different tastes, talents and inclinations. Different likes and dislikes in food abounded. One twin loved chocolate, while the other went mad for salty foods. One loved vegetables; the other only liked meat.

A pair of little girls also showed very different reactions to their mother's perfume. Mrs L explained, 'If I wear Shalimar I know she will be all over me, but Felicity will not. With Dior it is exactly the other way round.' Another, less well-off, family commented on the different reactions to the smell of cabbage and fish fingers!

However, there is no denying that along with all the differences similarities existed as well. Monozygotic twins were far more compatible than their dizygotic counterparts. From simple mannerisms, ways of walking and running, and to how they reasoned, their similarity and affinity could often be striking.

However, monozygotic twins showed degrees and variations in the strength of their link. For some mutual attachment virtually excluded attachment to anyone else, for others it didn't.

Together with reciprocally 'avoidant' Toby and Jack, Stanley and Martin probably represented the least 'twinned' end of the spectrum. During scans they behaved quite differently – one was very active and the other not. Preferential positions were noted, as well as preferential patterns of behavior: one constantly rubbed his face and bumped his head against the uterine wall, the other repeatedly pushed with his feet. So much so that Mrs G was perfectly capable of distinguishing their blows. 'Here comes Stanley!' she would say, and 'Yet one more kick from Martin!' Due to weight discrepancy the twins looked quite unlike at birth, though they were both very attractive with big black eyes, a slightly olive complexion and delicate but masculine features. Mrs G took real pleasure in caring for the boys and she breast-fed them until they were five months old. As time passed the twins began to look very similar, although Mrs G always noticed differences in them. One wanted a pacifier and the other only sucked his thumb. One took hours at the breast and the other ate voraciously in five minutes. One loved water and the other screamed when bathed. Differences continued with the introduction of solid foods. One loved fruit and the other mashed potatoes, and so on. Developmental milestones were also achieved at different moments. Furthermore, their temperamental inclinations were different. Stanley was cuddly and revelled in pushing his head against his mother's soft, curvy body. Martin was more outgoing and independent. Despite their tastes and inclinations continuing to remain quite distinct, there were also many affinities between them. Both found mutual proximity very soothing. They fought very little and shared most toys. Aided, perhaps, by different inclinations as well as by gentle natures, they also displayed minimal rivalry towards each other. Martin affirmed, 'I will not marry Mummy or Daddy. I will marry him.' Stanley declared, 'Me too! He is my best friend.' These twins were in fact also very popular with their peers. They were possibly the pair of monozygotic twins who blended best with other children. Their preference for each other, however, was undoubted. As Martin said, 'Other children are fun but Stanley is much more fun.' Nevertheless, it was interesting to note how their first drawings differed. Stanley, who had always loved his mother's curves, always drew big rounded circles with two smaller ones inside. Martin also drew big circles but with many small ones outside. Their mother commented, 'It shows that he is more outgoing. One is all inside, the other out.' Martin also liked to draw cars and trucks. Their handwriting also differed in later years. Stanley's letters were rounded and Martin's fairly pointed. Differences as well as similarities and affinities coexisted harmoniously in these two.

CHAPTER 12

CHANGES IN THE FAMILY

THE END OF THE TUNNEL

By the end of the second year of the twins' lives their families were beginning to see the light again. Sleepless nights, frantic activity, and endless fatigue were starting to recede. The twins were beginning to be a bit more independent and slightly more cognisant of the various dangers and perils surrounding them. By now they had reached that much-yearned-for stage when they started to play together and entertain themselves. Other forms of entertainment such as television and cartoons also gave caregivers a break. Parents also felt able to go out some evenings. Four couples with especially supportive alternative caregivers ventured as far as having short holidays alone. They all admitted to feeling 'strange' without the constant presence and noise of the twins. One mother remarked, 'Being away with my husband without the twins made me realise how much our life as a couple has changed forever. I needed a break and some freedom and intimacy, but I also missed the children. We are a family now and the twins are inextricably part of our existence.'

Twins were now generally 'fun' to be with. Bins still had to be emptied regularly, the shopping had to be done and diapers still had to be changed occasionally, but other more rewarding activities were also part of daily life. Parents could read stories to the twins and play games with them. Fathers took them out and could play a more distinctly 'paternal' role. They could also improvise football matches, and the twins – with their intrinsically well co-ordinated actions – made especially good sides. Mothers could venture out with the two on their own and were no longer virtually confined to their apartments. Everyone felt relieved with the newly acquired independence of the twins.

BACK IN SHAPE: SHAKING OFF DEPRESSION AND RESUMING WORK

This changed state of affairs introduced a more virtuous circle into the mothers' lives. They all began to look 'rejuvenated' at this stage. A new hairstyle, new clothes, a touch of make-up all began to reappear. Some mothers enrolled in gym classes.

One explained, 'So far I had to cancel myself. Until the twins were toddlers I had no choice. But now it's time to think about myself a bit too. My husband didn't want to pay for gym classes. We are such a big family now! But I exist too! All my friends came to my help. They all chipped in and gave me the subscription to a gym class as a birthday present. It's only two evenings a week. My husband complains because dinner is not ready. I couldn't care less! I deserve a break!'

All the mothers were beginning to get brief respites. In fact, except for those who had suffered a severe depression which had required various forms of medical help, they all felt lifted in their spirits. This in turn implied better care of themselves. While they had been in the middle of the hurricane none had had time to comb their hair or wear decent clothes. The twins invariably soiled everything with smelly stains of all kinds. Not that these aesthetic or cosmetic elements were the most important ones in helping mothers' moods, but they had their relevance.

Anthony and Adele had been very much wanted by their parents. Mrs R, a woman in her late thirties, worked as a nursery school teacher and she doted on children. However, a child of her own had never come. Both parents underwent all sorts of tests – she ovarian stimulation and he repeated sperm counts – until IVF was finally suggested. IVF was in fact tried seven times! Although the gestation was without complications throughout, the parents held their breath in apprehension till the very end. However, pregnancy was not kind to Mrs R's already rather prematurely aged physique. By twenty weeks she looked enormous and her body was covered with very visible stretch marks. Her legs were enormously swollen and broken capillaries and varicose veins began to appear. Her feet were also terribly swollen, so much so that she could no longer wear shoes. In the middle of the harsh winter she had to walk around in plastic flip-flops. Furthermore, her already poor eyesight got twice as bad. Everyone was dismayed by such a general physical collapse. What she resented most, though, was the catastrophe of her breasts. Whilst all other mothers complained about enormously enlarged breasts hers just became more and more slack. Nevertheless, during pregnancy Mrs R complained little about her altered appearance. All that mattered at that point was the health of the children. The twins were indeed healthy. They were born at term and their weight at birth was more than adequate. However, as they had moved into a podalic position a Caesarean had been inevitable. Mrs R's already tried body did not recover well from the operation. The incision took time to heal and caused her pain for months. She now walked around all bent over, holding her flabby abdomen with both hands. Her husband disappeared almost completely and this caused a lot of tension in their marriage.

When the children were one year old, Mrs R decided to go back to work even though she could have obtained further maternity leave. She explained her decision, saying, 'They need a mother, but not a dead one. Unless I go back to work I think I'll go out of my mind.' Mrs R was not the only mother to say something to that effect. Work did indeed bring some relevant improvement. However, just like the other nursery school teacher in the group, Mrs R could no longer stand working with children. She soon changed to an office job.

The big change in her life took place when the twins were two and a half and were regularly attending a local day care group. Mrs R admitted, 'I have being saving every penny I could. Now I am going to give myself a big present!' She had plastic surgery! In one fell swoop her breasts were lifted, her abdominals tightened, and quite a few wrinkles, stretch marks and broken capillaries were erased. Mrs R was elated. She rejoiced, 'I feel reborn!' She was not completely transformed: a beauty she never was and she continued not to be one. However, her self-esteem improved greatly and so did her marriage.

Not all mothers ended up under a plastic surgeon's miraculous scalpel. Mrs R was unique in that sense.

However, going back to work did wonders for everyone. By the time the twins entered nursery school, most mothers had done so; many, indeed, had actually resumed work well before then. From the very early days mothers had longed to get back to work. Besides purely economic considerations, their jobs gave them an opportunity for social contacts as well as for personal satisfaction. Not all jobs were particularly exciting, but even the humblest employment felt like a breath of fresh air compared to the endless, solitary and socially unappreciated routine of changing diapers and feeding two gaping mouths.

While the twins were still very young, a mother's homecoming was met with double demands and protests. This also applies to mothers of singletons, but two screaming infants after a day's work drove several mothers to tears. Furthermore, working mothers felt very guilty about leaving their baby twins.

IN THE PUBLIC EYE: THE IMPACT OF NURSERY SCHOOL ON PARENTS OF MONOZYGOTIC TWINS

Nursery school represented a big change. The twins were no longer babies and society now partly took charge of them. Mothers now felt less guilty about leaving the twins as the officialdom of nursery school[1] implied public approval and sanction.

When confronted with the more formal environment of nursery school, however, all the mothers began to worry about how they should foster the separate identities of their monozygotic twins. Teachers and schools now began to participate in the educational debate: whether twins should be separated to enhance individuality was the main argument (Gleenson *et al.* 1990; Hay 1991; Sandbank 1991; Preedy 1999). Various manuals also appeared in every household. Where once it had all been 'bonding' and idyllic closeness, it was now differentiation and reciprocal independence. A different bombardment from society had now begun. From 'Twins, how nice!' to 'Twins, what a problem!' Yet another anxiety had invaded their parents' lives.

When mothers went to pick up their children from nursery school they all seemed worried when they saw their twins emerge from the noisy crowd of children hugging and holding each other's hands. Most monozygotic twins immediately hugged each other and were invariably delighted to see each other again after a day in separate classes. To widespread parental dismay extreme stereotypes of twinning, usually involving tragic tales of entanglement, were also beginning to gain a certain notoriety at the time. The Gibbons twins,[2] with their secret language and anti-social behavior, were a favourite theme and a nightmare for many parents. They all started to look out for 'secret language' and other signs of anti-social behavior.

Besides the 'secret language' of the Gibbons twins other nightmares were evoked as well. The song 'Tsumani'[3] was mentioned. In one posh nursery school a 'friend' approached the elegant mother of one pair of twins and said, 'I was just thinking about you. Have you seen *Dead Ringers*?[4] It's a movie. It should be interesting. Someone was talking about twins and mentioned it. I thought I'd tell you.' Three other parents were advised to read *On the Black Hill*.[5]

Parents of dizygotic twins, on the other hand, seemed almost exclusively apprehensive about physical concerns.

Pressurised from all sides and barraged with relentless advice, parents of monozygotic twins tried different clothes and various other perceptual ruses in an attempt to camouflage the indisputable macroscopic similarities between twins. Often it was too late. The twins themselves now rebelled against different clothes and hairstyles. They looked at each other, and their simultaneous reactions were: 'I want my hair short like him' and 'I want my hair long just like his', or, 'I like her skirt' and 'I want trousers, too.' All mothers, except two, tried their best by turning a deaf ear to these frequent refrains. Nevertheless, almost unfailingly the twins' faces and body language gave away their true nature.

Parents were now keen to indicate any sign of distinction. Mothers showed elementary drawings. They all differed. A twin girl who was particularly outgoing only drew bright yellow suns. Her shy and reserved co-twin only drew grey and fairly shapeless circles. A boy drew all sorts of machinery. His co-twin only drew houses. One could well picture them having different handwriting as well as different careers later on (Rehmann 1979).

Verbal communication now favoured the open expression of differing tastes and thoughts. Some could be very profound. As a twin boy declared, 'We have the same face, but a different head.'

Despite what were often blatant displays of differences, all parents of monozygotic twins were anguished by the incessant social campaign, which almost advocated 'apartheid' in its zeal to foster diversity in monozygotic twins.

UNION AND DIVORCE

As with many major crises the arrival of the twins brought further unity to most families (Byng-Hall 1995). Having gone through so much together eventually reinforced most marriages. One father summed it up saying, 'Although I sometimes feel like an old man, I am happy that we made it. I never imagined anything like this. For about two years it felt like being in the middle of a hurricane. But we survived and life without them would be unthinkable now.' Before emerging from the tunnel all parents had gone through some pretty dark moments in their marriage.

The number of divorces and serious marital difficulties was very high in the sample, as other studies have also found (Hay *et al.* 1990). Parents of dizygotic twins suffered earlier and more acutely. Four marriages in this group eventually broke down and these parents are now divorced. Three couples of the monozygotic group are still facing a very uncertain outcome. By the admission of the parents only the tender age of the children still keeps them together. As one father said, 'It would be unfair to leave a woman alone with two young children, but our marriage is over.'

Sleepless nights and extreme fatigue were in all cases clearly important factors in exacerbating any existing friction. However, three out of four divorces concerned couples who had had lengthy fertility treatments and a particularly idealised view of parenthood. Clearly not all parents who have to resort to assisted reproduction go through these problems. Most continue to remain strongly united and move on to become excellent parents (Bryan and Higgins 1995; Golombok *et al.* 1995). This group as a whole, though, may be more subject to marital difficulties (Snowden and Mitchell 1981; Snowden *et al.* 1983). As previously mentioned, expectations can be enormous. Dreams and reality can be miles apart – especially so when the reality is twins.

Besides universal fatigue, separations seemed to stem from other reasons in the monozygotic group.

In one case the family had three older children. They all lived crammed together into three small rooms. The uncommon economic and physical strain brought about by the twins, maternal depression and social isolation were all too much in the end. Furthermore, the father could not tolerate that his wife, who was only thirty-three years old when the twins were born, had asked to be sterilised. This was contrary to his 'moral principles', and endless verbal abuse ensued. In the end the mother and all her children went to live with a female friend who was in a similarly unhappy condition.

In another case the parents had married very young. Their difficulties only started when the children were three and the husband became restless for sentimental/sexual encounters with other women. He explained, 'I have simply leaped out of childhood into parenthood.' These parents are now considering finalising their divorce.

The common denominator in the remaining two cases was the fact that the fathers had fled almost immediately after being told that their partners were expecting twins.

In one case pregnancy had not been planned, much less twins. The father met his moral obligation and got married, but clearly did not love his wife. When told that they were expecting twins, he took the news as a personal insult. He mumbled, 'I have been tricked into this!' His wife, on the other hand, probably sensing the bleak prospect of being abandoned with two babies, simply cried. After the twins were born their father was never around. There were hints during observations that he had set up another, more congenial family elsewhere.

The other father who immediately fled from the circumstances did so after making the sibylline statement, 'Twins are an aberration!' None of the hospital staff had time to ask him what he meant by that before he was gone.

Though any judgement may be premature, all of the twins involved seemed to find mutual solace and support in their co-twin's presence.

LOOKING BACKWARDS AND FORWARDS

Whilst in the middle of the initial maelstrom parents could only live from one day to the next. Now that the worst was over they could distance themselves from the former incredible hardships they had all gone through. Parents began to look backwards at the times gone by and forwards towards things to come.

There were some hints of nostalgia in this. Many regretted the fact that they had been too busy fighting for survival to fully enjoy the twins when they had been babies.

Ultrasound sessions were remembered as a particularly happy moment within an otherwise trying pregnancy. Whilst all parents had eagerly waited for a copy of the cassette containing the recording of the delivery, none of them had had the time, or indeed the energy, to look back at ultrasounds. Some parents now showed the video of the scans to the twins to help illustrate some simple biology lessons. When one mother pointed out, 'This was you and that was Jane', her twins only showed signs of restlessness and boredom. The cloudy and soundless grey images of the scans were merely glanced at. They had perhaps expected a cartoon.

More interesting were parental comments on the scans. Old memories were recalled in the context of their actual knowledge of the children. According to most parents the future temperament of the twins had first been glimpsed at through ultrasounds. They all declared that there was a clear continuity with post-natal behavior. 'She used to move a lot! Well, she is just the same now.' 'He was so jittery then and he is still very sensitive to anything new.' 'They have both remained the same. He moves all the time. She is very placid.' No parents ever doubted continuity between prenatal and post-natal temperament. Parents may have been right, but their recollections also seemed heavily influenced by their current knowledge of the twins.

ADDITIONS TO THE FAMILY: THE BIRTH OF ANOTHER CHILD

Whilst talking about pregnancy and ultrasounds, two couples mentioned that they were now planning to have another child. This was a big step after the chaotic situation they were only just emerging from. In a third case another child was a surprise. In all three families the twins had been the only children.

Another child was the exception rather than the rule. Most parents proclaimed that their reproductive efforts were over. The twins were beginning to give them great joys, but on the whole it had all been too much.

These three subsequent pregnancies were not studied with scans as the twins had been. However, contact was quite frequent as the mothers popped in to say hello on their way back from their routine check-ups at the clinic. All three mothers looked remarkably healthy and blooming compared to their first pregnancy.

They all continued working right up to the last minute, as they preferred to extend their maternity leave after the birth of the new child. Two had a Caesarean, but one successfully attempted natural childbirth.

Two days after their babies had been born, the mothers were moving about and talking about going home. They all breast-fed their healthy babies, and continued to do so for several months. When they left the hospital, the proud fathers came along to say goodbye to the obstetricians, but this time none risked dropping the baby.

When the twins were next observed, all their mothers remarked that it was an altogether different experience. One said, 'I can play and have fun with this one. It just was not possible with the twins. There was no energy or space left over for savouring any joys.' Another said, 'I delight in a very beautiful closeness with her. We even have one-to-one conversations. That was never possible with the twins.' The third remarked, 'When they are out at nursery school the silence is unbelievable. I am surprised I didn't go deaf with them! Nights too are incredibly peaceful now!'

However, they all seemed to miss at least some of the glamour and glory surrounding the birth of the twins. One, indeed, commented, 'You are completely anonymous with just one child. Nobody bothers looking at you. Unless they're twins, children are not an attraction in this society.'

DEATH OF A TWIN

Twins, especially monozygotic twins, are at increased risk until the age of two. Prematurity and other unknown factors make them more liable to suffer from various forms of disability and early death (Voss 1996). Twins are also almost twice as much at risk of dying of 'sudden infant death syndrome' (SIDS) or so-called 'cot death' (Beal 1983, 1989).

One family went through this shattering experience of early loss. One of their monozygotic twin boys died of SIDS when he was six months old. Some points of a more general nature, that could apply to the early death of any monozygotic twin, will be referred to here.

Both parents (hereafter called 'the Smiths') were young and the pregnancy was uncomplicated throughout. The twins were healthy at birth and were dismissed from hospital with their mother after five days. They continued to grow well and seemed to find mutual proximity highly soothing.

A desperate cry

One day I received a desperate phone call from Mrs Smith's sister who told me that Peter had died that night. She said that Mark, his co-twin, was under observation, but he seemed all right and would probably be dismissed within a day or so.

The relationship with Mrs Smith could no longer be purely professional. Mark was no longer a 'research case'. However, it would have been too cruel to stop the visits, unless Mrs Smith wanted to.

When visited ten days later Mrs Smith explained in detail what had happened. The twins had a slight cold that had been dragging on for days. They had their last feed at around 10 p.m. and had then fallen quietly asleep. Everything had seemed normal, and she and her husband also went to bed early. Mrs Smith was fast asleep when she suddenly heard a piercing cry. She ran to see the children. 'I immediately realised that something terrible had happened. Mark was yelling, as I had never heard him cry before. It was a desperate cry.' So she checked him first. But as soon as she turned towards Peter she realised that something was badly wrong. He looked cyanotic and was not breathing. 'He was still warm. I tried resuscitation and screamed for my husband to come. He called an ambulance. Probably it had only just happened. Then there was the rush to hospital, but nothing could be done. Peter was dead. Although this was clearly also due to the unusual surroundings and to our despair, Mark remained inconsolable throughout the night.' Mrs Smith was certain that he had sensed something wrong with Peter. As she said, 'I am sure they were used to each other's rhythms, including breathing. It must have been comforting for them to hear these regular, familiar noises. Possibly he sensed that his brother had stopped breathing and just screamed and screamed.' Though she was still waiting for the results of the autopsy the doctors were pretty certain that it had been cot death. This was confirmed a few days later.

Surviving death

On the same day Mrs Smith said that Mark seemed to look for Peter in various ways. She put a softball next to him and he turned and smiled briefly at it. Later she lay him on her bed. He immediately arched and looked behind him. She said, 'He really seems to be looking for something.' Then she picked him up and put him in front of the mirror. As soon as he saw his own reflection in the mirror Mark immediately brightened up. He smiled and gurgled and repeatedly touched it. Only after several failed attempts did he withdraw from the cold and rigid surface of the mirror and look back as if searching for something. Mark had possibly seen his absent brother for a fleeting moment in his reflection.

During the next visit a fortnight later, Mark happened to be placed in front of another mirror as his mother changed his diaper and wiped his bottom clean. This time Mark's gaze was completely blank (see Figure 12.1). Possibly the memory of his brother's appearance had by now faded from his mind. Long-term memory is generally considered to be short lived at this stage (Olson and Sherman 1983; Rovee-Collier 1987; Rovee-Collier et al. 1980; Rovee-Collier and Dufault 1991; Kupfermann 1991; Cohen and Eichenbaum 1993; Nelson 1994). Although it is hard to tell if Mark ever remembered, and missed his twin brother, he certainly never recovered his former contented expression.

The death of a child is the most tragic event that can possibly occur in any parent's life, but the death of a twin, furthermore monozygotic, brings with it additional anguish to what is already excruciating pain (Bryan 1983, 1992, 1999; Segal and Ream 1998; Woodward 1998).

Mrs Smith, who had always been very open about her feelings, now spoke about other aspects of the agony implicit in the death of a young twin. The survivor is a constant living reminder of the dead one. They would have been the same age and looked alike if he or she were still alive. Mrs Smith said, 'Life has to go on and it's none of Mark's fault, but whenever I look at him I also see Peter. When I rejoice for something Mark has done or achieved, at the same time I mourn for the other one.' Mrs Smith tried her best not to make Mark suffer too much for the death of his co-twin. Yet as she said, 'It is difficult when a young twin dies. You have no time or space left to fully express your despair, the other is still there with his vital needs. You are mourning for one whilst having to continue caring for the other. Smiles and tears of sorrow don't go well together.'

Mrs Smith also declared that she had become fearful and over-protective towards Mark. 'He is monozygotic, although I try hard not to think about it, the fear that he may just die like his brother is always lurking in the back of my mind. I can hardly sleep at night and for the moment I have placed his cot next to our bed.'

Although this was clearly not her major concern, Mrs Smith also explained how difficult it was to face people who had met her before with the twins.

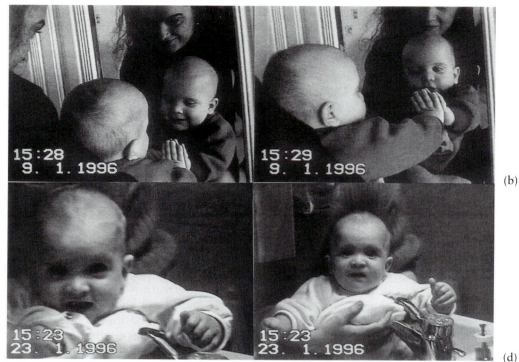

(a)   (b)   (c)   (d)

Figure 12.1 Death of a twin
The survivor of a pair of monozygotic twin boys is held by his mother. He is six months old.
(a–b) The other twin had died about twenty days before. The mother spontaneously puts the surviving twin in front of a mirror. He smiles immediately and tries to touch the face of his mirror image.
(c) Fourteen days later the surviving twin only shows a brief sign of recognition when put in front of a mirror. (Only his mirror image is showing in the picture.)
(d) Immediately an expression of bewilderment appears on his face and he pulls away from the mirror.

Many shrugged and said, 'You are lucky. At least you have one left. You are still very young, you can have another child.' As she said, 'But for me Peter was unique. Peter was Peter and Mark is Mark. They never were or ever will be interchangeable.'

Her husband reacted in a different way. He tried to push back his tears and act in a more traditionally 'masculine' way by adopting a 'life must go on' attitude. He didn't want to dwell on Peter's death in any open way. Mrs Smith became pregnant again two months after Peter had died. Her husband had wanted a 'replacement' child (Poznanski 1972; Bernabei and Levi 1976; Lewis and Page 1978; Lewis 1979; Bluglass 1980), in the illusory belief that this would relieve their unbearable pain. If possible this new pregnancy grieved Mrs Smith even more. When she told me the news she cried, 'How can I be expected to celebrate life whilst grieving at the same time. It's like violating his memory. Another child so soon feels like denying that Peter ever existed. It's like killing him a second time.' Her new gestation never brought her a minute of joy. She said, 'I can't help it, but I feel nothing for this one.

I cannot rejoice for its kicks, when I still remember those of Peter. His death is so recent and he was so young that I still carry his memory in my body. Maybe when I see this new baby I will feel something, but for the moment I am dead to any emotion.'

As term was approaching, Mrs Smith also worried a lot about Mark's reactions to the arrival of a baby. For quite a while her response was to over-indulge and over-protect Mark, who became a fat and fairly spoilt child.

When John was born Mrs Smith tried her best, but she could not form any strong attachment to him. He was skinny and dark, quite the opposite to what Peter had been. Her husband and her sister largely took over John's care. To deny his exist-ence seemed a way of freezing life at the time when Peter had still been there. Burst-ing into tears Mrs Smith admitted, 'I know this is terrible, but John was not there before Peter died. I feel I can't warm to anything that has happened since. Mark belongs to that past, but John does not.'

Peter's death had pushed her to do what she had been careful to avoid before. Mark had been 'twinned' by the cruel fate of his co-twin. Mrs Smith clung desper-ately to Mark in the illusory hope of keeping Peter alive. She said, 'Only when I see him do I find some joy. It's like having them both here again.' She now avoided referring to Mark by his name. It was always 'he' or 'him' or 'you' but never 'Mark'. Whilst Peter was alive Mrs Smith had tried to stress the differences between the twins. Now that Peter was gone she tried to erase all differences, including the fact that Mark continued in the unstoppable process of growing. Death had powerfully and inextricably united both twins in their mother's mind. However, one day, when Mark was two years old, Mrs Smith looked at her children. They both seemed mis-erable and depressed (Bernabei and Levi 1976; Bluglass 1980). They sat next to each other on a bench and did not move or play. Mrs Smith looked sadly at them and said, 'It's time for me to react now. I will never get over Peter's death. He will forever be engraved in my mind. But my pain is mine and should not reflect on them. My children look miserable. Mark is too fat. I have to do something about it. I owe it to my husband and to my children to try and make life less miserable for everyone.'

Mrs Smith had regained her strength and now needed to rebuild her life around her family. Visits had to stop. To continue would have risked becoming yet another constant reminder of the tragedy that had struck her life. As the bearer of the earli-est memories of Peter, the observer could also be used to continue stifling life in the fallacy of halting death.

Mrs Smith has been visited only briefly on two occasions since then. Mark seemed less depressed, although he still looked miserable. He had lost weight and seemed to enjoy John's company now. Apparently, at nursery school he liked playing with other children. Mrs Smith was also affectionate towards John and smiled whilst playing with him.

Mark will probably always be a twin in his parents' mind, and Peter's name is still inscribed on the wall where his cot used to be. Nothing will erase the tragedy that has struck this family, but the outcome seems more hopeful now.

CONCLUSION

Various disciplines are all contributing to help change fairly simplistic notions about twins. Behavioral sciences too can contribute to promote a different and more complex understanding. Following twins longitudinally as they emerge from their perilous first habitat until they finally enter the community of their peers can help to put each environment into perspective and dispel certain contemporary myths and prejudices. The roots of behavioral variation are to be found in prenatal life. Of course, we are only just beginning to see twins in a different light and to know more about their origins and their first environment. Ideas may have to be calibrated, certain aspects disregarded, and perspectives adjusted or changed altogether. Nevertheless, a much richer, less stereotyped and more realistic view of twins is beginning to emerge.

A UNIQUE NATURE AND A DIFFERENT UTERUS

Twins can hardly be equated to singletons. Their origin is particular and dissimilar. Furthermore, monozygotic twins are not equivalent to dizygotic ones. Deriving from the same zygote, and the consequent remarkable genetic sharing, distinguishes them from the start. Yet, at the same time, they themselves are not as 'identical' as previously thought. In addition they are not homogeneous. The timing of the 'twinning event' decides to what extent their intrauterine environment will differ from that of dizygotic twins.

The more they share the more they risk. We have seen that the clinical care of twins has been revolutionised by ultrasound diagnosis of placental and chorion type. Each possible combination has unique intrauterine environmental conditions and each is subject to different hazards. Clinically various types of twins are already handled distinctly. Some need intensive monitoring, others do not. Each twin fetus is also treated as an individual and monitored as such. One may suffer while the other does not. The notion of an unequal intrauterine existence now seems obvious to anyone dealing with the prenatal care of twins.

Unshared environmental factors have increasingly been evoked to explain the origins of individual differences between siblings in general. These often show remarkable behavioral differences that cannot be explained solely by the quota of genetic endowment they do not share (Plomin and Daniels 1987; Dunn 1988; Dunn and Plomin 1985, 1990, 1991). Though broadly speaking all twin fetuses inhabit the same uterus and grow and develop within its restricted boundaries, no twin experiences a totally identical intrauterine environment. Indeed, the primeval intrauterine milieu may well be the most unequal environment they will ever share in their entire existence. No twin emerges from intrauterine life as an 'identical' copy of its co-twin.

Singularity and chance characterise the intrauterine existence of twins (Thelen 1990). The intrauterine environment, far from being static, is subject to constant variance and shows innumerable individual differences even within such fundamentals as the placenta, the amniotic fluid and the umbilical cord (Alberts and Cramer 1988; Smootherman and Robinson 1988, 1989). The majority of twins do not share any of these macroscopic constituents. When they do the placenta is always unequally distributed, the quantity of amniotic fluid is not the same for both (except for those very rare monoamniotic pregnancies), and even in the extremely uncommon occurrence of a joint insertion their umbilical cords do not carry identical blood flows.

In any case, twins develop in different locations within the uterus and receive not only an unequal share of blood supply, nutrients and other substances, but of stimuli too. Not just macro- but also micro-environmental conditions vary both internally and externally from the start. The frequent weight discrepancy found in twins at birth is perhaps the most macroscopic evidence of such fortuitously unequal partaking. Even twins who are not overtly affected by their intrauterine environment will be shaped by it in an immeasurable number of subtle ways. Passing time may blur some of the more macroscopic differences created by such an environment, but other variations will never be erased.

The embryonic and fetal stages are very turbulent. Researchers from various disciplines now tend to adhere to a much more plastic view of developmental genetics and to underline the constant interplay between environment and genes from the earliest phases of our lives (Brauth *et al.* 1991; Elman *et al.* 1996).

Neuroscientists also indicate that no two individuals can ever be exactly alike as the processes of neuronal development ensure that our nervous systems are both topographically ordered and locally variant. Neural patterns, in their fine anatomical detail, are a product of local dynamics rather than predetermined instructions (Changeux 1983; Easter *et al.* 1985; Edelman 1987, 1992; Purves 1988; Brauth *et al.* 1991).

Studies that do not take the intrauterine environment into consideration, or regard it as equal or neutral, and regard everything prenatal as 'constitutional', clearly need to be evaluated with this in mind.

Investigations that take into account only one or a few macroscopic components also run the risk of falling into gross over-simplification. Just as a shared uterus does not mean an identical environment, so a single placenta or amniotic sac does not necessarily imply increased sharing.

Some of the most remarkable discrepancies in weight and appearance can be observed in those monochorionic twins suffering from feto-fetal or Twin-to-Twin Transfusion Syndrome. One twin may be small, incredibly skinny and pale, with a translucent and wrinkled skin, while the other is double its size, abnormally bloated and plethoric, with a strikingly thick purple-red epidermis. A lay person seeing the two infants would probably not only think that they were unrelated, but that they belonged to entirely different races. A single placenta, far from offering 'equal' opportunities, can produce very marked and often lethal inequalities.

A DIFFERENT PREGNANCY

Twin pregnancies can hardly be compared to their singleton counterparts (Price 1950; Benirschke and Kim 1973; Baldwin 1994).

The disproportionate decimation of the general population of 'twins' due to early fetal demise already distinguishes twin pregnancies from those of singletons. Many twins are conceived, far fewer are born. General maternal and fetal hazards are greater in twin pregnancies, which are all considered to be at risk:

> The twin fetus is affected not only by the innumerable intrauterine environmental influences of a single fetus but also by the interaction with the second fetus. At best it must compete for nutrition. At worst, it may be severely, even lethally, damaged by the co-twin.
>
> (Bryan 1993: 218)

Monozygotic and dizygotic pregnancies are also differentiated by other apparently superficial aspects. For instance, maternal age is usually higher for dizygotic twins. The numbers conceived by various techniques of assisted reproduction are rising at a staggering speed. This increase overwhelmingly, though not exclusively, concerns dizygotic twins.

Twins resulting from assisted reproduction are perhaps subject to greater, often quite unrealistic expectations. Traditionally conceived dizygotic twins can be unexpected, but often are not, there frequently being a family history of twins. Monozygotic twins are invariably a surprise, and sometimes an unwelcome one. The news that they are to give birth to monozygotic twins produces strong elation in many parents, who already seem to feel that their twin fetuses are sensational well before any social recognition of their 'phenomenal' nature has begun. A web of particular expectations, feelings, hopes and fantasies begins to be woven from the moment twins are diagnosed. Certainly singletons too are the subject of expectations and emotions from before they are born. However, anticipation and parental feelings are quite different for singletons and twins. Unequal labelling of twins starts very soon and a split between a 'good' and a 'bad' twin may already be established *in utero*. These may sound very trivial points but nevertheless, twins are not born in a vacuum. A different environment to that of singletons is already preparing itself to receive them once they are born.

DIFFERENT INTRAUTERINE BEHAVIOR

Fetal behavior has finally emerged from the misty and uncertain domain of mere meaning attribution. Perceived movements are no longer haphazardly interpreted as reflections of post-natal emotions. Thanks largely to the efforts of Prechtl and his co-workers (Prechtl 1985, 1989), fetal movements can now be reliably quantified and classified. Increasing knowledge may possibly further refine our present coding.

From the moment overt behavior starts, all twins are already dissimilar in their manifestations. All move differently, with distinct and non-coincidental cycles, and display distinct behavioral patterns, including different reactions to co-twin contact.

With advancing gestation the ruggedness and inequality of the intrauterine environment cancels the initially greater behavioral similarities between monozygotic twins. Furthermore, some individual consistency is attained. A relatively more active twin fetus generally shows a tendency to remain so at various stages during pregnancy. The same applies to a more or a less reactive one.

Rudimentary differences and apparently small asymmetries in the intrauterine sojourn of twins, with all the cascading effects they entail at such a particularly turbulent and sensitive stage, may paradoxically carry a greater weight in creating so-called 'constitutional' differences than other factors affecting us after birth (Elman *et al.* 1996). Seemingly trivial discrepancies in the intrauterine sojourn of monozygotic twins may have an explosive effect in putting even these apparently 'identical' individuals on behaviorally distinct and divergent paths.

All twin fetuses, within the limits of what they can perform, show preferential actions and reactions. The foundation stones of albeit elementary inclinations are laid during intrauterine life. Clearly, however, by inclination one does not mean complex or stabilised features at this stage.

Further disparities and complications can alter these flimsy trends. Only too many 'facts of life', including behavioral development, can later thwart, bury, dilute, enhance or inflate beyond recognition these primary tendencies. The incommensurably more complicated post-natal world can certainly disrupt and conceal in an unlimited cocktail what are fairly simplified proclivities. Nevertheless, behavioral propensities begin to dawn and behavioral uniqueness gains subsistence during pre-natal life (Gottlieb 1992; Elman *et al.* 1996).

Though we cannot yet measure in any comparable way behavioral manifestations occurring in the two 'different worlds' of the intrauterine and the post-natal environment, primeval inclinations should not be altogether disregarded. These phenomena do not cease to exist. Monozygotic twin fetuses are not behaviorally interchangeable. The limitations lie in our current capacity to measure and evaluate them.

Intrapair stimulation seems, perhaps, an irrelevant curiosity but we cannot rule out that it may have some long-lasting repercussions, albeit not clearly discernible. This apparently trivial factor not only differentiates twins from singletons but also differentiates between types of twins. Mutually evoked responses start earlier and are usually stronger in monochorionic–diamniotic twins compared to dichorionic twins. Monoamniotic twins rarely escape each other's blows, while the thicker membranes dividing twins with separate placentas buffer the intensity of their co-twin's blows. An increased intensity of reciprocal impacts could have a more disruptive effect on periodic cycling between activity and rest. Subtle effects of intrapair stimulation on the 'brain circuits' of twins cannot be ruled out either. Mutually evoked responses provide a wealth of additional sensory-motor feedback.

A DIVERSE START IN POST-NATAL LIFE

Twins have a more complex start compared to singletons. Besides the disproportionate number of Caesarean deliveries, many are born prematurely and/or growth-retarded. Some will continue to suffer from their disadvantaged beginning.

Once more, it is monochorionic–monozygotic twins who are particularly liable to perinatal complications.

Complications may continue to affect twins and their families unequally during the first year of their lives and often beyond that. Many twins are particularly fragile and liable to physical ailments. This clearly has repercussions on their parents too. Indispositions such as recurrent asthma or enterocolitis, delayed developmental milestones, and belated attainment of uninterrupted sleep all cause great parental distress. Again monochorionic–monozygotic twins stand out from the rest. Of course all these difficulties and the anxiety they cause can affect singletons as well. However, the exceptionally high frequency of these problems amongst twins makes them stand out from the general population.

A DIFFERENT POST-NATAL ENVIRONMENT

The home environment also distinguishes twins from singletons (Redshaw and Rutter 1991). The arrival of twins usually feels like a tornado hitting the house. Everybody's life is turned upside-down beyond their wildest dreams. Fathers are caught in the whirlwind immediately. A task force of helpers is called in whenever possible. Lack of uninterrupted sleep affects everyone. All the ponderous aspects of looking after any newborn child are exponentially increased when baby twins arrive. In ordinary circumstances, the parents of singletons derive pleasure and delight along with the more onerous duties involved, making the care of a newborn child not only tolerable but usually even enjoyable. Without these counterbalancing rewards our species would probably have become extinct long ago. These compensatory pleasures start late for most parents of twins. After a taste of the hardships involved in looking after twins, most parents decide that enough is enough.

Caring for two is quite unlike caring for one. It is also possibly less congruous to the human species. Just as the maternal body is not well adapted to the task of carrying two fetuses, so parental attention and care are ill-divided between two babies. In the animal world larger broods are generally born developmentally more advanced and independent, mature faster and do not require the same quality of interactions as the human child does. A newborn baby is initially totally dependent upon parental care for its survival. Full independence is acquired very late. The human infant is also an increasingly social creature requiring special attention and distinctive emotional interchanges. Many parents of twins feel quite inadequate, as they simply cannot provide two babies with all these requirements simultaneously. 'Choice' could possibly be viewed as an attempt to revert to a more customary dyadic condition. Besides the almost 'unnatural' amount of stress and fatigue connected with any twin birth, the high incidence of post-partum maternal depression further testifies perhaps to the relative unsuitability of our species to multiple pregnancies.

As pointed out repeatedly throughout this book, this does not necessarily imply psychological catastrophes. Quite simply the post-natal environmental conditions of twins differ in several significant ways from those of singletons. Mothering is different and so is fathering. Many twins survive and do quite well. Most of their parents also survive all the hardships. However, some do not. The gravity of marital difficulties is clearly recognised by the associations and foundations which care for the births of twins. Such organisations realise that there exists a very real need for assistance to help the families of twins surmount the problems they must face.

SINGULAR CIRCUMSTANCES

Once they are born and can be taken home twins are inevitably reunited and start to live an uncommonly shared life. During the first years of their lives twins are hardly ever apart.

Overwhelmingly, this enforced union is guided by purely pragmatic reasons. Twins soon end up sharing almost anything from feeding bottles and pacifiers, to clothes and cots. Singletons do not normally share so much time and such intimacy with another child of the same age. Nor do they usually have to compete for nourishment, interest and care with someone of the same age to the very day.

Siblings born nine months apart have been equated to twins (Segal 1999). However, although very close in age, they are inevitably already at significantly different stages of development and contend for attention of a different kind as a result of this. For instance, mothers display different facial expressions, and talk and gesture in specific ways when focusing on tiny babies compared to a nine-month-old baby whose vision, hearing and social development are quite different. 'Motherese' is finely tuned to the developmental changes in the infant (Stern 1985). Fathers begin to engage in rough and tumble with much more robust and participating nine-month-old babies. A nine-month-old whose mother became pregnant again straight after his or her birth may have never been breast-fed. However, if it were, by the time the other sibling is born it may already have teeth and be taking some solid foods. These may sound insignificant details, but we cannot rule out that they might be more important than they at first appear. Though siblings born a few months apart are the closest we can get to the shared lives of twins, the two circumstances cannot be equated.

The quality of maternal communication is also quite distinct with twins. Most interactions with the infants are characterised by brevity and dissociation between various forms of signalling.

Choice is also different between twins and between other siblings. Comparison is a constant feature with twins. One is always measured against the other. Intrauterine growth discrepancy may cause a bigger twin to be regarded as a vampire long before he or she is born, and some such labels stick for the rest of their lives.

Though some pairs are clearly more 'compatible' than others, each co-twin is a constant and important component of the post-natal environment. Individual idiosyncrasy is there from the start. The loudness of a twin's yells attests to their propensity to have their own needs taken into consideration above and beyond those of the other twin and his or her screams. Nevertheless, co-twins are always there. Long before signs of social recognition start to be consistently exchanged between them, twins begin to monitor each other. Later they imitate and 'learn' from each other. Though forced propinquity necessarily brings with it ferocious 'territorial' fights, twins also have to rely on each other to a rare degree. No singleton child experiences the same with a peer. The characteristics of mutual attachment distinguish twins from singletons.

It takes a long time before twins are in a position to go their separate ways. The entrance into the wider community of their peers is just a first small step. Even by that time no twin will have ever experienced the prevailing condition of being born and raised as a singleton.

Even early death distinguishes twins. When one dies the ghost of the dead co-twin continues to haunt the other – possibly for the rest of his or her life.

UNIQUE TWINS

Only birth fully brings out all the social consequences of being born as monozygotic twins.

Most monozygotic twins look quite unlike at birth. The majority, however, soon come to look very similar to each other. Many less visible, minute yet probably important differences have been created during prenatal life. Different behavior and distinct inclinations attest to this. However, unusual physical similarity in the end imprints the existence of most monozygotic twins.

Everyone immediately recognises most monozygotic twins as such. People stare at them and turn round when they pass in the street. Monozygotic twins are the centre of attraction from the start. This reflects on their numerous caregivers and has an impact on them too by quickly triggering the chain reaction of reinforced 'twinning' in them.

Parents are not driven by purely selfish motives in 'twinning' their monozygotic infants. From the very beginning twins begin shaping their environments too (Scarr and McCartney 1983). Parents also perceive and surrender to undoubted 'affinities' between their twins. Dizygotic twins can occasionally be very similar to monozygotic ones. However, generally monozygotic ones rebel less when made to sleep in the same cot; seek mutual proximity; seem more aware of each other's rhythms; and react with lower intensity to bodily manifestations, odours and substances. Parents, albeit unconsciously, often give in to the particular nature of monozygotic twins.

Many tolerate sleeping together long after what is considered normal. The twins themselves often yell if the other is not there. They hop into each other's bed whenever they can.

FREEDOM

Nursery school affords dizygotic twins their first opportunity to begin experiencing other peer relationships. The onset of nursery school certainly does not offer monozygotic twins many opportunities to undo their ties. At this early stage perhaps no other link can be stronger or more appealing than their mutual union.

Presumably only adolescence, with consequent mental and physical (including sexual) maturation, can offer most monozygotic twins real chances of separation. This delayed division may be particularly difficult by then.

However, not all aspects of the close link uniting many monozygotic twins should be discarded – far from it. Despite their generally unfavourable prenatal and post-natal start, many do quite well simply by relying on each other. The link uniting monozygotic twins is quite unusual. As soon as they can speak, many tell of joys unknown to the rest of us.

Monozygotic twins are a minority characterised by special and unique genetic and environmental features. Strong, distinctive intrapair dynamics prompt them to be a truly 'dissident minority' from very early on in life. Despite the powerful environmental pressures put on them, these twins often are perfectly able to manifest their different dispositions and to object to environmental measures enforcing separation.

Though not quite like the rest of us, most dizygotic twins in the end merge into the singleton majority. Monozygotic twins are often determined and proud to stick out in a crowd. Possibly we cannot enforce precepts on them which belong to the prevailing population. Some twins may want to stay together, others may not.

This work, by investigating many of the multifaceted aspects which all contribute to make twins what they are, may hopefully help to free them from many of the myths and prejudices still encumbering their lives. Twins are not hard-wired oddities resembling each other in all respects. Nor are they 'twin souls' bound together from conception and communicating with each other in paranormal ways. Superficial similarities and greater affinities can cloud even profound differences. Twins are simply related differently, thanks both to unusual genetic sharing and to uncommon environmental circumstances. Like any other social minority their own nature and nurture should be studied and respected for what it is. This includes investigating their roots and the possible nuances distinguishing different types and sub-types of twins.

A 'taxonomy' of all sub-types of twins is greatly needed and overwhelmingly absent from post-natal research into twins.[1] An improved knowledge of all these aspects could definitely refine our understanding.

Scientists trying to elucidate the mechanisms underlying their varied origin, clinicians assisting their perilous journey through pregnancy, and the many associations attempting to relieve the unbelievable burdens and anxieties parents of twins initially have to suffer, are all endeavouring to understand and help twins and their families in their own right.

EXPLANATORY NOTES

This section can be read separately from the rest of the book.

A fairly detailed analysis of all pairs of twins is necessary to understand how and on what basis various deductions have been made. The progressive sequence of the tables allows various aspects of each pair to be followed from conception to three years after birth. Twins have been divided into two groups according to zygosity.

Most parameters were derived from observational data and from detailed and independent evaluation of visual material by the main observer and the obstetricians before birth and by the observer and two psychologists after birth. If other particular criteria were applied, this will be specified in the text.

Subtler differences and nuances necessarily inherent to every pair could also be perceived from a careful examination of the data. Inevitably a selection of the material obtained has had to be made. Several clinical prenatal and perinatal parameters have been omitted. A summary of the results of the standardised developmental tests is reported. Given the numerous items considered, the Infant Behavioral Scale (Bayley 1969) has not been included. The focus is upon less closely investigated developmental and behavioral aspects.

Since most items in the tables are self-explanatory, only those which could cause confusion to the non-specialist reader will be explained. Brief comments stressing differences between the two groups are added.

Twins have been designated according to birth order throughout, the first born being Twin I and the second Twin II. The twin who died of SIDS at six months is not included, nor is he or any member of his family considered in any part of this section.

Table 1 Background

Maternal age was in accordance with epidemiological data, being higher (mean age = 35) in mothers of dizygotic twins than in those of monozygotic ones (mean age = 32).

Dizygotic twin pregnancies were both spontaneous (9) and the result of fertility treatments (6), either through ovarian stimulation (Clomid) or *in vitro* fertilisation (IVF). All monozygotic twin pregnancies were spontaneous.

Fathers were rarely present at the initial scan, therefore only maternal reactions to the news that they were expecting twins have been considered.

The high number (13) of mothers of dizygotic twins who were not surprised can be accounted for by two facts. Those who resorted to assisted reproduction knew that this carried a greater probability of twins. In other couples twins ran in the family and therefore the possibility had been considered.

Maternal reactions to the news were classified independently by two obstetricians and the main observer.

It may seem surprising that only two cases resulting from assisted reproduction expressed elation at this stage. This is probably because women who undergo fertility treatments are generally aware of the possibility of premature fetal loss and of the greater risks of a twin pregnancy. Most do not dare rejoice until their pregnancy has successfully run its course.

Gender is not disclosed during an early scan. Feminine genitalia are enlarged at this stage and could be mistaken for masculine ones, and vice versa. All the parents whose twins turned out to be opposite-sex expressed elation later when gender was revealed, normally between 15–20 weeks.

Table 2 Pregnancy

As explained earlier dizygotic twins are always dichorionic. Seventy per cent of monozygotic twins are monochorionic–diamniotic, 29 per cent are dichorionic and the remaining 1 per cent are monochorionic–monoamniotic.

In the monozygotic group twelve pairs were monochorionic–diamniotic, only one was dichorionic and two were monochorionic–monoamniotic.

Twin pregnancy and monozygosity were diagnosed during the same scan in every case, except one where two separate placentas meant it was not possible to ascertain that the twins were monozygotic until birth. Confirmation of chorionicity and zygosity was obtained at birth every time.

Maternal complications affected monozygotic pregnancies more frequently and more severely. Minor ailments have not been considered. Ten monozygotic pregnancies and eight dizygotic ones involved complications. In the monozygotic group nine cases required hospitalisation. The mean stay in hospital was seventeen days. In the dizygotic group five cases required hospitalisation. The mean stay in hospital was eighteen days.

Pre-eclampsia or toxaemia generally occurs in the latter half of pregnancy and is characterised by an acute and severe hypertension accompanied by edemas and proteinuria (the presence of proteins in the urine). This condition can lead to eclampsia, an even more severe form of hypertension with additional nephritis, sodium retention, convulsions and sometimes coma. Needless to say, careful monitoring is necessary in both cases.

Fetal complications were more common in the monozygotic group. Twelve monozygotic and eight dizygotic twins presented an alteration in the quantity of amniotic fluid. Seventeen monozygotic twins and one dizygotic twin had altered umbilical artery blood flows.

Altered amniotic fluid index (AFI) and pulsatility index (PI) are warning signs which prompt the clinician to search for further symptoms and intensify monitoring.

AFI gives an indication as to the quantity of amniotic fluid present in the amniotic sac. This may be within the normal range, increased (hydramnios) or decreased (oligohydramnios). If the AFI is increased or decreased in one or both sacs, the pregnancy is monitored more carefully and other indicators are assessed. However, an excess of amniotic fluid *per se* can contribute to trigger off a premature delivery in an already over-distended uterus.

Doppler studies evaluate placental vascular resistance using the umbilical artery pulsatility index (PI). This important index gives general information about fetal oxygenation and well-being. If the PI is altered in one or both twins, other signs of fetal distress are searched for. Cerebral blood flows, for instance, are measured and assessed. An increase in these is an indicator of initial fetal compromise. It is also a pointer to the 'intelligence' of fetal physiology. When the flow of blood and oxygen is limited, blood is diverted towards the more 'noble' and easily compromised areas of the brain, heart and adrenals (Thornburgh 1991). This directing of available oxygen towards the most delicate and precious components of the fetal body results in a visible increase in the cerebral blood flows, often best evaluated at the level of the carotid artery as it divides into its middle and cerebral branches. However, other tests are also carried out including a fetal biophysical profile, a kind of general check-up of multifarious fetal functions (Manning *et al.* 1980).

Table 3 Intrauterine behavior: activity levels

Table 4 Intrauterine behavior: reactivity levels

Intrauterine behavior in twin fetuses has been described at length in Chapter 3. Estimates of fetal behavior after weeks 20–22 are unreliable and, therefore, have not been included.

In Tables 3 and 4 the names of the more active and more reactive twin are given, thus rendering comparison with subsequent developmental and behavioral aspects possible. Birth order is indicated in Table 6.

In all but eight cases the more active twin displayed a tendency to remain the more active one throughout the period considered.

Reactivity was even more consistent. The more reactive twin remained so throughout. A dash indicates that intrapair stimulation had not started at the gestational age considered.

Table 5 Prenatal labels

Labels were considered such if repeated during a minimum of four separate encounters. Except in six cases (four monozygotic and two dizygotic), all twins were given prenatal labels.

Most labels in the monozygotic group (six pairs) were based on growth and/or clinical parameters. Monozygotic twins were also attributed a collective denomination more frequently (three pairs) compared to dizygotic twins (one pair).

Attributed and/or perceived movements led to differential labelling in four pairs in each group.

Gender-related issues ranging from intelligence, strength and chattiness, to sexiness and even sexual prowess(!) were reflected in the labels of four opposite-sex dizygotic cases.

Table 6 Birth

On average dizygotic twins were born at term (mean = 36 weeks 5 days). Monozygotic twins were born earlier (mean = 35 weeks 3 days).

Most twins were delivered by Caesarean section. The majority of Caesareans of monozygotic twins (9 out of 12) were prompted by fetal and/or maternal suffering. In such cases a careful assessment is generally made to determine whether the advantages of a premature operative delivery outweigh those of waiting.

Obstetricians are prepared for the eventuality of a premature delivery in monochorionic–monozygotic twins. Though this conduct is presently subject to debate, women are usually administered steroids starting from around week 29. These have been shown to accelerate pulmonary maturity, which is possibly the main determinant of the viability of a prematurely delivered baby.

The type of anaesthesia was largely a matter of maternal preference. Women known to be expecting monochorionic–monozygotic twins were able to discuss types of anaesthetic and decide which they preferred well before term. Since Caesareans did not require long planning, in most cases of dizygotic twins mothers simply came in on the day and so had fewer opportunities to discuss or think about anaesthetics.

Dizygotic twins on average had higher birthweights (mean birthweight = 2,528 g) than monozygotic ones (mean birthweight = 2,229 g).

Several cases (six monozygotic and three dizygotic) were markedly growth discordant. Intrapair birthweight differences ranged from 1,100 g to 400 g in such cases. In the monozygotic group the umbilical cord was found to have a velamentous or a marginal insertion in two growth-retarded cases and one artery in another case. The presence of one artery in the cord is generally detected prenatally with ultrasounds and colour Doppler. The umbilical cord was marginally inserted in one dizygotic pair who were markedly growth discordant.

Apgar scores give a quantitative estimate of the condition of an infant 1–5 minutes after birth. Scores are derived by assigning points to the quality of heart rate, respiratory effort, colour, muscle tone and reflexes. These are then expressed in scores out of 10.

Apgar scores were generally higher for dizygotic twins. Fifteen dizygotic twins reached the optimal score of 10 at the second evaluation, while only eight monozygotic twins were assigned this rating.

Second-born twins usually present lower Apgar scores, their delivery being generally more laborious.

Table 7 Perinatal period

Only eight dizygotic twins had to be kept in the NICU, compared to twenty-two monozygotic ones.

A stay in the NICU of 3–8 days usually indicates a period of observation.

Excessive weight loss and pronounced jaundice are fairly common problems linked with prematurity. Other complications, such as breathing irregularities, recurrent cardiac arrhythmia and cyanosis, recurrent hypoglycaemia and enteritis, all testify to the difficulties of the immature organism in dealing with the different requirements of post-natal life.

Respiratory distress syndrome (RDS) and necrotising enterocolitis (NEC) are possibly the most dreaded complications of prematurity. Both of these conditions can have long-term consequences and are often fatal.

RDS of the newborn can occur in the first days of life of premature infants and is characterised by respiratory distress, cyanosis, easy collapsibility of the alveoli (the 'air cells' of the lungs in which respiratory pathways terminate and through whose walls gases pass between air and blood), and loss of pulmonary surfactant (a substance secreted by alveolar cells and lining the alveolar surface which serves to maintain the stability of the alveolar mucous). A hyaline membrane (a layer of fibrinoid material lying on part or all of the pulmonary alveoli and causing damage to alveolar walls) coats the alveoli and alveolar ducts when the syndrome persists for more than a few hours.

NEC is a severe inflammation of the small intestine and colon, causing pathologic death of cells in such areas. Symptoms are abdominal distension, temperature instability, apnoea and blood in stools. Associated laboratory findings include anaemia, thrombocytopenia and electrolyte abnormalities.

Breast-feeding was unequally distributed amongst the groups. Nine mothers of monozygotic twins and four mothers of dizygotic pairs breast-fed their infants for at least ten days.

Pressures from the NICU were clearly strong on mothers of monozygotic twins. Out of nine breast-feeding mothers in this group, six had at least one twin in the NICU.

Table 8 Congenital anomalies and defects, and health problems during the first two years

Congenital anomalies and/or defects were present in three pairs of monozygotic twins and in none of the dizygotic group.

In case 2 the twins were discordant for a cardiac malformation. One presented transposition of the great arteries. In this malformation the aorta arises from the right ventricle and the pulmonary artery from the left ventricle and are thus 'transposed'. Heart surgery was performed twice in the neonatal period. The great arteries were switched over and each was relocated in its appropriate position. All went well.

Hypospadias is a congenital anomaly of the penis and urethra in which the urethra opens upon the ventral surface of the penis. The twins in case 4 needed surgery at six months and will possibly need some minor operation when six years old.

Congenital nystagmus is a continuous and rapid oscillatory movement of the eyeballs. Though these case 12 twins were highly intelligent, this anomaly did have cognitive/developmental repercussions. Problems in fine manipulation, fixation and many other consequences eventually lead to learning disabilities (principally reading and writing).

Fourteen monozygotic twins, but only four dizygotic ones were affected by health problems requiring medical intervention and/or investigation during the first two years. Colds or minor attacks of flu affected all twins and have not been considered.

Physical problems were less severe for dizygotic twins. One twin manifested a sudden and rapid enlargement of cranial circumference at five months. He was subjected to many examinations, including a TAC and an NMR. No apparent cause was detected and the enlargement ceased spontaneously. One twin suffered from impetigo, an acute infection of the skin, which was easily solved. Another twin had to be operated on at eight months for infantile hernia. Only one twin in this group had weight-gain problems and never recovered from his initial growth retardation.

In the monozygotic group all those twins (nine) who had had respiratory problems at birth manifested chest problems during the first two years. These ranged from bronchitis to bronchopneumonia and asthma. The two twins who had had severe intestinal problems at birth manifested recurrent colitis. Three twins who were growth retarded at birth and suffered from excessive weight loss requiring a stay in the NICU never recovered from their initial growth retardation. Finally, one monozygotic twin required lengthy examinations due to an enlargement of the cerebral ventricles. However, this problem went away spontaneously. She was well subsequently and did not show any signs of neurological compromise or developmental delay.

Table 9 Milestones

On average dizygotic twins were capable of sitting unsupported at 8.8 months and monozygotic ones at 9.31 months.

Dizygotic twins also walked earlier on average (12.98 months) than monozygotic ones (13.6 months).

Gross motor developmental milestones were all delayed in those monozygotic twins who were born prematurely and/or had problems at birth. Such delays only affected those dizygotic twins who had suffered from these same problems at birth. However, taking into account corrected ages (the difference between gestational age at birth and term), gross motor developmental milestones were not markedly delayed. Eventually, gross motor development was within the norm for all.

Monozygotic twins on average uttered their first words at 13.8 months and dizygotic ones at 14.1 months. The first sentence was vocalised on average at 22.6 months by monozygotic twins and at 22.9 months by dizygotic ones. Seven cases were delayed beyond 24 months in the utterance of the first sentence in the monozygotic group. In the dizygotic group eight cases were delayed. Maternal depression was probably a concurrent factor in all.

Table 10 Choice

Besides parental declarations, choice was evaluated longitudinally by careful and independent reading of the tapes. Criteria of evaluation included smiling, gazing, talking, picking up, cuddling and engaging in playful activities. Noting the consistency in directing these behavioral displays towards one twin rather than the other assessed intensity of choice.

Fourteen parents immediately voiced an open choice. These were equally divided between monozygotic and dizygotic twins.

All the monozygotic twins that were immediately chosen had quite dissimilar aspects at birth to their co-twin.

Parents of dizygotic twins who did not immediately express their choice denied it later. Denial concerned all (eight) pairs of opposite-sex twins.

Only the parents of two pairs of monozygotic twins denied any preference. Amongst mothers 'quieter' twins were popular in both groups (nine twins). Appearance was a distinguishing factor in only two cases. These twins looked very different at birth. Four mothers of monozygotic twins acted on a compensatory basis by preferring the twin who had been less favoured *in utero* and/or in the NICU.

This did not happen with mothers of dizygotic twins. Since most dizygotic twins had had untroubled gestations this element was less cogent. Gender played an important role in the choice of the elected dizygotic twins, but so did appearance. Male gender was overtly and strongly preferred by six mothers of opposite-sex dizygotic twins.

Six fathers of the monozygotic group reacted on a compensatory basis or on a 'one each' basis, choosing the twin their wives did not chose. Three fathers also preferred the quieter twin.

In the dizygotic group male gender was a real hit with fathers too: six fathers were openly biased towards boys.

Monozygotic twins aroused less extreme favouritism than their dizygotic counterparts. Only five mothers showed strong partiality. All these twins looked quite different from their co-twins at birth.

Eleven mothers and nine fathers of opposite-sex dizygotic twins displayed strong preferences. Gender dominated the issue. Only three fathers in the monozygotic group showed a strong preference. Several twins in both groups (nine monozygotic and ten dizygotic) were not chosen by either parent.

In the monozygotic group three rejected twins had less complicated beginnings, three were 'alert', two 'withdrawn' and one was 'too thin'. Six dizygotic twins were rejected because they were females, three for greater or inferior 'attractiveness' and one as 'less affectionate'.

Table 11 Maternal depression: concomitant and aggravating factors

Maternal depression was evaluated independently by the observer and the psychologists. The assessment was based on diagnostic criteria for detecting major depressive episodes, as propounded by the *Diagnostic and Statistical Manual of Mental Disorders* (DSM-IV) of the American Psychiatric Association (1994). Depression was accordingly diagnosed as 'mild', 'moderate' or 'severe'. All cases were free of psychotic features. The denomination 'very severe', although not included in DSM-IV, refers to those cases (four) which required psychiatric aid for over two years.

Only four mothers in each group were immune from depression. In the monozygotic group maternal depression was severe in six cases. Eight mothers of dizygotic twins were classified as very severely or severely depressed.

Only concomitant and possibly aggravating factors of maternal depression were taken into consideration. No one of these could be considered the single or principal cause. Lack of sleep and consequent fatigue clearly affected all mothers.

As can be evinced from Table 2, four mothers of monozygotic twins had to have fairly long stays in hospital (range 15–20 days) during pregnancy. These already seemed depressed prior to giving birth.

Women who had undergone assisted reproduction seemed especially liable to severe depression. Three of the four cases classified as very severely depressed had undergone fertility treatments.

Paternal involvement was classified as strong when the father was directly engaged in the care of the twins and also helped in various chores around the house. Fair involvement meant that the father generally helped with practical chores, but was initially less involved with the twins. A minimally involved father practically fled from the situation.

Many fathers (twelve) in both groups were strongly involved, but almost as many (six fathers of monozygotic and four of dizygotic twins) showed only minimal involvement.

Seven mothers with minimally involved companions were severely or very severely depressed. Only three women coped well with nearly absent fathers.

Ten mothers (five in each group) had no help from other caregivers. Six of these cases suffered severe or very severe depression. Only two mothers were quite happy to do without any help.

Three of the four very depressed mothers of the dizygotic group did not go back to work after the twins were born. All other severely depressed mothers in both groups (nine) either did not resume work, worked at home or only went back to work after the twins were one or older. They had all been employed before getting pregnant.

Most mothers (eleven in each group) frequently reported their altered physical shape as a cause of misery. Except for one mother, all took at least one year to regain their former silhouettes. After three years or more several women (nine) had still not got back to their previous shape. Most women (twenty-two) complained about protruding abdominal walls.

The rate of divorce and strong marital difficulties was very high. Parents of dizygotic twins suffered earlier and more acutely: four couples are already divorced; three of these had undergone assisted reproduction. The parents of three monozygotic pairs live separate lives, but are not divorced.

Table 12 Appearance

All dizygotic twins, except one pair, looked very different at birth.

Nine pairs of monozygotic twins had from different to very different appearance at birth. A birthweight discrepancy of at least 140 g (range 140–800 g) separated these twins. The six pairs of monozygotic twins who were very similar at birth also had minimal birthweight discrepancy (range 10–100 g).

The differences between most monozygotic twins reduced with time. At six months one pair classified as very different at birth looked similar, three more had very similar features but quite dissimilar height and weight. The situation was the same at one, two and three years. This latter, therefore, is the only data reported.

Only three pairs of monozygotic twins looked merely similar as opposed to very similar when the twins were three years old. Differences in weight and size persisted in these cases.

The only dizygotic twins similar at birth already looked different at six months.

Glamour was judged by the manifestations of occasional visitors to the family and/or of passers-by in the street. Loud exclamations of wonder, behavioral displays signalling amazement (from clapping of hands to indicating the twins repeatedly and excitedly), turning round to look at the twins, and approaching them were all considered as indicators of strong social glamour. Glamour was strong for most monozygotic pairs (thirteen) but only for two dizygotic ones.

Table 13 Twinning

All indicators of environmental enforcing were especially high in monozygotic twins.

The use of identical clothes was judged regular when repeated over at least two-thirds of the observations and occasional when recurring in fewer observations. At six months the use of identical clothes was occasional in five cases of the dizygotic group and regular in only one. Regular use was noted in eleven pairs of monozygotic twins and occasional use in the other three pairs. Two of these pairs were growth discordant. The situation in both groups was unchanged at one year. This data, therefore, has been omitted.

After two years all families of dizygotic twins had stopped dressing the twins the same. Nine pairs of monozygotic twins continued to be dressed identically at the age of two. When the twins were three years old six families persisted in buying identical clothes.

Hairstyles were the same for thirteen monozygotic pairs at age two and for twelve at age three. Only three pairs of dizygotic twins had the same hairstyle when two years old, and only two pairs when three years old.

Eight pairs of monozygotic twins were always called with a joint name. For seven others a joint name was only used occasionally (not more than twice per observation). Only two pairs of dizygotic twins were regularly named jointly.

Toy duplication was assessed (at six months, one, two and three years) as 'most' when more than fifteen identical toys could be counted; 'several' when there were 5–15; and 'few' when five or less identical toys were noted. Ten pairs of monozygotic twins had most toys duplicated at all considered ages. Dizygotic twins, except for one pair, either had few (five) or no (nine) identical toys.

Praising of joint activities was determined to be present when more than ten such actions were acclaimed during each observation and such behavior was spread over two-thirds of the observations. Twelve monozygotic pairs were regularly acclaimed for joint behavior. Only three dizygotic pairs were equally approved.

Labels were considered such when repeated over at least two-thirds of all observations. All but one pair of twins had regular labels. This pair was physically and behaviorally extremely similar and had been labelled identical prenatally. Contrasting was more accentuated and clear-cut in all cases of monozygotic twins. The qualification 'less so' was used for eight dizygotic twins, but for none of the monozygotic ones. Five monozygotic and three dizygotic twins had labels denoting a complete split between a 'good' and a 'bad' twin. Prenatal labels persisted, albeit with some variation, in four cases (nos 3, 5, 7 and 26).

Table 14 Intrapair dynamics

Monozygotic twins on average started giving out initial mutual social signs slightly earlier (3.6 months) than dizygotic ones (4.3 months).

Twins were classified as 'strong' imitators if six episodes of mutual mimicry could be noted during each observation, as 'mild' if three such episodes occurred and as 'minimal' if only one occurred. At a longitudinal reading strong, mild and minimal imitators had to be classified as such during at least two-thirds of the observations, starting from one year onwards. Those that did not fit in with this parameter were moved down to the next category. This criterion, unless otherwise specified, has also been applied to all other behavioral manifestations evaluated here.

No dizygotic twin was a strong imitator. Twelve pairs of monozygotic twins could be classified as strong imitators.

When practising for verbal communication the twins exchanged some verbal babble, nodded or acted in accordance to what had been 'said', and often laughed. This type of 'secret language', albeit in a transitory form, was noted in thirteen cases of monozygotic twins and in eight cases of dizygotic ones.

Twins were classified as strongly dominant if at least six episodes of domineering behavior could be noted during each observation and as mildly dominant if no more than two such displays were observed. In nine pairs of monozygotic twins one child was classified strongly dominant. Only four dizygotic twins were consistently strongly dominant.

Fights were observed to be 'regular' (meaning more than once during each visit) in six pairs of monozygotic twins and 'occasional' (not more than once during each observation) in the remaining nine pairs. Fights were regular in eleven pairs of dizygotic twins.

Rivalry was appraised on verbal and behavioral displays from two years old onwards. Strong rivalry implied six or more exhibitions and mild at least one per observation. Rivalry was classified as minimal if it could only be noted in one-third or less of the observations. Ten dizygotic pairs displayed strong competitiveness. Strong rivalry could only be observed in two pairs of monozygotic twins.

Strong and regular ganging up, which here means acting together not always with 'innocent' intents and with great accompanying fun was evaluated from two years onwards. Ganging up was marked in eleven cases of monozygotic twins and only in one dizygotic pair.

'Telepathic' phenomena consisted in expressing the need or distress of the other in its presence, crying when the other was hurt but not present or playing jointly in separate rooms without being able to see what the other was doing. They were all occasional instances and were observed in seven cases of monozygotic pairs and in none of the dizygotic group.

The habit of sharing the same cot, and later the same bed, also differentiated monozygotic and dizygotic twins. Since sharing the same bed continued until the twins were three years old, the ages of one and two years have been omitted.

Only four dizygotic pairs shared their cots during the first six months and just one pair continued to share the same bed occasionally at three years. Nine pairs of monozygotic twins shared the same cot during the first six months. Four pairs regularly slept in the same bed when three years old. For six other pairs, although formally having separate beds, sleeping together was 'tolerated' by their parents.

Mutual masturbatory/exploratory activities of some kind were observed in ten pairs of monozygotic twins from the age of two. Masturbation meant fondling each other's genitals (covered or uncovered) and/or French kissing. Masturbatory activities of this kind were frequent (noted more than once per observation) in eight cases and sporadic (noted only once per observation) in two cases. Only one dizygotic pair openly engaged in these activities.

Table 15 Attachment

Attachment was evaluated in the home environment by a psychologist, who had no prior acquaintance with the families, during a special session when twins were between twelve and fifteen months old.

The sequence of episodes of separations and reunions generally used for singletons was followed. In addition the reactions of the twins were appraised in all various possible combinations, both leaving them together and separating them.

Evaluation was aimed at establishing the quality of attachment to the mother, to each other, and finally to each other compared to their attachment towards their mother.

Six monozygotic pairs and five dizygotic ones were assessed as securely attached to their mother. Five monozygotic and five dizygotic pairs were classified as insecure–avoidant and insecure–ambivalent respectively. The remainder were discordant in their reactions.

In nine pairs of monozygotic twins the main attachment figure was evaluated to be the co-twin, in three the mother and in four cases the reactions were discordant (one twin was more strongly attached to its mother and the other to its co-twin).

In twelve pairs of dizygotic twins the main attachment figure was evaluated to be the mother. In the remaining three pairs the twins were discordant.

Table 16 Tests: higher scorers on Bayley scales

Table 17 Tests: home observation for measurement of the environment

A psychologist with no prior knowledge of their prenatal and perinatal history administered developmental tests (Bayley Scales of Infant Development 1969) to the twins at six months, one, two and three years.

The same psychologist also completed an evaluation of the home environment using the HOME assessment when the twins were one year old (Caldwell and Bradley 1984). HOME was used again when the twins were three years old. However, on this occasion the home environment was assessed independently for each twin in order to appraise non-shared environmental factors between the two.

For a description of the tests readers should refer to the original publications.

The accent of this work has been on intrapair relationships throughout. Therefore, in Table 16 the twin who obtained the higher score at each age is reported.

Three twins in each group consistently performed better in the Mental Development Index and the Physical Development Index. Four monozygotic and eight dizygotic twins performed better in either MDI or PDI. This indicates greater intrapair differences amongst dizygotic twins.

Looking back at the history of higher-scoring twins some interesting elements emerge. Curiously, all but one of them were more reactive *in utero*. Prenatal and post-natal suffering, birthweight and Apgar scores, whilst affecting twins as a general population, were not of absolute predictive value of better intrapair scores. Choice, on the other hand, seemed very relevant. Three of those who achieved higher results in both tests had been chosen by both parents and the remaining three by one. Only three of the twins scoring higher than their co-twins in one test had been rejected by both parents.

Table 17 gives an itemised evaluation of the home environment. The appraisal of three cases of dizygotic twins differed notably from the impressions of the main observer and of the other psychologist who had independently viewed the video material. Possibly these families were 'on their best behavior' with a stranger in the house.

It is interesting to note how evaluations differed for each group.

Monozygotic twins, despite strong initial difficulties, received better environmental care. Provision of play materials was the exception. Exhausted parents of dizygotic twins gave them less attention, but lots of toys.

Differential appraisal of the home environment for each twin, when three years old, is not summarised in table form. However, choice was again the overriding element which favoured better care of one twin. All twins who were favoured by both parents were granted upper-fourth parental responsivity, acceptance, involvement and variety of stimulation. On the other hand, all 'rejected' twins were given lowest-half attention. Besides organisation which generally was equanimous for all, only toys were appraised to be numerically within the same range for 'rejected' and 'chosen' co-twins.

Table 1 Background

Mz twins	Parental age		Profession		Siblings	Conception type	Twins in family	Maternal	
	Mother	Father	Mother	Father				Surprise	Reaction
Case 1	30	30	Visiting professor	Assistant professor	No	Spontaneous	No	Yes	Elation
Case 2	33	34	Cleaner	Traffic warden	3	Spontaneous	No	Yes	Despair
Case 3	22	24	Computer programmer	Decorator	No	Spontaneous	No	Yes	Elation
Case 4	32	39	Executive	Advertising agent	No	Spontaneous	No	Yes	Elation
Case 5	34	38	Civil servant	Truck driver	No	Spontaneous	Yes	Yes	Mixed
Case 6	33	35	Architect	Architect	No	Spontaneous	No	Yes	Mixed
Case 7	23	28	Hairdresser	Clerk	No	Spontaneous	No	Yes	Elation
Case 8	36	40	Housewife	Contractor	1	Spontaneous	No	Yes	Mixed
Case 9	34	38	Bank clerk	Sales representative	No	Spontaneous	No	Yes	Positive
Case 10	33	35	Housewife	Builder	3	Spontaneous	No	Yes	Despair
Case 11	34	37	Clerk	Bank manager	No	Spontaneous	No	No	Elation
Case 12	30	38	Secretary	Physiotherapist	No	Spontaneous	Yes	Yes	Elation
Case 13	34	40	Fashion designer	Bank manager	No	Spontaneous	No	Yes	Mixed
Case 14	33	36	Lawyer	Doctor	No	Spontaneous	No	Yes	Positive
Case 15	35	37	Clerk	Bank clerk	No	Spontaneous	No	Yes	Despair

Dz twins	Parental age		Profession		Siblings	Conception type	Twins in family	Maternal	
	Mother	Father	Mother	Father				Surprise	Reaction
Case 16	35	36	Hairdresser	Clerk	1	Spontaneous	No	Yes	Despair
Case 17	34	35	Teacher	Bank manager	No	IVF	No	No	Elation
Case 18	37	45	Nursery school teacher	Railway worker	No	IVF	No	No	Positive
Case 19	33	37	Teacher	Architect	1	Spontaneous	Yes	No	Despair
Case 20	36	36	Nursery school teacher	Policeman	No	IVF	No	No	Positive
Case 21	37	37	Family business	Family business	No	Spontaneous	Yes	No	Despair
Case 22	37	38	Bank clerk	Civil servant	1	Spontaneous	Yes	No	Despair
Case 23	36	42	Qualified nurse	Family business	No	Clomid	No	No	Positive
Case 24	38	38	Qualified nurse	Builder	1	Spontaneous	Yes	No	Despair
Case 25	37	38	Teacher	Manager	1	Spontaneous	Yes	No	Despair
Case 26	32	43	Designer	Executive	No	Spontaneous	Yes	No	Elation
Case 27	36	45	Interpreter	Sales manager	No	IVF	No	No	Positive
Case 28	36	30	Physiotherapist	Doctor	No	Spontaneous	No	Yes	Despair
Case 29	29	32	Secretary	Computer programmer	1	Spontaneous	Yes	No	Despair
Case 30	30	40	Bank clerk	Mechanic	No	Clomid	No	No	Elation

Table 2 Pregnancy

Mz twins	Placental and amnion type	Maternal complications	Hospitalisation
Case 1	MC DA	Pre-eclampsia 6 m.	20 days
Case 2	MC DA	Pre-eclampsia 7 m.	20 days
Case 3	MC DA	No	No
Case 4	MC DA	Mild hypertension	No
Case 5	MC DA	Pre-eclampsia 6 m.	15 days
Case 6	MC DA	No	No
Case 7	MC DA	No	No
Case 8	MC DA	Pre-eclampsia 7 m.	21 days
Case 9	DC	No	No
Case 10	MC DA	Contractions 3 m. and kidney stones 7 m.	10 days at 7 m.
Case 11	MC DA	Threatened premature labour 3 + 5 m.	15 days at 5 m.
Case 12	MC DA	No	No
Case 13	MC DA	Threatened premature labour 7 m.	20 days
Case 14	MC MA	Kidney stones 4 m.	10 days
Case 15	MC MA	Threatened premature labour 6 m.	20 days

Dz twins	Placental and amnion type	Maternal complications	Hospitalisation
Case 16	DC	No	No
Case 17	DC	Threatened premature labour 7 m.	20 days
Case 18	DC	No	No
Case 19	DC	No	No
Case 20	DC	No	No
Case 21	DC	Bleeding 2 m.	No
Case 22	DC	No	No
Case 23	DC	Hypertension 7 m.	10 days
Case 24	DC	Gestational diabetes 7 m.	No
Case 25	DC	Contractions plus hypertension 6 m.	20 days
Case 26	DC	Hypertension 7 m.	15 days
Case 27	DC	No	No
Case 28	DC	Threatened premature labour 7 m.	23 days
Case 29	DC	Contractions	No
Case 30	DC	No	No

MC: monochorionic
DC: dichorionic
MA: monoamniotic
H: hydramnios
Oligo.: oligohydramnios

Amniotic fluid index		Pulsatility index	
Twin I	Twin II	Twin I	Twin II
Regular	H 30 w.	Pathologic 30 w.	Borderline 27, 28, 29 w.
Regular	Regular	Borderline 29, 30, 32 w.	Regular
H 34 w.	H 34 w.	Regular	Regular
H 20, 24, 28 w.	Regular	Regular	Regular
Regular	Regular	Regular	Regular
Regular	Regular	Borderline 35 w.	Pathologic 35 w.
Regular	Regular	Regular	Regular
H 28, 32 w.	H 28, 32 w.	Borderline 32 w.	Regular
Regular	Regular	Regular	Regular
Regular	Regular	Pathologic 32 w.	Borderline 32 w.
Regular	Regular	Pathologic 35 w.	Pathologic 35 w.
Regular	Regular	Borderline 35 w.	Pathologic 35 w.
H 20, 24, 28 w.	H 20, 24 w.	Regular	Borderline 32 w.
H 24, 26, 28, 30 w.	H 24, 26, 28, 30 w.	Borderline 30, 32 w.	Pathologic 32 w.
H 26, 28, 30, 32 w.	H 26, 28, 30, 32 w.	Borderline 34 w.	Pathologic 35 w.

Amniotic fluid index		Pulsatility index	
Twin I	Twin II	Twin I	Twin II
Regular	Regular	Regular	Regular
H 28, 32 w.	Oligo. 28, 32 w.	Regular	Regular
Regular	Regular	Regular	Regular
H 28, 32, 36 w.	Regular	Regular	Regular
Regular	Regular	Regular	Regular
H 20, 24, 28, 32 w.	Regular	Regular	Regular
Regular	Regular	Regular	Regular
H 20, 24, 28 w.	Regular	Regular	Regular
H 28, 32 w.	Regular	Regular	Regular
Regular	Regular	Regular	Regular
Regular	Regular	Regular	Regular
H 34 w.	Regular	Regular	Regular
Regular	Regular	Regular	Regular
Regular	Regular	Regular	Regular
Oligo. 34 w.	Regular	Regular	Regular

Table 3 Intrauterine behavior: activity levels.

Weeks: Mz twins	10/11 More active	12/13 More active	14/15 More active	16/18 More active	19/20 More active
Case 1	Victor	Greg	Victor	Victor	Greg
Case 2	Valerie	Valerie	Valerie	Valerie	Valerie
Case 3	Ian	Ian	Ian	Ian	Ian
Case 4	Fred	Fred	Fred	Fred	Fred
Case 5	Alex	Alex	Alex	Alex	Alex
Case 6	Jack	Jack	Jack	Jack	Jack
Case 7	Stanley	Stanley	Stanley	Stanley	Stanley
Case 8	Mary	Mary	Mary	Mary	Mary
Case 9	Eileen	Frances	equal	Eileen	Frances
Case 10	Wes	Stephen	Stephen	Stephen	Wes
Case 11	Felicity	Felicity	Felicity	Felicity	Felicity
Case 12	Adrian	Adrian	Adrian	Adrian	Adrian
Case 13	Henry	Henry	Henry	Henry	Henry
Case 14	Diane	Fiona	Fiona	Fiona	Fiona
Case 15	Veronique	Veronique	Veronique	Veronique	Veronique

Weeks: Dz twins	10/11 More active	12/13 More active	14/15 More active	16/18 More active	19/20 More active
Case 16	Bruce	Bruce	Marlon	Marlon	Marlon
Case 17	Eric	Eric	Eric	Eric	Eric
Case 18	Anthony	Anthony	Anthony	Anthony	Anthony
Case 19	Bill	Bill	Bill	Bill	Bill
Case 20	Fernanda	Fernanda	Fernanda	Fernanda	Fernanda
Case 21	Sharon	Sharon	Sharon	Sharon	Sharon
Case 22	Stuart	Stuart	Stuart	Stuart	Stuart
Case 23	Sean	Sean	Sean	Sean	Sean
Case 24	Liv	Liv	Liv	Liv	Liv
Case 25	Jane	Jane	Jane	Jane	Jane
Case 26	Antonia	Antonia	Antonia	Antonia	Antonia
Case 27	Tom	Julia	Tom	Tom	Tom
Case 28	Dina	Dina	Dina	Dina	Mark
Case 29	Lenny	Lenny	Lenny	Lenny	Lenny
Case 30	Bella	Bella	Bella	Martha	Martha

Table 4 Intrauterine behavior: reactivity levels

Weeks: Mz twins	10/11 More reactive	12/13 More reactive	14/15 More reactive	16/18 More reactive	19/20 More reactive
Case 1	—	Victor	Victor	Victor	Victor
Case 2	—	Valerie	Valerie	Valerie	Valerie
Case 3	—	Damien	Damien	Damien	Damien
Case 4	—	Paul	Paul	Paul	Paul
Case 5	—	Phil	Phil	Phil	Phil
Case 6	—	Jack	Jack	Jack	Jack
Case 7	—	Stanley	Stanley	Stanley	Stanley
Case 8	—	Mary	Mary	Mary	Mary
Case 9	—	—	Equal level	Equal level	Equal level
Case 10	—	Stephen	Stephen	Stephen	Stephen
Case 11	—	Giorgia	Giorgia	Giorgia	Giorgia
Case 12	—	Adrian	Adrian	Adrian	Adrian
Case 13	—	Nick	Nick	Nick	Nick
Case 14	Diane	Diane	Diane	Diane	Diane
Case 15	Veronique	Veronique	Veronique	Veronique	Veronique

Weeks: Dz twins	10/11 More reactive	12/13 More reactive	14/15 More reactive	16/18 More reactive	19/20 More reactive
Case 16	—	—	Bruce	Bruce	Bruce
Case 17	—	Eric	Eric	Eric	Eric
Case 18	—	—	Anthony	Anthony	Anthony
Case 19	—	—	Matt	Matt	Matt
Case 20	—	—	Vivian	Vivian	Vivian
Case 21	—	Maurice	Maurice	Maurice	Maurice
Case 22	—	—	Stuart	Stuart	Stuart
Case 23	—	—	Carol	Carol	Carol
Case 24	—	—	Liv	Liv	Liv
Case 25	—	—	Rebecca	Rebecca	Rebecca
Case 26	—	Antonia	Antonia	Antonia	Antonia
Case 27	—	—	Julia	Julia	Julia
Case 28	—	—	Dina	Dina	Dina
Case 29	—	Lenny	Lenny	Lenny	Lenny
Case 30	—	—	Bella	Bella	Bella

Table 5 Prenatal labels

Mz twins	Gender		Label		Dz twins	Gender		Label	
	Twin I	Twin II	Twin I	Twin II		Twin I	Twin II	Twin I	Twin II
Case 1	M	M	—	—	Case 16	M	M	Fatty	Thin
Case 2	F	F	Pest	Pest	Case 17	M	M	Pest	Calm
Case 3	M	M	Hooligan	Quiet	Case 18	M	F	Intelligent	Tardy
Case 4	M	M	Active	Jittery	Case 19	M	M	—	—
Case 5	M	M	Vampire	Victim	Case 20	F	F	Pest	Plague
Case 6	M	M	—	—	Case 21	M	F	Intelligent	Calm
Case 7	M	M	Fatty	Finicky	Case 22	M	M	Bigger	Smaller
Case 8	F	F	Good eater	Bad	Case 23	M	F	Bright	Dull
Case 9	F	F	Identical	Identical	Case 24	M	F	Crafty	Victim
Case 10	M	M	Poor thing	Thief	Case 25	F	F	Pest	Pest
Case 11	F	F	—	—	Case 26	M	F	Stud	Sexy
Case 12	M	M	Lovely	Lovely	Case 27	M	F	—	—
Case 13	M	M	Big eater	Agitated	Case 28	M	F	Strong	Chatty
Case 14	F	F	—	—	Case 29	F	M	Big eater	Skinny
Case 15	F	F	Big	Small	Case 30	F	F	Good	Pest

Table 6 Birth

Mz twins	Birth order		Delivery		Reason for Caesarean	Anaesthesia	Birthweight (grams)		Umbilical cord		Apgar	
	1st	2nd	Week	Type			Twin I	Twin II	Twin I	Twin II	Twin I	Twin II
Case 1	Greg	Victor	30	Caesarean	Fetal/maternal suffering	Total	970	1,600	1 artery	Normal	3 + 4	3 + 5
Case 2	Rachel	Valerie	36	Caesarean	Maternal suffering	Total	2,630	2,700	Normal	Normal	6 + 9	8 + 9
Case 3	Ian	Damien	37	Induced		No	2,240	2,320	Normal	Normal	7 + 9	8 + 10
Case 4	Fred	Paul	36	Caesarean	Fetal malpresentation	Total	2,320	2,310	Normal	Normal	4 + 9	5 + 9
Case 5	Alex	Phil	35	Caesarean	Maternal suffering	Total	2,100	1,300	Normal	VI	5 + 8	3 + 7
Case 6	Toby	Jack	37	Induced		No	2,660	2,800	Normal	Normal	9 + 10	8 + 10
Case 7	Stanley	Martin	37	Induced		No	2,720	2,500	Normal	Normal	9 + 10	8 + 10
Case 8	Linda	Mary	37	Caesarean	Fetal/maternal suffering	Total	2,930	2,430	Normal	Normal	7 + 8	6 + 9
Case 9	Eileen	Frances	36	Caesarean	Fetal malpresentation	Epidural	2,760	2,700	Normal	Normal	9 + 10	8 + 10
Case 10	Wes	Stephen	34	Caesarean	Fetal suffering	Total	1,900	2,570	Normal	Normal	5 + 7	6 + 9
Case 11	Giorgia	Felicity	35	Caesarean	Fetal suffering	Total	2,200	2,300	Normal	Normal	6 + 9	5 + 7
Case 12	Adrian	Arthur	35	Caesarean	Fetal suffering	Total	2,060	2,540	MI	Normal	8 + 10	7 + 10
Case 13	Henry	Nick	38	Caesarean	Fetal malpresentation	Epidural	2,500	1,900	Normal	Normal	6 + 8	4 + 7
Case 14	Fiona	Diane	32	Caesarean	Fetal suffering	Epidural	1,730	1,800	Normal	Normal	6 + 9	5 + 9
Case 15	Audrey	Veronique	35	Caesarean	Fetal suffering	Epidural	1,860	1,530	Normal	Normal	4 + 6	3 + 7

Dz twins	Birth order		Delivery		Reason for Caesarean	Anaesthesia	Birthweight (grams)		Umbilical cord		Apgar	
	1st	2nd	Week	Type			Twin I	Twin II	Twin I	Twin II	Twin I	Twin II
Case 16	Marlon	Bruce	37	Caesarean	Fetal malpresentation	Total	3,000	2,600	Normal	Normal	7 + 10	8 + 9
Case 17	Eric	Michel	33	Caesarean	Broken waters	Total	1,700	1,870	Normal	Normal	9 + 10	8 + 9
Case 18	Anthony	Adele	36	Caesarean	Fetal malpresentation	Total	2,720	2,750	Normal	Normal	7 + 9	8 + 10
Case 19	Matt	Bill	37	Caesarean	Fetal malpresentation	Total	2,420	2,670	Normal	Normal	6 + 8	5 + 7
Case 20	Vivian	Fernanda	37	Caesarean	Maternal choice	Total	2,270	2,550	Normal	Normal	8 + 10	5 + 9
Case 21	Maurice	Sharon	35	Caesarean	Broken waters	Total	1,830	1,990	Normal	Normal	5 + 7	4 + 8
Case 22	Stuart	Donald	36	Caesarean	Fetal malpresentation	Total	2,470	2,730	Normal	Normal	8 + 10	7 + 10
Case 23	Sean	Carol	37	Caesarean	Fetal malpresentation	Total	3,000	2,700	Normal	Normal	7 + 10	8 + 10
Case 24	Leo	Liv	38	Spontaneous		No	3,480	3,450	Normal	Normal	9 + 10	9 + 10
Case 25	Jane	Rebecca	36	Spontaneous		Epidural	2,890	2,530	Normal	Normal	9 + 10	8 + 10
Case 26	Agustin	Antonia	38	Caesarean	Fetal malpresentation	Total	2,500	2,340	Normal	Normal	5 + 7	5 + 8
Case 27	Tom	Julia	37	Caesarean	Maternal choice	Total	2,940	2,690	Normal	Normal	5 + 7	5 + 8
Case 28	Mark	Dina	38	Spontaneous		No	2,700	2,450	Normal	Normal	6 + 10	6 + 10
Case 29	Claire	Lenny	36	Spontaneous		No	2,660	1,560	Normal	MI	8 + 10	6 + 8
Case 30	Martha	Bella	37	Caesarean	Fetal malpresentation	Total	2,430	1,970	Normal	Normal	6 + 8	4 + 7

VI: Velamentous insertion
MI: Marginal insertion

Table 7 Perinatal period

Mz twins	Twin I	Twin II	Days in NICU		Complications		Breast-feeding
			Twin I	Twin II	Twin I	Twin II	
Case 1	Greg	Victor	60	60	Respiratory distress syndrome	Respiratory distress syndrome	—
Case 2	Rachel	Valerie	13	10	Cardiac arrhythmias, cyanosis and cardiac surgery	Hypoglycaemia	6 months mixed
Case 3	Ian	Damien	1	4	—	Recurrent cyanosis	25 days mixed
Case 4	Fred	Paul	15	15	Excessive weight loss	Excessive weight loss	45 days mixed
Case 5	Alex	Phil	2	21	—	Excessive weight loss	—
Case 6	Toby	Jack	0	0	—	—	—
Case 7	Stanley	Martin	0	0	—	—	5 months
Case 8	Linda	Mary	6	6	Breathing irregularities	Pronounced jaundice	—
Case 9	Eileen	Frances	0	0	—	—	5 months
Case 10	Wes	Stephen	15	0	Excessive weight loss	—	4 months
Case 11	Giorgia	Felicity	2	2	—	—	—
Case 12	Adrian	Arthur	2	2	—	—	6 months mixed
Case 13	Henry	Nick	0	25	—	Enteritis and excessive weight loss	—
Case 14	Fiona	Diane	57	50	Necrotising enterocolitis	Breathing irregularities	2 months mixed
Case 15	Audrey	Veronique	21	35	Excessive weight loss	Breathing irregularities and weight loss	21 days

Dz twins	Twin I	Twin II	Days in NICU		Complications		Breast-feeding
			Twin I	Twin II	Twin I	Twin II	
Case 16	Marlon	Bruce	0	0	—	—	—
Case 17	Eric	Michel	30	21	Jaundice and enteritis	Excessive weight loss	—
Case 18	Anthony	Adele	7	0	Recurrent hypoglycaemia	—	15 days
Case 19	Matt	Bill	0	0	—	—	—
Case 20	Vivian	Fernanda	0	4	—	Weight loss	10 days
Case 21	Maurice	Sharon	3	3	—	—	—
Case 22	Stuart	Donald	0	0	—	—	2 days
Case 23	Sean	Carol	0	0	—	—	10 months mixed
Case 24	Leo	Liv	0	0	—	—	—
Case 25	Jane	Rebecca	0	0	—	—	6 months mixed
Case 26	Agustin	Antonia	0	0	—	—	—
Case 27	Tom	Julia	0	0	—	—	—
Case 28	Mark	Dina	0	0	—	—	—
Case 29	Claire	Lenny	0	30	—	Enterocolitis and excessive weight loss	—
Case 30	Martha	Bella	0	20	—	Weight loss and breathing irregularities	—

Table 8 Congenital anomalies and defects, and health problems during the first two years

Mz twins	Congenital anomalies and defects	Health problems	
		Twin I	Twin II
Case 1	—	Bronchopneumonia 11 m. and 22 m., and asthma	Asthma and insufficient weight gain
Case 2	Cardiac anomaly Twin I	—	—
Case 3	—	Recurrent bronchitis	Bronchopneumonia 24 m.
Case 4	Congenital hypospadias	—	—
Case 5	—	—	—
Case 6	—	—	—
Case 7	—	Recurrent asthmatic bronchitis	—
Case 8	—	—	—
Case 9	—	Insufficient weight gain	—
Case 10	—	—	—
Case 11	—	—	Dilatation cerebral ventricles (transitory) at 6 m.
Case 12	Congenital nystagmus	—	—
Case 13	—	—	Bronchopneumonia 9 m. and recurrent colitis
Case 14	—	Recurrent colitis	Recurrent bronchitis and asthma
Case 15	—	Insufficient weight gain	Recurrent bronchitis and insufficient weight gain

Dz twins	Congenital anomalies and defects	Health problems	
		Twin I	Twin II
Case 16	—	—	—
Case 17	—	—	—
Case 18	—	Enlargement cranic circumference (transitory) at 5 m.	—
Case 19	—	—	—
Case 20	—	—	—
Case 21	—	—	—
Case 22	—	—	—
Case 23	—	—	—
Case 24	—	—	Impetigo 4 m.
Case 25	—	—	—
Case 26	—	—	Infantile hernia 8 m.
Case 27	—	—	—
Case 28	—	—	—
Case 29	—	—	Insufficient weight gain
Case 30	—	—	—

Table 9 Milestones (age in months)

| Mz twins | Twin I | Twin II | Gross motor development | | | | Language development | | | |
| | | | Sitting | | Walking | | First words | | First sentence | |
			Twin I	Twin II	Twin I	Twin II	Twin I	Twin II	Twin I	Twin II
Case 1	Greg	Victor	11	10	17	16	16	18	26	26
Case 2	Rachel	Valerie	10	9	15	15	14	14	23	23
Case 3	Ian	Damien	8	8	12	12	12	12.5	19.5	20
Case 4	Fred	Paul	9	9	12	12	12.5	13	20	20.5
Case 5	Alex	Phil	9	9	12	12.5	13	13	20	20
Case 6	Toby	Jack	9	9.5	12	12.5	13	13	21	21.5
Case 7	Stanley	Martin	8.5	8	13	13	15	14	24	24
Case 8	Linda	Mary	9	9	13	13	12	14	21	25
Case 9	Eileen	Frances	10	10	14	14	15	15	25	25
Case 10	Wes	Stephen	10	10	12	12	13	13.5	21	21
Case 11	Giorgia	Felicity	10	10	15	15	16	16	24	24
Case 12	Adrian	Arthur	8	8	13	13	12	12	21	21.5
Case 13	Henry	Nick	9	9	12.5	12	14.5	13	24	22.5
Case 14	Fiona	Diane	10	11	16	15	12.5	12.5	23	23
Case 15	Audrey	Veronique	10	9.5	15	15	16	16	25	25

(continued)

Table 9 (continued)

Dz twins	Twin I	Twin II	Gross motor development				Language development			
			Sitting		Walking		First words		First sentence	
			Twin I	Twin II	Twin I	Twin II	Twin I	Twin II	Twin I	Twin II
Case 16	Marlon	Bruce	8	8	12	12	13	13	22.5	22
Case 17	Eric	Michel	10	10	14	16	12	14	20	23
Case 18	Anthony	Adele	9	9	14	14	14	15	23	24
Case 19	Matt	Bill	8	8.5	14	13	16	15.5	25	25
Case 20	Vivian	Fernanda	9	9	14	13	12	12.5	21	21.5
Case 21	Maurice	Sharon	10	10	13	14	16	17	25	26
Case 22	Stuart	Donald	8	9	13	14	15	15	24	25
Case 23	Sean	Carol	9	9	11.5	12	16.5	16	24.5	24
Case 24	Leo	Liv	9	9.5	13.5	12	14	14.5	24	24
Case 25	Jane	Rebecca	8	8.5	12	12.5	15	15.5	23	23
Case 26	Agustin	Antonia	9	9.5	13	11.5	15	12	24	20
Case 27	Tom	Julia	8	8	12	14	15	14.5	23	22.5
Case 28	Mark	Dina	9	9	13	12	15	12	25	22
Case 29	Claire	Lenny	9	8	13	13	14	12	23	19.5
Case 30	Martha	Bella	8	8	12	13	12.5	12.5	20	20

Table 10 Choice

	Choice			Apparent motives		Intensity of choice		Rejected twins
Mz twins	Maternal	Paternal	Expression	Maternal	Paternal	Maternal	Paternal	
Case 1	Greg	Victor	Immediate	Quieter	1 each, compensatory	Strong	Mild	—
Case 2	Valerie	Rachel	Delayed	Quieter	More attractive	Mild	Mild	—
Case 3	Damien	Damien	Delayed	Quieter; cuddly	Quieter; cuddly	Mild	Mild	Ian
Case 4	Paul	Paul	Delayed	Quieter; cuddly	Quieter; cuddly	Mild	Mild	Fred
Case 5	Phil	Alex	Immediate	Smaller; less favoured *in utero*	1 each, compensatory	Strong	Mild	—
Case 6	Toby	Jack	Immediate	Quieter; cuddly	More attractive	Strong	Strong	—
Case 7	Stanley	Stanley	Immediate	Smaller; less favoured *in utero*	Smaller; less favoured *in utero*	Mild	Mild	Martin
Case 8	Linda	Linda	Denied	Fatter (mother obese)	Looks like mother	Strong	Strong	Mary
Case 9	Eileen	Frances	Denied	1 each, no apparent motive	1 each, no apparent motive	Very mild	Very mild	—
Case 10	Wes	Wes	Delayed	More outgoing	More outgoing	Mild	Mild	Stephen
Case 11	Giorgia	Felicity	Delayed	Quieter; cuddly	1 each, compensatory	Mild	Mild	—
Case 12	Adrian	Adrian	Immediate	More alert	More alert; fun	Mild	Mild	Arthur
Case 13	Henry	Henry	Immediate	Less alert	Less alert	Strong	Strong	Nick
Case 14	Fiona	Fiona	Delayed	Post-natal complications	Post-natal complications	Mild	Mild	Diane
Case 15	Veronique	Veronique	Immediate	Smaller; less favoured *in utero*	Smaller; less favoured *in utero*	Mild	Mild	Audrey

	Choice			Apparent motives		Intensity of choice		Rejected twins
Dz twins	Maternal	Paternal	Expression	Maternal	Paternal	Maternal	Paternal	
Case 16	Bruce	Bruce	Immediate	Less attractive	Less attractive	Strong	Mild	Marlon
Case 17	Michel	Eric	Immediate	Quieter	More fun	Mild	Strong	—
Case 18	Anthony	Anthony	Denied	Gender	Gender	Strong	Strong	Adele
Case 19	Matt	Matt	Immediate	Less attractive; quieter	Less attractive; quieter	Strong	Mild	Bill
Case 20	Vivian	Fernanda	Immediate	More affectionate	1 each split, compensatory	Mild	Mild	—
Case 21	Maurice	Maurice	Denied	Gender	Gender	Strong	Strong	Sharon
Case 22	Stuart	Stuart	Immediate	More attractive	More attractive	Strong	Mild	Donald
Case 23	Sean	Sean	Denied	Gender	Gender	Strong	Strong	Carol
Case 24	Leo	Liv	Denied	Gender	Gender	Strong	Mild	—
Case 25	Jane	Rebecca	Immediate	Quieter	1 each split, compensatory	Mild	Mild	—
Case 26	Agustin	Agustin	Denied	Gender	Gender	Strong	Strong	Antonia
Case 27	Tom	Tom	Denied	Gender	Gender	Strong	Mild	Julia
Case 28	Mark	Mark	Denied	Gender	Gender	Strong	Strong	Dina
Case 29	Claire	Lenny	Delayed	Less attractive; quieter	More fun	Mild	Mild	—
Case 30	Martha	Martha	Immediate	More affectionate	More affectionate	Strong	Mild	Bella

Table 11 Maternal depression. concomitant and aggravating factors

Mz twins	Maternal depression	Paternal involvement	Other caregivers	Resumed work	Back in shape	Main physical complaints	Marital difficulties
Case 1	Severe	Strong	—	6 m. at home	No	None	—
Case 2	Severe	Minimal	—	No	2 years	Abdomen	Separation
Case 3	—	Strong	Maternal grandmother	1 year	18 m.	Abdomen	Separation
Case 4	—	Fair	Qualified nurse and Philippine domestic	6 m. part time	1 year	Abdomen	—
Case 5	Severe	Minimal	Grandmothers	1 year	1 year	Abdomen	Strong
Case 6	Mild	Fair	Maternal grandmother and Philippine domestic	1 year	1 year	Thighs	—
Case 7	—	Strong	—	3 years	2 years	Abdomen	—
Case 8	Mild	Fair	Maternal grandparents	No	No	None	Mild
Case 9	Severe	Minimal	Maternal grandparents	2 years part time	No	Abdomen	Separation
Case 10	Mild	Minimal	—	No	No	Abdomen, thighs	Strong
Case 11	Mild	Strong	Maternal grandmother	No	1 year	Breasts	—
Case 12	—	Strong	Maternal grandfather	1 year part time	No	None	—
Case 13	Severe	Minimal	Paternal grandmother	2 years	1 year	Abdomen	Strong
Case 14	Moderate	Minimal	Maternal sister	1 year part time	1 year	Abdomen	Strong
Case 15	Severe	Fair	—	No	No	Abdomen	Strong

Dz twins	Maternal depression	Paternal involvement	Other caregivers	Resumed work	Back in shape	Main physical complaints	Marital difficulties
Case 16	—	Strong	Neighbour	2 years	1 year	Breasts	—
Case 17	Mild	Strong	Maternal grandmother	1 year part time	18 m.	Abdomen	Mild
Case 18	Severe	Fair	Maternal grandfather	1 year part time	2 years	Abdomen, breasts	Strong
Case 19	Severe	Minimal	Maternal grandmother (occasional)	2 years part time	1 year	Abdomen	Strong
Case 20	Severe	Strong	—	1 year part time	2 years	Abdomen	Divorce
Case 21	Very severe	Minimal	—	No	2 years	Abdomen	Divorce
Case 22	Severe	Strong	Maternal grandmother and Philippine domestic	1 year	1 year	Abdomen	Strong
Case 23	Very severe	Fair	Maternal and paternal grandparents	2 years part time	3 years	Abdomen, hair loss	Divorce
Case 24	—	Strong	—	18 m. part time	No	None	—
Case 25	Moderate	Fair	Maternal grandmother	1 year part time	1 year	Abdomen	—
Case 26	—	Strong	Philippine domestic and au pair	6 m.	6 m.	None	—
Case 27	Very severe	Fair	—	No	No	Abdomen	Mild
Case 28	Very severe	Minimal	Maternal grandmother (occasional)	No	No	Abdomen	Divorce
Case 29	—	Strong	—	No	2 years	Abdomen	—
Case 30	Moderate	Minimal	Maternal grandmother	1 year part time	2 years	Abdomen	Strong

Table 12 Appearance

Mz twins	Birthweight (grams)		Difference I–II	Appearance			Social glamour
	Twin I	Twin II		At birth	At 6 months	At 3 years	
Case 1	970	1,600	−630	Very different	Similar	Very similar	Strong
Case 2	2,630	2,700	−70	Very similar	Very similar	Very similar	Strong
Case 3	2,240	2,320	−80	Very similar	Very similar	Very similar	Strong
Case 4	2,320	2,310	10	Very similar	Very similar	Very similar	Strong
Case 5	2,100	1,300	800	Different	Very similar	Very similar	Strong
Case 6	2,660	2,800	−140	Very different	Very similar	Very similar	Strong
Case 7	2,720	2,500	220	Different	Very similar	Very similar	Strong
Case 8	2,930	2,430	500	Very different	Different weight, size	Different weight, size	Mild
Case 9	2,760	2,700	60	Very similar	Very similar	Very similar	Strong
Case 10	1,900	2,570	−670	Different	Very similar	Very similar	Strong
Case 11	2,200	2,300	−100	Very similar	Very similar	Very similar	Strong
Case 12	2,060	2,540	−480	Different	Very similar	Very similar	Strong
Case 13	2,500	1,900	600	Different	Different weight, size	Different weight, size	Strong
Case 14	1,730	1,800	−70	Very similar	Very similar	Very similar	Strong
Case 15	1,860	1,530	330	Different	Different weight, size	Different weight, size	Mild

Dz twins	Birthweight (grams)		Difference I–II	Appearance			Social glamour
	Twin I	Twin II		At birth	At 6 months	At 3 years	
Case 16	3,000	2,600	400	Very different	Very different	Very different	Strong
Case 17	1,700	1,870	−170	Similar	Different	Different	Strong
Case 18	2,720	2,750	−30	Very different	Very different	Very different	Minimal
Case 19	2,420	2,670	−250	Very different	Very different	Very different	Minimal
Case 20	2,270	2,550	−280	Very different	Very different	Very different	Minimal
Case 21	1,830	1,990	−160	Very different	Very different	Very different	Minimal
Case 22	2,470	2,730	−260	Very different	Very different	Very different	Minimal
Case 23	3,000	2,700	300	Very different	Very different	Very different	Minimal
Case 24	3,480	3,450	30	Very different	Very different	Very different	Minimal
Case 25	2,890	2,530	360	Very different	Very different	Very different	Minimal
Case 26	2,500	2,340	160	Very different	Very different	Very different	Minimal
Case 27	2,940	2,690	250	Very different	Very different	Very different	Minimal
Case 28	2,700	2,450	250	Very different	Very different	Very different	Minimal
Case 29	2,660	1,560	1,100	Very different	Very different	Very different	Minimal
Case 30	2,430	1,970	460	Very different	Very different	Very different	Minimal

Table 13 Twinning

Mz twins	Twin I	Twin II	Identical clothes		
			At 6 months	At 2 years	At 3 years
Case 1	Greg	Victor	Occasional	Occasional	Occasional
Case 2	Rachel	Valerie	Occasional	Occasional	Occasional
Case 3	Ian	Damien	Regular	Different colours	Different colours
Case 4	Fred	Paul	Regular	Regular	Different colours
Case 5	Alex	Phil	Regular	Regular	Regular
Case 6	Toby	Jack	Regular	Regular	Different colours
Case 7	Stanley	Martin	Regular	Regular	Different colours
Case 8	Linda	Mary	Regular	Regular	Regular
Case 9	Eileen	Frances	Different colours	Different colours	Different colours
Case 10	Wes	Stephen	Regular	Regular	Regular
Case 11	Giorgia	Felicity	Regular	Regular	Regular
Case 12	Adrian	Arthur	Regular	Regular	Regular
Case 13	Henry	Nick	Regular	Occasional	Occasional
Case 14	Fiona	Diane	Regular	Regular	Regular
Case 15	Audrey	Veronique	Occasional	Occasional	Occasional
Dz twins	Twin I	Twin II	Identical clothes		
			At 6 months	At 2 years	At 3 years
Case 16	Marlon	Bruce	Occasional	—	—
Case 17	Eric	Michel	Regular	Occasional	—
Case 18	Anthony	Adele	No	—	—
Case 19	Matt	Bill	No	—	—
Case 20	Vivian	Fernanda	Occasional	—	—
Case 21	Maurice	Sharon	No	—	—
Case 22	Stuart	Donald	No	—	—
Case 23	Sean	Carol	No	—	—
Case 24	Leo	Liv	No	—	—
Case 25	Jane	Rebecca	Occasional	—	—
Case 26	Agustin	Antonia	Occasional	—	—
Case 27	Tom	Julia	No	—	—
Case 28	Mark	Dina	No	—	—
Case 29	Claire	Lenny	No	—	—
Case 30	Martha	Bella	Occasional	—	—

| Hairstyle | | Use of joint name | Same toys | Praise of joint activity | Labels | |
At 2 years	At 3 years				Twin I	Twin II
Same	Same	Regular	Most	Yes	Good	Bad
Same	Same	Occasional	Few	Yes	Terrible	Good
Different	Same	Occasional	Several	No	Terrible	Good
Same	Different	Occasional	Most	No	Daring	Shy
Same	Same	Regular	Most	Yes	Vampire	Victim
Same	Same	Occasional	Most	Yes	Ugly	Attractive
Same	Different	Occasional	Most	Yes	Cuddly	Outgoing
Same	Same	Regular	Several	Yes	Good	Bad
Same	Same	Regular	Most	Yes	—	—
Same	Same	Regular	Few	Yes	Outgoing	Shy
Same	Same	Regular	Most	Yes	Outgoing	Shy
Same	Same	Regular	Most	Yes	Outgoing	Shy
Different	Different	Occasional	Several	Yes	Cuddly	Indifferent
Same	Same	Regular	Most	Yes	Alert	Quiet
Same	Same	Occasional	Most	No	Alert	Quiet

| Hairstyle | | Use of joint name | Same toys | Praise of joint activity | Labels | |
At 2 years	At 3 years				Twin I	Twin II
Different	Different	Occasional	Few	No	Attractive	Less so
Same	Different	Regular	Several	Yes	Quiet	Alert
Different	Different	—	None	No	Alert	Less so
Different	Different	—	Few	No	Less so	Alert
Same	Same	Occasional	Few	No	Good	Nasty
Different	Different	—	None	No	Funny	Dull
Different	Different	—	None	No	Attractive	Less so
Different	Different	—	None	No	Good	Witch
Different	Different	—	None	No	Good	Seductive
Same	Same	Occasional	Few	Yes	Good	Less so
Different	Different	Occasional	None	Yes	Good	Seductive
Different	Different	—	None	No	Good	Less so
Different	Different	—	None	No	Alert	Less so
Different	Different	—	None	No	Less so	Alert
Different	Different	Regular	Few	No	Good	Nasty

Table 14 Intrapair dynamics

Mz twins	Twin I	Twin II	Mutual social signalling	Imitation	Secret language	Dominant twin	Degree of dominance
Case 1	Greg	Victor	3 m.	Strong	Yes	Victor	Strong
Case 2	Rachel	Valerie	5 m.	Strong	Yes	Rachel	Strong
Case 3	Ian	Damien	3 m.	Strong	Yes	Ian	Strong
Case 4	Fred	Paul	3 m.	Strong	Yes	Fred	Strong
Case 5	Alex	Phil	3 m.	Strong	Yes	Phil	Strong
Case 6	Toby	Jack	5 m.	Mild	Yes	Jack	Mild
Case 7	Stanley	Martin	3 m.	Strong	No	Stanley	Mild
Case 8	Linda	Mary	4 m.	Mild	Yes	Linda	Strong
Case 9	Eileen	Frances	3 m.	Strong	Yes	Neither	Mild
Case 10	Wes	Stephen	3 m.	Strong	Yes	Stephen	Strong
Case 11	Giorgia	Felicity	4 m.	Strong	Yes	Giorgia	Mild
Case 12	Adrian	Arthur	3 m.	Strong	Yes	Adrian	Strong
Case 13	Henry	Nick	5 m.	Strong	Yes	Henry	Strong
Case 14	Fiona	Diane	4 m.	Mild	No	Neither	Mild
Case 15	Audrey	Veronique	3 m.	Strong	Yes	Audrey	Mild

Dz twins	Twin I	Twin II	Mutual social signalling	Imitation	Secret language	Dominant twin	Degree of dominance
Case 16	Marlon	Bruce	5 m.	Minimal	No	Marlon	Mild
Case 17	Eric	Michel	3 m.	Mild	Yes	Eric	Strong
Case 18	Anthony	Adele	5 m.	Minimal	No	Anthony	Strong
Case 19	Matt	Bill	5 m.	Minimal	No	Matt	Mild
Case 20	Vivian	Fernanda	4 m.	Minimal	No	Fernanda	Mild
Case 21	Maurice	Sharon	3 m.	Mild	Yes	Maurice	Mild
Case 22	Stuart	Donald	5 m.	Minimal	Yes	Stuart	Mild
Case 23	Sean	Claire	5 m.	Minimal	Yes	Sean	Mild
Case 24	Leo	Liv	3 m.	Minimal	Yes	Leo	Mild
Case 25	Jane	Rebecca	4 m.	Mild	No	Rebecca	Mild
Case 26	Agustin	Antonia	5 m.	Minimal	Yes	Antonia	Strong
Case 27	Tom	Julia	5 m.	Mild	Yes	Tom	Mild
Case 28	Matt	Dina	5 m.	Minimal	No	Dina	Mild
Case 29	Claire	Lenny	3 m.	Minimal	Yes	Lenny	Strong
Case 30	Martha	Bella	5 m.	Minimal	No	Martha	Mild

Fights	Rivalry	Ganging up	Telepathy	Shared cot	Shared bed at 3 years	Mutual masturbation	
						Type	Frequency
Occasional	Minimal	Strong	Yes	Yes	Regular	Fondling and French kissing	Frequent
Regular	Minimal	Strong	No	Yes	Regular	Fondling and French kissing	Frequent
Regular	Minimal	Strong	Yes	Yes	Regular	Fondling	Frequent
Regular	Minimal	Strong	No	No	No	—	—
Regular	Minimal	Strong	Yes	Yes	Tolerated	French kissing	Frequent
Regular	Strong	Minimal	No	No	No	—	—
Occasional	Minimal	Minimal	Yes	Yes	Tolerated	Fondling and French kissing	Frequent
Occasional	Strong	Mild	No	Yes	Tolerated	Fondling and French kissing	Sporadic
Occasional	Minimal	Strong	Yes	Yes	Regular	Fondling and French kissing	Sporadic
Occasional	Minimal	Strong	No	No	Tolerated	—	—
Occasional	Minimal	Strong	No	Yes	Tolerated	Fondling and French kissing	Frequent
Regular	Minimal	Strong	Yes	Yes	Tolerated	Fondling and French kissing	Frequent
Occasional	Minimal	Strong	No	No	No	—	—
Occasional	Minimal	Mild	No	No	No	—	—
Occasional	Minimal	Strong	Yes	No	No	Fondling	Frequent

Fights	Rivalry	Ganging up	Telepathy	Shared cot	Shared bed at 3 years	Mutual masturbation	
						Type	Frequency
Regular	Mild	Minimal	No	No	No	—	—
Regular	Strong	Strong	No	Yes	Tolerated	Fondling and French kissing	Frequent
Regular	Strong	Minimal	No	No	No	—	—
Regular	Strong	Minimal	No	No	No	—	—
Regular	Strong	Minimal	No	No	No	—	—
Occasional	Mild	Minimal	No	Yes	No	—	—
Regular	Strong	Minimal	No	No	No	—	—
Occasional	Mild	Minimal	No	No	No	—	—
Regular	Mild	Minimal	No	Yes	No	—	—
Regular	Mild	Mild	No	No	No	—	—
Regular	Strong	Minimal	No	Yes	No	—	—
Occasional	Strong	Minimal	No	No	No	—	—
Occasional	Strong	Minimal	No	No	No	—	—
Regular	Strong	Minimal	No	No	No	—	—
Regular	Strong	Minimal	No	No	No	—	—

Table 15 Attachment

Mz twins	Twin I	Twin II	Attachment to mother		Main attachment figure	
			Twin I	Twin II	Twin I	Twin II
Case 1	Greg	Victor	Insecure–avoidant	Insecure–avoidant	Co-twin	Co-twin
Case 2	Rachel	Valerie	Insecure–ambivalent	Insecure–ambivalent	Mother	Mother
Case 3	Ian	Damien	Insecure–avoidant	Insecure–avoidant	Co-twin	Co-twin
Case 4	Fred	Paul	Secure	Secure	Co-twin	Mother
Case 5	Alex	Phil	Insecure–avoidant	Insecure–avoidant	Co-twin	Co-twin
Case 6	Toby	Jack	Secure	Secure	Mother	Mother
Case 7	Stanley	Martin	Secure	Secure	Co-twin	Co-twin
Case 8	Linda	Mary	Insecure–ambivalent	Insecure–avoidant	Mother	Co-twin
Case 9	Eileen	Frances	Insecure–avoidant	Insecure–avoidant	Co-twin	Co-twin
Case 10	Wes	Stephen	Secure	Secure	Mother	Mother
Case 11	Giorgia	Felicity	Insecure–ambivalent	Insecure–avoidant	Co-twin	Co-twin
Case 12	Adrian	Arthur	Secure	Secure	Co-twin	Co-twin
Case 13	Henry	Nick	Insecure–ambivalent	Insecure–avoidant	Mother	Co-twin
Case 14	Fiona	Diane	Secure	Secure	Co-twin	Co-twin
Case 15	Audrey	Veronique	Insecure–avoidant	Insecure–avoidant	Co-twin	Co-twin

Dz twins	Twin I	Twin II	Attachment to mother		Main attachment figure	
			Twin I	Twin II	Twin I	Twin II
Case 16	Marlon	Bruce	Secure	Secure	Mother	Mother
Case 17	Eric	Michel	Insecure–ambivalent	Insecure–avoidant	Mother	Co-twin
Case 18	Anthony	Adele	Insecure–ambivalent	Insecure–ambivalent	Mother	Mother
Case 19	Matt	Bill	Insecure–ambivalent	Insecure avoidant	Mother	Co-twin
Case 20	Vivian	Fernanda	Insecure–ambivalent	Insecure–ambivalent	Mother	Mother
Case 21	Maurice	Sharon	Insecure–ambivalent	Disorganised	Mother	Co-twin
Case 22	Stuart	Donald	Insecure–ambivalent	Insecure–avoidant	Mother	Mother
Case 23	Sean	Carol	Insecure–ambivalent	Insecure–avoidant	Mother	Mother
Case 24	Leo	Liv	Secure	Secure	Mother	Mother
Case 25	Jane	Rebecca	Secure	Secure	Mother	Mother
Case 26	Agustin	Antonia	Insecure–ambivalent	Secure	Mother	Mother
Case 27	Tom	Julia	Insecure–ambivalent	Insecure–ambivalent	Mother	Mother
Case 28	Mark	Dina	Insecure–ambivalent	Insecure–avoidant	Mother	Mother
Case 29	Claire	Lenny	Secure	Secure	Mother	Mother
Case 30	Martha	Bella	Secure	Secure	Mother	Mother

Table 16 Tests: higher scorers on Bayley scales

Mz twins	Twin I	Twin II	Mental development index (MDI)				Physical development index (PDI)			
			6 months	1 year	2 years	30 months	6 months	1 year	2 years	30 months
Case 1	Greg	Victor	Victor	Victor	Victor	Victor	Victor	Victor	Victor	Victor
Case 2	Rachel	Valerie	Same	Valerie	Same	Same	Valerie	Valerie	Valerie	Valerie
Case 3	Ian	Damien	Same	Damien	Ian	Ian	Ian	Damien	Ian	Ian
Case 4	Fred	Paul	Same	Paul	Fred	Fred	Same	Paul	Fred	Fred
Case 5	Alex	Phil	Alex	Phil	Alex	Alex	Alex	Same	Phil	Phil
Case 6	Toby	Jack	Jack	Toby	Jack	Jack	Jack	Same	Jack	Jack
Case 7	Stanley	Martin	Martin	Martin	Martin	Martin	Martin	Martin	Same	Same
Case 8	Linda	Mary	Mary	Mary	Mary	Mary	Same	Mary	Mary	Mary
Case 9	Eileen	Frances	Same	Eileen	Same	Same	Same	Frances	Same	Same
Case 10	Wes	Stephen	Wes	Wes	Wes	Wes	Wes	Wes	Wes	Wes
Case 11	Giorgia	Felicity	Giorgia	Giorgia	Giorgia	Giorgia	Giorgia	Giorgia	Giorgia	Giorgia
Case 12	Adrian	Arthur	Adrian	Adrian	Adrian	Adrian	Arthur	Same	Adrian	Adrian
Case 13	Henry	Nick	Henry	Nick	Nick	Nick	Henry	Same	Nick	Nick
Case 14	Fiona	Diane	Same	Diane	Fiona	Fiona	Fiona	Same	Fiona	Fiona
Case 15	Audrey	Veronique	Audrey	Veronique	Audrey	Audrey	Veronique	Audrey	Audrey	Audrey

Dz twins	Twin I	Twin II	Mental development index (MDI)				Physical development index (PDI)			
			6 months	1 year	2 years	30 months	6 months	1 year	2 years	30 months
Case 16	Marlon	Bruce	Bruce	Bruce	Bruce	Bruce	Bruce	Marlon	Marlon	Marlon
Case 17	Eric	Michel	Same	Same	Eric	Eric	Eric	Same	Same	Same
Case 18	Anthony	Adele	Anthony	Anthony	Anthony	Anthony	Adele	Same	Anthony	Anthony
Case 19	Matt	Bill	Matt	Bill	Matt	Matt	Bill	Same	Same	Same
Case 20	Vivian	Fernanda	Vivian	Same	Vivian	Vivian	Vivian	Vivian	Vivian	Vivian
Case 21	Maurice	Sharon	Sharon	Maurice	Maurice	Maurice	Maurice	Maurice	Maurice	Maurice
Case 22	Stuart	Donald	Stuart	Donald	Donald	Donald	Same	Stuart	Stuart	Stuart
Case 23	Sean	Carol	Carol	Carol	Sean	Sean	Carol	Carol	Sean	Sean
Case 24	Leo	Liv	Same	Leo	Liv	Liv	Same	Same	Same	Same
Case 25	Jane	Rebecca	Rebecca	Rebecca	Rebecca	Rebecca	Rebecca	Jane	Jane	Jane
Case 26	Agustin	Antonia	Antonia	Antonia	Antonia	Antonia	Antonia	Agustin	Antonia	Antonia
Case 27	Tom	Julia	Julia	Julia	Julia	Julia	Tom	Tom	Tom	Tom
Case 28	Mark	Dina	Dina	Dina	Dina	Dina	Dina	Dina	Dina	Dina
Case 29	Claire	Lenny	Lenny	Lenny	Lenny	Lenny	Lenny	Lenny	Lenny	Lenny
Case 30	Martha	Bella	Martha	Martha	Martha	Martha	Martha	Martha	Martha	Martha

Table 17 Tests: home observation for measurement of the environment

Mz twins	Parental responsivity	Acceptance	Organisation	Involvement	Play materials	Variety of stimulation
Case 1	Lowest-middle	Lowest-middle	Lowest-middle	Lowest-middle	Lowest-middle	Lowest-middle
Case 2	Lowest-middle	Middle-half	Lowest-middle	Lowest-middle	Lowest-middle	Lowest-middle
Case 3	Upper-fourth	Upper-fourth	Lowest-middle	Upper-fourth	Upper-fourth	Upper-fourth
Case 4	Upper-fourth	Upper-fourth	Upper-fourth	Middle-half	Upper-fourth	Upper-fourth
Case 5	Middle-half	Middle-half	Upper-fourth	Middle-half	Middle-half	Middle-half
Case 6	Upper-fourth	Upper-fourth	Upper-fourth	Upper-fourth	Upper-fourth	Upper-fourth
Case 7	Upper-fourth	Upper-fourth	Upper-fourth	Upper-fourth	Upper-fourth	Upper-fourth
Case 8	Middle-half	Middle-half	Middle-half	Middle-half	Upper-fourth	Middle-half
Case 9	Middle-half	Middle-half	Upper-fourth	Upper-fourth	Upper-fourth	Upper-fourth
Case 10	Middle-half	Middle-half	Lowest-middle	Middle-half	Lowest-middle	Middle-half
Case 11	Upper-fourth	Middle-half	Upper-fourth	Middle-half	Upper-fourth	Middle-half
Case 12	Upper-fourth	Upper-fourth	Middle-half	Upper-fourth	Middle-half	Upper-fourth
Case 13	Lowest-middle	Lowest-middle	Middle-half	Middle-half	Upper-fourth	Lowest-middle
Case 14	Upper-fourth	Upper-fourth	Upper-fourth	Upper-fourth	Upper-fourth	Upper-fourth
Case 15	Middle-half	Middle-half	Lowest-middle	Middle-half	Lowest-middle	Middle-half

Dz twins	Parental responsivity	Acceptance	Organisation	Involvement	Play materials	Variety of stimulation
Case 16	Upper-fourth	Upper-fourth	Middle-half	Upper-fourth	Middle-half	Upper-fourth
Case 17	Middle-half	Upper-fourth	Middle-half	Upper-fourth	Upper-fourth	Middle-half
Case 18	Lowest-middle	Middle-half	Upper-fourth	Lowest-middle	Upper-fourth	Lowest-middle
Case 19	Lowest-middle	Lowest-middle	Upper-fourth	Lowest-middle	Upper-fourth	Lowest-middle
Case 20	Lowest-middle	Lowest-middle	Middle-half	Middle-half	Upper-fourth	Lowest-middle
Case 21	Lowest-middle	Lowest-middle	Lowest-middle	Lowest-middle	Lowest-middle	Lowest-middle
Case 22	Middle-half	Lowest-middle	Middle-half	Middle-half	Middle-half	Lowest-middle
Case 23	Lowest-middle	Lowest-middle	Upper-fourth	Lowest-middle	Upper-fourth	Lowest-middle
Case 24	Upper-fourth	Lowest-middle	Lowest-middle	Upper-fourth	Lowest-middle	Lowest-middle
Case 25	Middle-half	Upper-fourth	Upper-fourth	Middle-half	Upper-fourth	Middle-half
Case 26	Upper-fourth	Upper-fourth	Upper-fourth	Middle-half	Upper-fourth	Upper-fourth
Case 27	Lowest-middle	Lowest-middle	Middle-half	Lowest-middle	Middle-half	Lowest-middle
Case 28	Lowest-middle	Lowest-middle	Upper-fourth	Lowest-middle	Upper-fourth	Lowest-middle
Case 29	Upper-fourth	Upper-fourth	Middle-half	Upper-fourth	Upper-fourth	Upper-fourth
Case 30	Middle-half	Middle-half	Middle-half	Upper-fourth	Middle-half	Middle-half

NOTES

1 BIOLOGY OF TWINNING

1 For an excellent account of all the varieties of twins, as well as the extent of variance in the intrauterine environment, see Baldwin (1994).
2 It is customary in obstetrics to refer to gestational age, deriving an approximate date of conception from the date of the last menstrual period. Whilst women rarely know with precision when conception took place, most of them remember the precise date of their last menstrual period. Therefore, fetal age or number of weeks always refers to gestational age here. Conceptual age is only commonly used in embryology.

3 INTRAUTERINE BEHAVIOR

1 The complete nerve cell is called a neuron. Most neurons are composed of a cell body, of long processes called axons (along which electrical impulses are conducted), and of dendrites. Dendrites are spidery processes protruding from the cell body, on which large numbers of incoming axons terminate.
2 The junction between the terminal of an axon and the dendrite or cell body of the next neuron in the chain is called a synapse. The signal is transmitted across the minute gap between the two by a chemical transmitter substance secreted by the axon terminal whenever impulses arrive along the axon. The cell body of neurons varies enormously in shape and size and neurons can thus be subdivided into hundreds of types (Blakemore 1998). Equally the nature of the transmitter substances can vary. Besides neurons, the second broad type of cells in the brain are glia (meaning 'glue') cells. These serve a variety of supportive functions, but do not transmit impulses.
3 During neural development, parallel to the protracted span of dendritic growth and synapse refinement, at least one other essential process, myelination, needs to be mentioned. The axons of most neurons are progressively shielded with a fatty substance called myelin that acts as an electrical insulator. Myelination permits an increase in the speed of transmission of electrical signals as well as preventing leaking out of the ions responsible for their transmission.
4 The proportions between feet and femur length are measured when dwarfism is suspected.
5 The remaining portion of the brain after the cerebral hemispheres and cerebellum have been removed.
6 Though research with animals has contributed greatly to our knowledge of fetal development, reference here will principally be made to the human fetus.

5 STILL IN HOSPITAL: BIRTH AND SOON AFTER BIRTH

1   A cheesy deposit on the skin of the fetus that protects it from the macerative effects of the amniotic fluid and facilitates the passage through the birth channel.

2   For reasons of simplicity and clarity, unless otherwise stated, only monozygotic and dizygotic twins will be referred to. Chorion and amnion type of monozygotic twins or sex split of dizygotic twins will not be specified each time.

3   The literature on the impact of the NICU, and of prematurity on parents and their infants, is extensive. Readers interested in psychological/developmental aspects related to these topics can refer to the following works: Richards (1978, 1979, 1983, 1989), Klaus and Kennell (1983, 1993), Field (1990a, 1990b), and to textbooks: Field *et al.* (1980), Davies *et al.* (1983), Field and Sostek (1983), Lester and Tronick (1990), Affleck *et al.* (1991).

6 BACK HOME

1   Most families residing in large urban areas in Italy, such as Milan, live in apartments. Detached or semi-detached houses are the exception rather than the rule. Living in an apartment, unless it is on the ground floor, necessarily means using an elevator or stairs. Elevators are often too small for a double pram; stairs are an obvious problem.

8 'TWINNING'

1   Though dizygotic twins are usually considered to share 50 per cent of their genes, members of some pairs of dizygotic twins share genes for a greater number of traits than others and therefore resemble each other more. Some are virtually indistinguishable from monozygotic twins and only serological analyses can reveal their true 'nature'.

9 BECOMING 'TWINNED' – THE COUPLE EFFECT

1   The expressing of need or distress of the other twin in its presence; crying when the other, though not present, was hurt; and playing jointly while in separate rooms and unable to see what the co-twin was doing.

2   Fondling each other's genitals, French kissing and engaging in conduct resembling intercourse.

12 CHANGES IN THE FAMILY

1   Whilst pre-nursery school day care is generally only available to low-income families and to families where both parents work, in Italy nursery school is state-provided and accessible to all.

2   Marjory Wallace's book *The Silent Twins* (Wallace 1986) recounts the true story of June

and Jennifer Gibbons, a pair of coloured monozygotic twins. All the worst-case scenarios for twins, such as extreme isolation, barrier-forming secret language, mutual entanglement, and madness leading to imprisonment and to the death of one twin, are epitomised in their tragic case.

3   Recently a Welsh pop group, The Manic Street Preachers, have written an acclaimed song, 'Tsunami', inspired by the Gibbons twins' dire story.

4   *Dead Ringers*, 1988, by David Cronenberg is a film depicting the perverse relationship of monozygotic twin gynaecologists. The symbiotic balance between the brothers is suddenly upset by the eruption into their lives of a woman. As always the twins share everything, including her. When one twin realises that he does not want to share this object of love with his co-twin, they are both ultimately confronted with the deadly threat of separation. Both twins are eventually sucked into an inexorable vortex of mutual destruction.

5   *On the Black Hill* (Chatwin 1982) is a novel describing the secluded life of monozygotic twin men who prove to be 'constitutionally' inseparable. The now eighty-year-old twins recollect their bachelor lives in which any chances of joy, possibilities of romance, and ultimately of separation were all stifled by the barriers their union created and the stiff-necked pride and bigotry characterising their temperaments.

CONCLUSION

1   For an excellent account of twin studies, see Wright (1997) and Segal (1999).

BIBLIOGRAPHY

Achiron, R., N. Rosen and H. Zakut (1987) 'Pathophysiologic mechanism of hydramnios development in twin transfusion syndrome. A case report.' *Journal of Reproductive Medicine*, 32: 305–308.

Acker, D.B. and B.P. Sachs (1989) 'Twin gestation and labor.' In: W.R. Cohen, D.B. Acker and E.A. Friedman (eds) *Management of Labor* (2nd edn). Rockville, Md.: Aspen Publications.

Adams, D.M. and F.A. Chervenak (1992) 'Multifetal pregnancies: epidemiology, clinical characteristics, and management.' In: E.A. Reece *et al.* (eds) *Medicine of the Fetus and Mother*. Philadelphia, Pa.: J.B. Lippincott.

Affleck, G., H. Tennen and J. Rowe (1991) *Infants in Crisis: How Parents Cope with Newborn Intensive Care and its Aftermath*. New York: Springer-Verlag.

Aicardi, J. (1992) *Diseases of the Nervous System in Childhood* (2nd edn). Cambridge, UK: Mac Keith Press.

Ainsworth, M.D.S. *et al.* (1978) *Patterns of Attachment: A Psychological Study of the Strange Situation*. Hillsdale, N.J.: Erlbaum.

Alberman, E.D. (1964) 'Cerebral palsy in twins.' *Guys Hospital Report*, 113: 285–295.

Alberts, J.R. (1981) 'Ontogeny of olfaction: reciprocal roles of sensation and behaviour in the development of perception.' In: R.N. Aslin, J.R. Alberts and M.R. Petersen (eds) *The Development of Perception: Psychobiological Perspectives*. New York: Academic Press.

Alberts, J.R. and C.P. Cramer (1988) 'Ecology and experience. Sources of means and meaning of developmental change.' In: E.M. Blass (ed.) *Handbook of Behavioral Neurobiology*. Vol. 9: *Developmental Psychobiology and Behavioral Ecology*. New York: Plenum Press.

Alexander, G.M. and M. Hines (1994) 'Gender labels and play styles: Their relative contribution to children's selection of playmates.' *Child Development*, 65: 869–879.

Allen, G. (1978) 'The parity effect and fertility in mothers of twins.' In: W.E. Nance (ed.) *Twin Research: Biology and Epidemiology. Progress in Clinical and Biological Research*, 24B: 89–97.

Allen, G. and P. Parisi (1990) 'Trends in monozygotic and dizygotic twinning rates by maternal age and parity.' *Acta Geneticae Medicae et Gemellologiae*, 39: 317–328.

Alm, I. (1953) 'The long term prognosis of prematurely born children.' *Acta Paediatrica*, 42: 9–116.

Al Mufti, W. and O. Bomsel-Helmreich (1979) 'Etude expérimentale de la surmaturité ovocytaire et ses conséquences chez les rongeurs.' *Contraception, Fertility and Sexuality*, 7: 845–847.

Als, H. (1994) 'Individualized developmental care for the very low-birth-weight preterm infant. Medical and neurofunctional effects.' *JAMA*, 272: 853–858.

American Psychiatric Association (1994) *Diagnostic and Statistical Manual of Mental Disorders* (4th edn): *DSM-IV*. Washington, DC: American Psychiatric Association.

Amiel-Tison, C. and R. Korobkin (1993) 'Neurologic problems.' In: M.H. Klaus and A.A. Fanaroff (eds) *Care of the High-risk Neonate* (4th edn). Philadelphia, Pa.: W.B. Saunders.

Anand, K.J.S. and P.R. Hickey (1988) 'Pain in the neonate and fetus.' *New England Journal of Medicine*, 318: 1398–1399.

Anand, K.J.S. and P.J. McGrath (1993) *Pain in Neonates*. Amsterdam: Elsevier.

Anastasiow, N.J. and S. Harel (1993) *At-Risk Infants: Interventions, Families and Research.* Baltimore, Md.: Paul H. Brookes.

Anders, T.F., A. Sadeh and A. Viaja Appareddy (1995) 'Normal sleep in neonates and children.' In: R. Ferber and M. Kryger (eds) *Principles and Practice of Sleep Medicine in the Child*. Philadelphia, Pa.: W.B: Saunders.

Anderson, A. and B. Anderson (1990) 'Toward a substantive theory of mother–twin attachment.' *American Journal of Maternal and Child Nursing*, 15: 373–378.

Arabin, B., U. Gembruch and J. van Eyck (1995) 'Intrauterine behavior.' In: L.G. Keith *et al.* (eds) *Multiple Pregnancy: Epidemiology, Gestation and Perinatal Outcome*. New York: The Parthenon Publishing Group.

Arbib, M.A., P. Erdi and J. Szentàgothay (1998) 'Chapter 2. A Structural Overview.' In: M.A. Arbib, P. Erdi and J. Szentàgothay (eds) *Neural Organization, Structure, Function and Dynamics*. Cambridge, Mass.: MIT Press.

Archer, J. (1992) 'Childhood gender roles: Social context and organization.' In: H. McGurk (ed.) *Childhood Social Development: Contemporary Perspectives*. Howe, UK: Erlbaum.

Arduini, A. *et al.* (1986) 'Modification of ultraradian and circadian rhythms of fetal heart rate after fetal-maternal adrenal gland suppression: A double bind study.' *Prenatal Diagnosis*, 6: 409–417.

Arduini, A. *et al.* (1987) 'Loss of circadian rhythms of fetal behavior in a totally adrenalectomized pregnant woman.' *Gynecological and Obstetrical Investigations*, 23: 226–229.

Arnold, S.J. (1987) 'Genetic correlation and the evolution of physiology.' In: M.E. Feder *et al.* (eds) *New Directions in Ecological Physiology*. Cambridge: Cambridge University Press.

Artal, R. (1980) 'Fetal adrenal medulla.' *Clinical Obstetrics and Gynecology*, 23: 825–836.

Asher, P. and F.E. Schonell (1950) 'A survey of 400 cases of cerebral palsy in childhood.' *Archives of Diseases in Childhood*, 25: 360–379.

Asher, S.R. and J.D. Coie (1992) *Peer Rejection in Childhood* (2nd edn). Cambridge: Cambridge University Press.

Aslin, R.N., D.B. Pisoni and P.W. Jusczyck (1983) 'Auditory development and speech perception in infancy.' In: P.H. Mussen (ed.) *Handbook of Child Psychology*, Vol. 2 (4th edn) [M.M. Haith and J.J. Campos vol. eds]. New York: John Wiley.

Atkinson, J. (1984) 'Human visual development over the first 6 months of life: A review and a hypothesis.' *Human Neurobiology*, 3: 61–74.

Bajora, R., J. Wiggleworth and N.M. Fisk (1995) 'Angioarchitecture of monochorionic placentas in relation to the twin–twin transfusion syndrome.' *American Journal of Obstetrics and Gynecology*, 172: 856–863.

Bakker, P. (1987) 'Autonomous language in twins.' *Acta Geneticae Medicae et Gemellologiae*, 36: 233–238.

Baldwin, V.J. (1994) *Pathology of Multiple Pregnancy*. New York: Springer-Verlag.

Balogh, R.D. and R.H. Porter (1986) 'Olfactory preferences resulting from mere exposure in human neonates.' *Infant Behavioral Development*, 9: 395–401.

Bank, S.P. and M.D. Kahn (1997) *The Sibling Bond*. New York: Basic Books.

Banks, M.S. and P. Salapatek (1983) 'Infant visual perception.' In: P.H. Mussen (ed.) *Handbook of Child Psychology*, Vol. 2 (4th edn) [M.M. Haith and J.J. Campos vol. eds]. New York: John Wiley.

Barnett, M.A. (1990) 'Empathy and related responses in children.' In: N. Eisenberg and J. Strayer (eds) *Empathy and its Development* (1st paperback edn). Cambridge: Cambridge University Press.

Baron-Cohen, S., H. Tager-Flusberg and D.J. Cohen (1993) *Understanding Other Minds: Perspectives from Autism.* Oxford: Oxford University Press.

Barrs, V.A., B.R. Benacerraf and F.D. Frigoletto (1985) 'Sonographic determination of chorion type in twin gestation.' *American Journal of Obstetrics and Gynecology,* 179: 779–783.

Bartoshuk, L.M. and G.K. Beauchamp (1994) 'Chemical senses.' *Annual Review of Psychology,* 45: 419–449.

Bateson, P. (1991) *The Development and Integration of Behavior.* Cambridge: Cambridge University Press.

Bayley, D.B. Jr. *et al.* (1993) 'Social interactions of toddlers and preschoolers in same-age and mixed-age play groups.' *Journal of Applied Developmental Psychology,* 14: 261–275.

Bayley, N. (1969) *Manual for the Bayley Scales of Infant Development.* New York: The Psychological Corporation.

Beal, S. (1983) 'Some epidemiological factors about sudden infant death syndrome (SIDS) in South Australia.' In: J.T. Tildon, L.M. Roeder and A. Steinschneider (eds) *Sudden Infant Death Syndrome.* New York: Academic Press.

—— (1989) 'Sudden infant death syndrome in twins.' *Pediatrics,* 100: 735–760.

Bekoff, M. (1981) 'Mammalian sibling interactions. Genes, facilitative environments and the coefficient of familiarity.' In: D.J. Gubernick and P.H. Klopfer (eds) *Parental Care in Mammals.* New York: Plenum Press.

Bekoff, M., J.A. Byers and A. Bekoff (1980) 'Prenatal motility and postnatal play: functional continuity.' *Developmental Psychobiology,* 13: 225–228.

Benacerraf, B.R. (1998) *Ultrasound of Fetal Syndromes.* Philadelphia, Pa.: Churchill Livingstone.

Bendon, R.W. and T. Siddiqi (1989) 'Acute twin-to-twin in utero transfusion.' *Pediatric Pathology,* 9: 591–598.

Benirschke, K. (1961) 'Accurate recording of twin placentation: a plea to the obstetrician.' *Obstetrics and Gynecology,* 18: 334–347.

—— (1972) 'Origin and significance of twinning.' *Clinics in Obstetrics and Gynecology,* 15: 220–235.

—— (1992) 'The contribution of placental anastomoses to prenatal twin damage.' *Human Pathology,* 23: 1319–1320.

—— (1998) 'Twinning: biology and placentation.' In: A. Monteagudo and I.E. Timor-Tritsch (eds) *Ultrasound and Multifetal Pregnancy.* New York: The Parthenon Publishing Group.

Benirschke, K. and P. Kaufmann (1995) 'Multiple pregnancy.' In: K. Benirschke and P. Kaufmann (eds) *Pathology of the Human Placenta* (3rd edn). New York: Springer-Verlag.

Benirschke, K. and C.K. Kim (1973) 'Multiple pregnancy.' *New England Journal of Medicine,* 288: 1276–1284, 1329–1336.

Bennett, D.E. and P. Slade (1991) 'Infants born at risk: consequences for maternal postpartum adjustment.' *British Journal of Medical Psychology,* 64: 159–172.

Benson, M.J. (1992) 'Beyond the reaction range concept: A developmental, contextual, and situational model of the heredity environment interplay.' *Human Relations,* 45: 937–956.

Benson, P.B. *et al.* (1987) 'Foetal heart rate and maternal emotional state.' *British Journal of Medical Psychology,* 60: 151–154.

Berg, W.K. and K.M. Berg (1987) 'Psychophysiological development in infancy: State, startle, and attention.' In: J. Osofsky (ed.) *Handbook of Infant Development* (2nd edn). New York: John Wiley.

Bernabei, P. and G. Levi (1976) 'Psychopathologic problems in twins during childhood.' *Acta Geneticae Medicae et Gemellologiae,* 25: 381–383.

Bernstein, B.A. (1980) 'Siblings of twins.' *Psychoanalytic Study of the Child,* 35: 135–154.

Besinger, R.E. and N.J. Carlson (1995) 'The physiology of preterm labor.' In: L.G. Keith *et al.* (eds) *Multiple Pregnancy: Epidemiology, Gestation and Perinatal Outcome.* New York: The Parthenon Publishing Group.

Bick, E. (1964) 'Notes on infant observation in psycho-analytic training.' *International Journal of Psycho-Analysis*, 45: 484–486.

Bieber, F.R. *et al.* (1981) 'Genetic studies of an acardiac monster, evidence of polar body twinning in man.' *Science*, 214: 775–777.

Billings, P.R., J. Beckwith and J.S. Alper (1992) 'The genetic analysis of human behavior: A new era?' *Social Sciences and Medicine*, 35: 227–238.

Birksted-Breen, D. (1975) *The Birth of a First Child*. London: Tavistock.

—— (1981) *Talking with Mothers*. London: Jill Norman.

—— (1986) 'The experience of having a baby: a developmental view.' *Free Associations*, 33: 22–35.

Birnholz, J.C. and B.B. Benacerraf (1983) 'The development of the human fetal hearing.' *Science*, 222: 516–518.

Birnholz, J.C., J.C. Stephens and M. Faria (1978) 'Fetal movement patterns: a possible means of defining neurologic developmental milestones in utero.' *American Journal of Roentgenology*, 130: 537–540.

Bizzi, E. *et al.* (1994) 'Does the nervous system use equilibrium-point control to guide single and multiple joint movements?' In: P. Cordo and S. Harnad (eds) *Movement Control*. Cambridge: Cambridge University Press.

Bjorrkqvist, K., K.M.J. Lagerspetz and A. Kaukiainen (1992) 'Do girls manipulate and boys fight? Developmental trends in regard to direct and indirect aggression.' *Aggressive Behavior*, 18: 117–127.

Blaffer Hardy, S. (1999) *Mother Nature*. London: Chatto & Windus.

Blakemore, C. (1991) 'Sensitive and vulnerable periods in the development of the visual system.' In: *The Childhood Environment and Adult Disease. Ciba Foundation Symposium 156*. Chichester: John Wiley.

—— (1998) 'How the environment helps to build the brain.' In: B. Cartledge (ed.) *Mind, Brain and the Environment*. Oxford: Oxford University Press.

Blass, E.M. and M.H. Teicher (1980) 'Suckling.' *Science*, 210: 15–22.

Bleker, O.P., J. Oosting and D.J. Hemrika (1988) 'On the cause of the retardation of fetal growth in multiple gestations.' *Acta Geneticae Medicae et Gemellologiae*, 37: 41–46.

Bleker, O.P., H. Wolf and J. Oosting (1995) 'The placental cause of fetal growth retardation in twin gestations.' *Acta Geneticae Medicae et Gemellologiae*, 44: 103–106.

Blickstein, I. and M. Lancet (1988) 'The growth discordant twin.' *Obstetrics and Gynecology*, 43: 509–515.

Blickstein, I. *et al.* (1987) 'Characterization of the growth-discordant twin.' *Obstetrics and Gynecology*, 70: 11–16.

Bloom, L. (1993) *The Transition from Infancy to Language*. Cambridge: Cambridge University Press.

Bluglass, K. (1980) 'Psychiatric morbidity after cot death.' *Practitioner*, 224: 533–539.

Blurton-Jones, N. (1972) *Ethological Studies of Child Behaviour*. Cambridge: Cambridge University Press.

Boklage, C.E. (1981) 'On the timing of monozygotic twinning events.' In: L. Gedda, P. Parisi and W.E. Nance (eds) *Twin Research 3: Twin Biology and Multiple Pregnancy. Special Issue of Progress in Clinical and Biological Research*, 69A: 155–165.

—— (1990) 'Survival probability of human conceptions from fertilization to term.' *International Journal of Fertility*, 35: 75–94.

—— (1995) 'The frequency and survival probability of natural twin conceptions.' In: L.G. Keith *et al.* (eds) *Multiple Pregnancy: Epidemiology, Gestation and Perinatal Outcome*. New York: The Parthenon Publishing Group.

Bomsel-Helmreich, O. and W. Al Mufti (1991) 'Zygosité et déterminisme des grossesses gémellaires et multiples.' In: E. Papiernick-Berkhauer and J.C. Pons (eds) *Les Grossesses Multiples*. Paris: Doin.

—— (1995) 'The mechanism of monozygosity and double ovulation.' In: L.G. Keith *et al.* (eds) *Multiple Pregnancy: Epidemiology, Gestation and Perinatal Outcome.* New York: The Parthenon Publishing Group.

Bomsel-Helmreich, O. and E. Papiernick (1976) 'Delayed ovulation and monozygotic twinning.' *Acta Geneticae Medicae et Gemellologiae*, 25: 73–76.

Boothe, R.G. (1988) 'Visual development: Central neural aspects.' In: E. Meisami and P.S. Timiras (eds) *Handbook of Human Growth and Developmental Biology*, Vol. 1. Boca Raton, Fla: CRC Press.

Botting, B., I. Macdonald-Davis and A. Macfarlane (1987) 'Recent trends in the incidence of multiple births and their mortality.' *Archives of Diseases in Childhood*, 62: 941–950.

Bouchard, T.J. (1984) 'Twins reared together and apart: What do they tell us about human diversity.' In: S.S. Fox (ed.) *The Chemical and Biological Basis of Individuality.* New York: Plenum Press.

Bouchard, T.J. and M. McCue (1981) 'Familial studies of intelligence: A review.' *Science*, 212: 1055–1059.

Bouchard, T.J. Jr. (1994) 'Genes, environment and personality.' *Science*, 2664: 1700–1701.

Bouchard, T.J. Jr. *et al.* (1990) 'A source of human psychological differences: the Minnesota study of twins reared apart.' *Science*, 250: 223–228.

Bourgeois, J.P. and P. Rakic (1993) 'Changing of synaptic density in the primary visual cortex of rhesus monkey from fetal to adult stage.' *Journal of Neurosciences*, 13: 2801–2802.

Bourgeois, J.P., P.S. Goldman-Rakic and P. Rakic (1994) 'Synaptogenesis in the prefrontal cortex of rhesus monkey.' *Cerebral Cortex*, 4: 78–96.

Bourne, S. (1968) 'The psychological effects of stillbirth on women and their doctors.' *Journal of the Royal College of General Practitioners,* 16: 103–112.

—— (1983) 'Psychological impact of stillbirth.' *Practitioner*, 227: 53–60.

Bowlby, J. (1969) *Attachment and Loss.* Vol. 1: *Attachment.* New York: Basic Books.

—— (1973) *Attachment and Loss.* Vol. 2: *Separation.* New York: Basic Books.

—— (1980) *Attachment and Loss.* Vol. 3: *Loss, Sadness and Depression.* New York: Basic Books.

Boysson-Bardies, B. (1999) *How Language Comes to Children.* Cambridge, Mass.: MIT Press.

Bracken, H. von (1934a) 'Psychologische Untersuchungen an Zwillingen.' *Archives für die gesamte Psychologie*, 97: 97–105.

—— (1934b) 'Mutual intimacy in twins. Types of social structure in pairs of identical and fraternal twins.' *Character and Personality*, 2: 203–209.

Bradley, R.M. (1972) 'Development of the taste bud and gustatory papillae in human fetuses.' In: J. Bosna (ed.) *Third Symposium on Oral Sensation and Perception: The Mouth of the Infant.* Springfield, Ill.: Thomas.

Braken, M.B. (1979) 'Oral contraception and twinning: an epidemiologic study.' *American Journal of Obstetrics and Gynecology*, 133: 432–434.

Brauth, S.E., W.S. Hall and R.J. Dooling (1991) *Plasticity in Development.* Cambridge, Mass.: MIT Press.

Brazelton, T.B. (1974) 'The origins of reciprocity: The early mother–infant interaction.' In: M. Lewis and L.A. Rosenblum (eds) *The Effect of the Infant on its Caregiver.* New York: Wiley.

Broadbent, B. (1985) 'Twin trauma.' *Nursing Times*, 28: 28–30.

Bromley, B.R. and B.R. Benacerraf (1995) 'Using the number of yolk sacs to determine amnionicity in early first trimester monochorionic twins.' *Journal of Ultrasound Medicine*, 14: 415–419.

Bronfenbrenner, U. (1972) 'Is 80% of intelligence genetically determined?' In: U. Bronfenbrenner (ed.) *Influences on Human Development.* Hillsdale, Ill.: Dryden.

—— (1979) *The Ecology of Human Development. Experiments by Nature and Design.* Cambridge, Mass.: Harvard University Press.

Bronstein, P. (1984) 'Differences in mothers' and fathers' behaviours towards children: A cross-cultural comparison.' *Developmental Psychology*, 6: 995–1003.

Bruer, J.T., (1999) *The Myth of the First Three Years*. New York: Free Press.

Bryan, E.M. (1977) 'Twins are a handful. How can we help?' *Maternal and Child Health*, 1: 348–353.

—— (1983) 'The loss of a twin.' *Maternal and Child Health*, May: 201–206, 218.

—— (1986) 'Are they identical? The importance of determining zygosity in twins.' *Maternal and Child Health*, 11: 171–176.

—— (1989) 'The response of mothers to selective fetocide.' *Ethical Problems in Reproductive Medicine*, 1: 28–30.

—— (1992) *Twins and Higher Multiple Births. A Guide to their Nature and Nurture*. London: Edward Arnold.

—— (1993) 'Prenatal and perinatal influences on twin children: implications for behavioral studies.' In: T.J. Bouchard Jr. and P. Propping (eds) *Twins as a Tool of Behavioral Genetics*. Chichester: John Wiley.

—— (1994)'Problems surrounding selective fetocide.' In: L. Abramsky and J. Chapel (eds) *The Human Side of Prenatal Diagnosis*. Oxford: Chapman and Hall.

—— (1999) 'The death of a twin.' In: A. Sandbank (ed.) *Twin and Triplet Psychology*. London: Routledge.

Bryan, E.M. and R. Higgins (1995) *Infertility, New Choices, New Dilemmas*. London: Penguin Books.

Bryan, E.M., J. Little and J. Burn (1987) 'Congenital anomalies in twins.' *Balliere's Clinics in Obstetrics and Gynecology*, 1: 697–721.

Bsat, F.A. and M.F.A. Seoud (1987) 'Superfetation secondary to ovulation induction with clomiphene citrate: a case report.' *Fertility and Sterility*, 47: 516–517.

Buckler, J.M.H. (1999) 'Growth and development of twins.' In: A. Sandbank (ed.) *Twin and Triplet Psychology*. London: Routledge.

Bulmer, M.G. (1970) *The Biology of Twinning in Man*. Oxford: Clarendon Press.

Burlingham, D. (1949) 'Twins as a gang in miniature.' In: K. Eissler (ed.) *Searchlights on Delinquency*. London: Imago.

—— (1952) *Twins: A Study of Three Pairs of Identical Twins*. New York: International Press.

Burnham, D.H. and M.B. Harris (1992) 'Effects of real gender and labeled gender on adults' perceptions of infants.' *Journal of Genetic Psychology*, 153: 165–183.

Burns, G.L. and A. Farina (1992) 'The role of physical attractiveness in adjustment.' *Genetic, Social, and General Psychology Monographs*, 118: 157–194.

Busnel, M.C. *et al.* (1986) 'Perception et acquisition auditves prénatales.' In: B. Blanc and J.M. Thoulon (eds) *Médécine Périnatale*. Paris: Arnette.

Busnel, M.C., C. Granier-Deferre and J.P Lecanuet (1992) 'Fetal audition.' In: G. Turkewitz (ed.) *Developmental Psychobiology, Annals of the New York Academy of Science*, 662.

Byng-Hall, J. (1995) *Rewriting Family Scripts*. London: The Guilford Press.

Caldwell, B.M. and R.H. Bradley (1984) *Home Observation for Measurement of the Environment (HOME)*. Little Rock: University of Arkansas.

Camaioni, L. (1993) 'The development of intentional communication: A re-analysis.' In: J. Nadel and L. Camaioni (eds) *New Perspectives in Early Communicative Development*. London: Routledge.

Campbell, D.M., A.J. Campbell and I. McGillivray (1974) 'Maternal characteristics of women having twin pregnancies.' *Journal of Biosocial Science*, 6: 463–470.

Campbell, D.M. *et al.* (1987) 'Does the use of oral contraception depress DZ twinning rates?' *Acta Geneticae Medicae et Gemellologiae*, 36: 409–415.

Campbell, S., A.E. Reading and D.N. Cox (1982) 'Ultrasound scanning in pregnancy: the short-term psychological effects of early time scans.' *Journal of Psychosomatic Obstetrics and Gynecology*, 1: 57–60.

Carlson, D.B. and R.C. Labarba (1979) 'Maternal emotionality during pregnancy and reproductive outcome: A review of the literature.' *International Journal of Behavioral Development*, 2: 343–376.

Carr, S.R., M.P. Aronson and C.R. Coustan (1990) 'Survival rates of monoamniotic twins do
not decrease after 30 weeks' gestation.' *American Journal of Obstetrics and Gynecology*,
163: 719–722.

Casey, M.L. and P.C. MacDonald (1993) 'Placental endocrinology.' In: C.W.G. Redman, I.L.
Sargent and P.M. Starkey (eds) *The Human Placenta: A Guide for Clinicians and Scientists.* Oxford: Blackwell Scientific Publications.

Cetrulo, C. (1986) 'The controversy of mode of delivery in twins: the intrapartum management of twin gestation.' *Seminars in Perinatology*, 23: 533–548.

Changeux, J.P. (1983) *L'Homme neuronal.* Paris: Fayard.

Charlesworth, R. and W.W. Hartup (1967) 'Positive social reinforcement in the nursery
school peer group.' *Child Development*, 38: 993–1002.

Chatwin, B. (1982) *On the Black Hill.* London: Jonathan Cape.

Chauhan, S.P. and W.E. Roberts (1996) 'Intrapartum management.' In: S.A. Gall (ed.) *Multiple Pregnancy and Delivery.* St Louis, Mo.: Mosby Year Book.

Cheng Y.J., C.J. Chen and C. Chang (1986) 'Twinning rates in Taiwan.' *Acta Geneticae
Medicae et Gemellologiae*, 35: 52.

Chernoch, J.M. and R.H. Porter (1985) 'Recognition of maternal axillary odors by infants.'
Child Development, 56: 1593–1598.

Chevernak, F.A. (1986) 'The controversy of mode of delivery in twins: the intrapartum management of twin gestation.' *Seminars in Perinatology*, 10: 44–49.

—— (1995) 'The optimum route of delivery.' In: L.G. Keith *et al.* (eds) *Multiple Pregnancy: Epidemiology, Gestation and Perinatal Outcome.* New York: The Parthenon Publishing Group.

Chomsky, N. (1988) *Language and Problems of Knowledge.* Cambridge, Mass.: MIT Press.

Clark, P.M. and Z. Dickman (1984) 'Features of interaction in infant twins.' *Acta Geneticae
Medicae et Gemellologiae*, 33: 151–159.

Cohen, N.J. and H. Eichenbaum (1993) *Memory, Amnesia and the Hippocampal System.*
Cambridge, Mass.: MIT Press.

Coie, J.D. and A.H.N. Cillessen (1993) 'Peer rejection: Origins and effects on children's development.' *Current Directions in Psychological Science*, 2: 89–92.

Collaer, M. and M. Hines (1995) 'Human behavioral sex differences: A role for gonadal hormones during early development?' *Psychological Bulletin*, 118: 55–107.

Coltrane, S. (1996) *Family Man: Fatherhood, Housework, and Gender Equity.* New York:
Oxford University Press.

Corney, G. (1975) 'Mythology and customs associated with twins.' In: I. MacGillivray, P.P.S.
Nylander and G. Corney (eds) *Human Multiple Reproduction.* London: W.B. Saunders.

Corsaro, W.A. (1985) *Friendship and Peer Culture in the Early Years.* Norwood, N.J.: Ablex.

Crook, C. (1987) 'Taste and olfaction.' In: P. Salapatek and L. Cohen (eds) *Handbook of
Infant Perception*, Vol. 1. Orlando, Fla: Academic Press.

Crowther, C.A. (1999) 'Multiple pregnancy.' In: D.K. James, P.J. Steer, C.P. Weiner and B.
Gonik (eds) *High Risk Pregnancy.* London: Harcourt Brace and Co. Ltd.

Damasio, A.R. (1999) *The Feeling of What Happens. Body and Emotion in the Making of
Consciousness.* New York: Harcourt Brace and Co. Ltd.

Danskin, F.H. and J.P. Nielson (1989) 'Twin transfusion syndrome: What are appropriate criteria?' *American Journal of Obstetrics and Gynecology*, 161: 365–369.

Davies, J.A., M.P.M. Richards and N.R.C. Roberton (1983) *Parent–Baby Attachment in Premature Infants.* New York: St Martin's Press.

Davis, E.A. (1937) *The Development of Linguistic Skill in Twins, Singletons with Siblings,
and Only Children from Five to Ten Years.* Monograph 14, Institute of Child Welfare.
Minneapolis: University of Minnesota.

Daw, N.W. (1995) *Visual Development*. New York: Plenum Press.

Dawes, G.S. (1984) 'Fetal physiology and behavior: Changing direction. 1954–1983' *Journal of Developmental Physiology*, 6: 259–265.

—— (1986) 'The central control of fetal behaviour.' *European Journal of Obstetrics and Gynecology and Reproductive Biology*, 21: 341–346.

Day, E.J. (1932) 'The development of language in twins: A comparison of twins and single children.' *Child Development*, 3: 179–199.

DeCasper, A.J. and W.P. Fifer (1980) 'Of human bonding: newborns prefer their mother's voice.' *Science*, 208: 1174–1176.

DeCasper, A.J. and P.A. Prescott (1984) 'Human newborns' perception of male voices: Preference, discrimination and reinforcing value.' *Developmental Psychobiology*, 17: 481–491.

De Lia, J.E. *et al.* (1995) 'Fetoscopic laser ablation of placental vessels in severe previable twin–twin transfusion syndrome.' *American Journal of Obstetrics and Gynecology*, 172: 1202–1211.

Derom, C. *et al.* (1991) 'Zygosity testing at birth: A plea to the obstetrician.' *Journal of Perinatal Medicine*, 19 (suppl.): 234–240.

Derom, R. *et al.* (1987) 'Increased monozygotic twinning rate after ovulation induction.' *Lancet*, 8544 (May 30): 1236–1238.

De Snoo, K. (1937) 'Das trinkende Kind im Uterus.' *Monatsschrift fuer Geburt und Gyneakologie*, 105: 88.

Diamond, K., W. LeFurgy and S. Blass (1993) 'Attitude of preschool children toward their peers with disabilities: A year-long investigation in integrated classrooms.' *Journal of Genetic Psychology*, 154: 215–221.

Dickerson, P. (1981) 'Early postpartum separation and attachment in twins.' *Journal of Obstetric Gynecologic and Neonatal Nursing*, 10: 120–127.

Dodd, B. and S. McEvey (1994) 'Twin language or phonological disorder?' *Child Language*, 21: 273–289.

Drachman, D.B. and A.J. Coulombre (1962) 'Experimental clubfoot and arthrogryposis multiplex congenita.' *The Lancet*, 2: 523–526.

Drachman, D.B. and L. Sokoloff (1966) 'The role of movement in embryonic joint development.' *Developmental Biology*, 14: 401–420.

Dreyfus-Brisac, C. (1968) 'Sleep ontogenesis in early human prematurity from 24–27 weeks of conceptual age.' *Developmental Psychobiology*, 2: 162–169.

—— (1970) 'Ontogenesis of sleep in human prematures after 32 weeks post-conceptional age.' *Developmental Psychobiology*, 8: 91–121.

—— (1979) 'Ontogenesis of brain bioelectrical activity and sleep organization in neonates and infants.' In: F. Falkner and J.M. Tanner (eds) *Human Growth*. Vol. 3: *Neurobiology and Nutrition*. New York: Plenum Press.

Dubowitz, L.S.M. *et al.* (1980) 'Visual function in the preterm and full-term newborn infant.' *Developmental Medicine and Child Neurology*, 22: 465–475.

Dunn, J. (1983) 'Sibling relationships in early childhood.' *Child Development*, 54: 787–811.

—— (1985) *Sisters and Brothers*. Cambridge, Mass.: Harvard University Press.

—— (1988) *The Beginnings of Social Understanding*. Cambridge, Mass.: Harvard University Press.

—— (1993) *Young Children's Close Relationships: Beyond Attachment*. London: Sage.

—— (1995) *From One Child to Two*. New York: Fawcett Columbine.

Dunn, J. and C. Kendrick (1982) *Siblings: Love, Envy and Understanding*. Cambridge, Mass.: Harvard University Press.

Dunn, J. and S. McGuire (1992) 'Sibling and peer relationships in childhood.' *Journal of Child Psychology and Psychiatry*, 33: 67–105.

Dunn, J. and R. Plomin (1985) 'Differential experiences of siblings in the same family.' *Developmental Psychology*, 21: 747–760.

—— (1990) *Separate Lives: Why Siblings are so Different.* New York: Basic Books.

—— (1991) 'Why are siblings so different? The significance of differences in sibling experiences within the family.' *Family Process,* 30: 271–283.

Dunsford, I. *et al.* (1953) 'A human blood-group chimera.' *British Medical Journal,* 2: 81.

Easter, S.S. *et al.* (1985) 'The changing views of neuronal specificity.' *Science,* 230: 507–511.

Eckerman, C.O. and S.M. Didow (1988) 'Lessons drawn from observing young peers together.' *Acta Pediatrica Scandinavica,* 77: 55–70.

—— (1996) 'Nonverbal imitation and toddlers' mastery of verbal means of achieving coordinated action.' *Developmental Psychology,* 32: 141–152.

Eckerman, C.O., C.C. Davis and S.M. Didow (1989) 'Toddlers' emerging ways of achieving social coordination with a peer.' *Child Development,* 60: 440–453.

Edelman, G.M. (1987) *Neural Darwinism: The Theory of Neuronal Group Selection.* New York: Basic Books.

—— (1992) *Bright Air, Brilliant Fire.* New York: Basic Books.

Ehret, G. (1988) 'Auditory development: Psychophysical and behavioral aspects.' In: E. Meisani and P.S. Timiras (eds) *Handbook of Human Growth and Developmental Biology,* Vol. 1. Boca Raton, Fla: CRC Press.

Eibl-Eibesfeldt, I. (1975) *Ethology* (2nd edn). New York: Holt, Rinehart and Winston.

Eisenberg, N. and P.H. Mussen (1989) *The Roots of Prosocial Behaviour in Children.* Cambridge Studies in Social and Emotional Development. Cambridge: Cambridge University Press.

Eliot, L. (1999) *What's Going On In There? How the Brain and Mind Develop in the First Five Years of Life.* New York: Bantam Books.

Elliott, J.P., M.A. Urig and W.H. Clewell (1991) 'Aggressive therapeutic amniocentesis for treatment of twin–twin transfusion syndrome.' *Obstetrics and Gynecology,* 77: 537–540.

Elman, J.L. *et al.* (1996) *Rethinking Innateness. A Connectionist Perspective on Development.* Cambridge, Mass.: MIT Press.

Emde, R.N. *et al.* (1992) 'Temperament, emotion and cognition at fourteen months: The MacArthur longitudinal twin study.' *Child Development,* 63: 1437–1455.

Eyer, D.E. (1992) *Mother–infant Bonding: A Scientific Fiction.* New Haven, Conn.: Yale University Press.

Fanaroff, A.A. and R.J. Martin (1992) 'Obstetric management of multiple gestation.' In: A.A. Fanaroff and R.J. Martin (eds) *Neonatal–Perinatal Medicine,* Vol. 1 (5th edn). St Louis, Mo.: Mosby Year Book.

Farmer, P. (1996) *Two or the Book of Twins and Doubles.* London: Virago Press.

Ferreira, A.J. (1965) 'Emotional factors in prenatal environment.' *Journal of Nervous and Mental Diseases,* 141 (1): 109–117.

Field, T.M. (1990a) 'Neonatal stress and coping in intensive care.' *Journal of Infant Mental Health,* 11: 57–65.

—— (1990b) 'Alleviating stress in newborn infants in the intensive care unit.' *Clinics in Perinatology,* 17: 1–9.

Field, T.M. *et al.* (1980) *High-Risk Infants and Children: Adult and Peer Interactions.* New York: Academic Press.

Field, T.M. and A. Sostek (1983) *Infants Born at Risk.* New York: Grune and Stratton.

Fisk, N.M. and E.M. Bryan (1993) 'Routine prenatal determination of chorionicity in multiple gestation: A plea to the obstetrician.' *British Journal of Obstetrics and Gynecology,* 100: 975–977.

Fleming, A.D., W.F. Rayburn and N.T. Mandsager (1990) 'Perinatal outcomes of twin pregnancies at term.' *Journal of Reproductive Medicine,* 35: 88–92.

Folgman, R. (1976) 'Monoamniotic twins.' *Acta Geneticae Medicae et Gemellologiae,* 26: 62–65.

Foot, H.C., M.J. Morgan and R.H. Shute (1990) 'Children's helping relations: An overview.'

In: H.C. Foot, M.J. Morgan and R.H. Shute (eds) *Children Helping Children*. New York: John Wiley.

Forssberg, H. (1985) 'Spinal locomotor functions and descending control.' In: B. Sjolund and B. Bjorklund (eds) *Brainstem Control of Spinal Mechanisms*. Amsterdam: Elsevier.

Frazer, J.G. ([1922] 1932) *The Golden Bough: A Study in Magic and Religion* (3rd edn). London: Macmillan.

Freud, S. (1905) 'Infantile sexuality.' In: S. Freud, *Three Essays on Sexuality*. Standard edn, Vol. VII. London: Hogarth Press.

Friedman, R. and B. Gradstein (1992) *Surviving Pregnancy Loss* (2nd edn). Toronto: Little Brown.

Frith, P. (1989) *Autism: Explaining the Enigma*. Oxford: Blackwell.

Frontisi-Ducroux, F. (1992) 'Les Grecs, le double et les jumeaux.' *Topique*, 50: 239–262.

Fuster, J.A. (1999) *Memory in the Cerebral Cortex*. Cambridge, Mass.: MIT Press.

Gagnon, R. (1989) 'Stimulation of human fetuses with sound and vibration.' *Seminars in Perinatology*, 13: 353–355.

Galenson, E. and H. Rophie (1971) 'The impact of early sexual discovery on mood, defensive organization and symbolization.' *The Psychoanalytic Study of the Child*, 26: 195–216.

—— (1974) 'The emergence of genital awareness during the second year of life.' In: R.C. Friedman (ed.) *Sex Differences in Behavior*. New York: Wiley.

Galton, F. (1875) 'The history of twins as a criterion of the relative powers of nature and nurture.' *Journal of the Anthropological Institute of Great Britain and Ireland*, 5: 391–406.

Gandelman, R. (1992) 'Origin and function of embryonic behavior.' In: R. Gandelman (ed.) *The Psychobiology of Behavioral Development*. Oxford: Oxford University Press.

Gandevia, S.C. and D. Burke (1994) 'Does the nervous system depend on kinesthetic information to control natural limb movements?' In: P. Cordo and S. Harnad (eds) *Movement Control*. Cambridge: Cambridge University Press.

Gardner, M.O. and K.D. Wenstrom (1996) 'Maternal adaptation.' In: S.A. Gall (ed.) *Multiple Pregnancy and Delivery*. St Louis, Mo.: Mosby Year Book.

Garvey, C. (1984) *Children's Talk*. London: Fontana.

—— (1990) *Play*. Cambridge, Mass.: Harvard University Press.

Gedda, L. (1961) *Twins in History and Science*. Springfield, Ill.: Charles Thomas.

Gedda, L., D. Casa and M. Milani-Coparetti (1980) 'La diagnosi di zigotismo nei gemelli: esperimenti con cani poliziotti.' *Rivista di Biologia*, 73 (1): 95–97.

Gélis, J. (1991) 'Deux enfants d'une meme ventrée: Introduction à l'histoire des naissances gémellaires.' In: E. Papiernik-Berkhauer and J. Pons (eds) *Les Grossesses Multiples*. Paris: Doin.

George, C. and M. Main (1980) 'Abused children: Their rejection of peers and caregivers.' In: T. Martini-Field *et al.* (eds) *High-Risk Infants and Children*. New York: Academic Press.

Ghai, V. and D. Vidyasagar (1988) 'Morbidity and mortality factors in twins. An epidemiologic approach.' *Clinics in Perinatology*, 15: 123–140.

Giannakoulopoulos, H., W. Sepulveda, P. Kourtis, V. Glover and N.M. Fisk (1994) 'Fetal plasma cortisol and fl-endorphin response to intrauterine needling.' *Lancet*, 344: 77–81.

Gilbert, K.R. and L.S. Smart (1992) *Coping with Infant or Fetal Loss*. Psychosocial Stress Series No. 22. New York: Bruner Mazel.

Gilligan, C. (1982) *In a Different Voice: Psychological Theory and Women's Development*. Cambridge, Mass.: Harvard University Press.

Glass, L. and M.C. Mackey (1988) *From Clocks to Chaos. The Rhythms of Life*. Princeton, N.J.: Princeton University Press.

Gleeson, C. *et al.* (1990) 'Twins in school: An Australian-wide program.' *Acta Geneticae Medicae et Gemellologiae*, 39: 231–244.

Goffman, E. (1959) *The Presentation of Self in Everyday Life*. London: Penguin Books.

—— (1961) *Encounters*. Indianapolis, Ind.: Bobbs-Merrill.

—— (1963) *Behavior in Public Places*. New York: The Free Press.

—— (1967) *Interaction Ritual*. Garden City, N.Y.: Anchor Books.

Golombok, S. *et al.* (1995) 'Families created by the new reproductive technologies: Quality of parenting and social and emotional development of the children.' *Child Development*, 67: 218–235.

Gopnik, A., A.M. Meltzoff and P.K. Kuhl (1999) *The Scientist in The Crib*. New York: William Morrow.

Goshen-Gottstein, E.R. (1980) 'The mothering of twins, triplets and quadruplets.' *Psychiatry*, 43: 189–204.

—— (1981) 'Differential maternal socialization of opposite-sexed twins, triplets and quadruplets.' *Child Development*, 52: 1255–1264.

Gottlieb, G. (1992) *Individual Development and Evolution: The Genesis of Novel Behavior*. New York: Oxford University Press.

Gould, S.J. (1996) *The Mismeasure of Man* (2nd edn). New York: W.W. Norton.

Greenberg, M., D. Cicchetti and E.M. Cummings (eds) (1990) *Attachment in the Preschool Years: Theory, Research and Intervention*. Chicago, Ill.: Chicago University Press.

Grillner, S. and M.L. Shik (1973) 'On the descending control of the lumbosacral spinal cord from the "mesencephalic locomotor region".' *Acta Physiologica Scandinavica*, 87: 320–333.

Gromada, K. (1981) 'Maternal–infant attachment: The first steps in individualizing twins.' *American Journal of Maternal and Child Nursing*, 6: 129–134.

Groothuis, J.R. (1985) 'Twins and twin families: A practical guide to outpatient management.' *Clinics in Perinatology*, 12: 459–474.

Groothuis, J.R. *et al.* (1982) 'Increased child abuse in families with twins.' *Pediatrics*, 70: 769–763.

Hagay, Z.J. *et al.* (1986) 'Management and outcome of multiple pregnancies complicated by antenatal death of one fetus.' *Journal of Reproductive Medicine*, 31 (8): 717–720.

Hall, E.T. (1959) *The Silent Language*. Garden City, N.Y.: Doubleday and Co.

Hall, J.G. (1996) 'Twins and twinning.' *American Journal of Medical Genetics*, 61: 202–204.

Hall, J.G. and E. Lopez-Rangell (1996) 'Embryologic development and monozygotic twinning.' *Acta Geneticae Medicae et Gemellologiae*, 45: 53–57.

Halpin, Z.T. (1991) 'Kin recognition cues of vertebrates.' In: P.G. Hepper (ed.) *Kin Recognition*. Cambridge: Cambridge University Press.

Hamburger, V. and R.W. Oppenheim (1982) 'Naturally occurring cell death in vertebrates.' *Comments in Neuroscience*, 1: 39–55.

Hamilton, J.A. and P.N. Harberger (1992) *Postpartum Psychiatric Illness. A Picture Puzzle*. Philadelphia, Pa.: University of Pennsylvania Press.

Hamilton, W.J., J.D. Boyd and H.W. Mossman (1978) *Human Embryology* (4th edn, by the Late W.J. Hamilton and H.W. Mossman). London: The Macmillan Press.

Harris, M. (1969) *On Understanding Infants*. London: Dickens Press.

Hartup, W.W. (1974) 'Aggression in childhood: Developmental perspectives.' *American Psychologist*, 29: 336–341.

—— (1983) 'Peer relations.' In: P.H. Mussen (ed.) *Handbook of Child Psychology*. Vol. IV: *Socialization, Personality and Social Development* (4th edn). New York: John Wiley.

Hartup, W.W. and J. deWitt (1974) 'The development of aggression. Problems and perspectives.' In: J. deWitt and W.W. Hartup (eds) *Determinants and Origins of Aggressive Behavior*. The Hague: Mouton.

Hay, D.A. (1987) 'Early influences on the school social adjustments of twins.' *Acta Geneticae Medicae et Gemellologiae*, 36: 239–248.

—— (1991) *Twins in School. La Trobe Twins Study*. Department of Psychology, La Trobe University, Melbourne, Australia: Australian Multiple Births Association Inc.

Hay, D.A., R. McIndoe and P.J. O'Brien (1988) 'The older sibling of twins.' *Australian Journal of the Early Child,* 13: 25–28.

Hay, D.A. and P.J. O'Brien (1987) 'The role of parental attitudes in the development of temperament in twins at home, school and test situations.' *Acta Geneticae Medicae et Gemellologiae,* 33: 191–204.

Hay, D.A. and H.S. Ross (1981) 'Development in preschool twins.' *Acta Geneticae Medicae et Gemellologiae,* 36: 213–223.

Hay, D.A. and H.S. Ross (1982) 'The social nature of early conflict.' *Child Development,* 53: 105–113.

Hay, D.A. *et al.* (1990) 'What information should the multiple birth family receive before, during and after the birth?' *Acta Geneticae Medicae et Gemollologiae,* 39: 259–269.

Heidrich, S.M. and M.S. Cranley (1989) 'Effect of fetal movement, ultrasound scans, and amniocentesis on maternal–fetal attachment.' *Nursing Research,* 38 (2): 81–84.

Hepper, P.G. (1988a) 'Adaptive fetal learning: Prenatal exposure to garlic effects and postnatal preferences.' *Animal Behavior,* 36: 935–936.

—— (1988b) 'The discrimination of human odor by the dog.' *Perception,* 17: 549–554.

—— (1990) 'Foetal olfaction.' In: D.W. Macdonald, D. Muller-Schwarze and S.E. Natynczuck (eds) *Chemical Signals in Vertebrates V.* Oxford: Oxford University Press.

—— (1991) 'Recognizing kin: Ontogeny and classification.' In: P.G. Hepper (ed.) *Kin Recognition.* Cambridge: Cambridge University Press.

—— (1992) 'Fetal psychology. An embryonic science.' In: J.G. Nijhuis (ed.) *Fetal Behavior: Developmental and Perinatal Aspects.* Oxford: Oxford University Press.

Hepper, P.G. and S. Shadidullah (1992) 'Habituation in normal and Down syndrome fetuses.' *Quarterly Journal of Experimental Psychology,* 37: 112–115.

Hepper, P.G., R. White and S. Shadidullah (1991) 'The development of fetal responsiveness to external auditory stimulation.' *Abstracts of the British Psychological Society,* 45: 30.

Herschkowitz, N. (1988) 'Brain development in the fetus, neonate and infant.' *Biology of the Neonate,* 54: 1–19.

Hertzberg, B.S., A.B. Kurtz and H.Y. Choy (1987) 'Significance of membrane thickness in the sonographic evaluation of twin gestations.' *American Journal of Roentgenology,* 148: 151–153.

Higonnet, A. (1998) *Pictures of Innocence.* London: Thames and Hudson.

Hill, L.M. *et al.* (1996) 'Sonographic determination of first trimester twin chorionicity and amnionicity.' *Journal of Clinical Ultrasound,* 24: 305–308.

Hill-Goldsmith, H. *et al.* (1987) 'Roundtable: What is Temperament? Four Approaches.' *Child Development,* 58: 505–529.

Hinde, R.A. (1968) 'Dichotomies in the study of development.' In: J.M. Thoday and A.S. Parkes (eds) *Genetic and Environmental Influences on Behavior.* Edinburgh: Oliver and Boyd.

—— (1982) *Ethology: Its Nature and Relation with Other Sciences.* Oxford: Oxford University Press.

—— (1983) 'Ethology and child development.' In: M.M. Haith and J.J. Campos (eds) *Handbook of Child Psychology.* Vol. 2: *Infancy and Developmental Psychobiology* (4th edn). New York: Wiley.

—— (1988) *Individuals, Relationships and Culture.* Themes in the Social Sciences Series. Cambridge: Cambridge University Press.

Hinton, P.R. (1993) *The Psychology of Interpersonal Perception.* London: Routledge.

Hobson, P. (1993) *Autism and the Development of the Mind.* Hillsdale, N.J.: Lawrence Erlbaum Associates.

Hofer, M.A. (1988) 'On the nature and function of prenatal behavior.' In: W.P. Smootherman and S. Robinson (eds) *Behavior of the Fetus.* Cladwell, N.J.: Telford Press.

Horgan, J. (1999) *The Undiscovered Mind.* New York: The Free Press.

Howes, C. (1985) 'Sharing fantasy: Social pretend play in toddlers.' *Child Development*, 56: 1253–1258.

Hutt, S.J. and C. Hutt (1970) *Direct Observation and Measurement of Behavior*. Springfield, Ill.: Thomas.

Huttenlocher, P.R. (1990) 'Morphometric study of human cerebral cortex development.' *Neuropsychologia*, 28: 517–527.

Huttenlocher, P.R. and C. de Courten (1987) 'The development of synapses in the striate cortex of man.' *Human Neurobiology*, 6: 1–9.

Ianniruberto, A. and E. Tajani (1981) 'Ultrasonographic study of fetal movements.' *Seminars in Perinatology*, 5: 175–181.

Istvan, J. (1986) 'Stress, anxiety, and birth outcome: A critical review of the evidence.' *Psychological Bulletin*, 100: 331–348.

Jacoby, A. (1988) 'Mothers' views about information and advice in pregnancy and childbirth: Findings from a national study.' *Midwifery*, 4: 103–110.

Jeanty, P. *et al.* (1981) 'The vanishing twin.' *Ultrasons*, 2: 225–231.

Joffe, J.M. (1978) 'Hormonal mediation of the effects of prenatal stress on offspring behavior.' In: G. Gottlieb (ed.) *Studies on the Development of Behavior and the Nervous System*. Vol. 4. New York: Academic Press.

Johnson, M.H. (1990) 'Cortical maturation and the development of visual attention in early infancy.' *Journal of Cognitive Neuroscience*, 2: 81–95.

—— (1994) 'Brain and cognitive development in infancy.' *Current Opinions in Neurobiology*, 4: 218–225.

Johnson, M.H. and J. Morton (1991) *Biology and Cognitive Development: The Case of Face Recognition*. Oxford: Blackwell.

Johnson-Laird, P.N. and R.M.J. Byrne (1991) *Deduction*. London: Erlbaum.

Jones, C.T. (1986) 'The significance of the placenta in monitoring fetal state.' In: H. Ludwig and K. Thomsen (eds) *Gynecology and Obstetrics*. Berlin: Springer-Verlag.

—— (1988) 'Pathways of signalling between foetus and placenta: role of catecholamine metabolism and action in the placenta of the sheep.' In: D. Dhalstrom (ed.) *Progress in Catecholamine Research. Part A. Aspects and Peripheral Mechanisms*. New York: Alan Liss.

—— (1989) 'Endocrine mechanisms of communication between the placenta and fetus.' In: E.V. Cosmi and G.C. Di Renzo (eds) *Proceedings of the XI European Congress of Perinatal Medicine*. London: Harewood.

—— (1993) 'Endocrine and metabolic interaction between placenta and fetus: Pathways of maternal–fetal communication.' In: C.W.G. Redman, I.L. Sargent and P.M. Starkey (eds) *The Human Placenta: A Guide for Clinicians and Scientists*. Oxford: Blackwell Scientific Publications.

Jones, C.T., W. Gu and T.J. Parer (1989) 'The control of the output of corticotrophin releasing hormone from the sheep placenta.' *Journal of Developmental Physiology*, 11: 121–134.

Josse, D. and M. Robin (1986) 'Some aspects of mother–child relationships following the birth of twins.' *Early Child Development and Care*, 26: 1–18.

Jou, J.H. *et al.* (1993) 'Doppler sonographic detection of reverse twin–twin transfusion after intrauterine death of the donor.' *Journal of Ultrasound Medicine*, 3: 307–309.

Kagan, J. (1994) *Galen's Prophecy. Temperament in Human Nature*. London: Free Association Books.

—— (1998) *Three Seductive Ideas*. Cambridge, Mass.: Harvard University Press.

Kagan, J., R.B. Kearsley and P.R. Zelazo (1978) *Infancy: Its Place in Human Development*. Cambridge, Mass.: Harvard University Press.

Karras Sokol, D. *et al.* (1995) 'Intrapair differences in personality and cognitive ability among young monozygotic twins distinguished by chorion type.' *Behavior Genetics*, 25 (5): 457–465.

Keenan, E.O. (1974) 'Conversational competence in children.' *Journal of Child Language,* 1: 163–183.

Keenan, E.O. and E. Klein (1975) 'Coherency in children's discourse.' *Journal of Psycholinguistic Research,* 4: 365–380.

Keet, M.P., A.M. Jaroszewicz and C.J. Lombard (1986) 'Follow-up study of physical growth of monozygous twins with discordant within-pair birth weights.' *Pediatrics,* 77: 336–344.

Keith, L.G. *et al.* (1995) In: L.G. Keith *et al.* (eds) *Multiple Pregnancy: Epidemiology, Gestation and Perinatal Outcome.* New York: The Parthenon Publishing Group.

Kelley, H.H. (1971) *Attribution in Social Interaction.* Morristown, N.J.: General Learning Press.

Kelly, D.D. (1991) 'Sexual differentiation of the nervous system.' In: E.R. Kandel, J.H. Schwartz and T.M. Jessell (eds) *Principles of Neural Science* (3rd edn). Amsterdam: Elsevier.

Kelso, J.A.S., J.P. Sholz and G. Schoner (1986) 'Non-equilibrium phase transitions in coordinated biological motion: Critical fluctuations.' *Physics Letters,* 118: 279–284.

Kemp, V.H. and C.K. Page (1987) 'Maternal prenatal attachment in normal and high-risk pregnancies.' *Journal of Obstetrics, Gynecology and Neonatal Nursing,* 16: 179–184.

Kim, C.C. *et al.* (1969) 'Social interaction of like-sex twins and singletons in relation to intelligence, language and physical development.' *Journal of Genetics and Psychology,* 114: 203–214.

Kindermann, T.A. (1995) 'Distinguishing "buddies" from "bystanders": The study of children's development within natural peer contexts.' In: T.A. Kindermann and J. Valsiner (eds) *Development of Person–Context Relations.* Hillsdale, N.J.: Erlbaum.

Kirk, E.P. (1984) 'Psychological effects and management of perinatal loss.' *American Journal of Obstetrics and Gynecology,* 149: 46–51.

Kittinger, G.W. (1974) 'Feto-maternal production and transfer of cortisol in the rhesus (Macaca mulatta).' *Steroids,* 23: 229–243.

Kitzinger, S. (1988) *The Experience of Childbirth* (5th edn). London: Penguin Books.

Klaus, M.H. and J.H. Kennell (1970) 'Mothers separated from their newborn infants.' *Pediatric Clinics of North America,* 17: 1015–1037.

—— (1983) 'An evaluation of interventions in the premature nursery.' In: A.J. Davies, M.P.M. Richards and N.R.C. Roberton (eds) *Parent–Baby Attachment in Premature Infants.* London: Croom Helm.

—— (1993) 'Care of the parents.' In: M.H. Klaus and A.A. Fanaroff (eds) *Care of the High-Risk Neonate.* Philadelphia, Pa.: W.B. Saunders.

Kleeman, J.M. (1975) 'Genital self-stimulation in infant and toddler girls.' In: I.M. Marcus and J.J. Francis (eds) *Masturbation from Infancy to Senescence.* New York: International Universities Press.

Koch, H. (1966) *Twins and Twin Relations.* Chicago, Ill.: Chicago University Press.

Kochenour, N.K. (1992) 'Obstetric management of multiple gestation.' In: A.A. Fanaroff and R.J. Martin (eds) *Neonatal–Perinatal Medicine,* Vol. 1 (5th edn). St. Louis, Mo.: Mosby Year Book.

Kohlberg, L. and E. Ziegler (1967) 'The impact of cognitive maturity on the development of sex-roles attitudes in the years 4–8.' *Genetic Psychology Monographs,* 75: 84–165.

Koluchova, J. (1972) 'Severe deprivation in twins: a case study.' *Journal of Child Psychology and Psychiatry,* 13: 107–114.

—— (1976) 'The further development of twins after severe and prolonged separation.' *Journal of Child Psychology and Psychiatry,* 17: 181–188.

Kopin, I.J., G. Eisenhofer and D. Goldstein (1989) 'Adrenergic response following recognition of stress.' In: S. Breznitz and O. Zinder (eds) *Molecular Biology of Stress.* New York: Alan R. Liss.

Koziel, S.M. (1998) 'Effect of disparities in birthweight on differences in postnatal growth of monozygotic and dizygotic twins.' *Annals of Human Biology,* 25: 159–168.

Kumar, R. and I.F. Brockington (1988) *Motherhood and Mental Illness 2: Causes and Consequences*. London: Wright.

Kupfermann, I. (1991) 'Learning and memory.' In: E. Kandell, J.H. Schwartz and T.M. Jessell (eds) *Principles of Neural Science* (3rd edn). New York: Elsevier.

Kurtz, A.B. *et al.* (1992) 'Twin pregnancies: accuracy of first-trimester abdominal US in predicting chorionicity and amnionicity.' *Radiology*, 185: 759–762.

LaMantia, R. and P. Rakic (1990) 'Axon overproduction and elimination in the corpus callosum of the developing rhesus monkey.' *Journal of Neuroscience*, 10 (7): 2156–2175.

Lamb, M.E. (1997) *The Role of Father in Child Development* (3rd edn). New York: Wiley.

Landy, H. *et al.* (1986) 'The vanishing twin. Ultrasonographic assessment of fetal disappearance in the first trimester.' *American Journal of Obstetrics and Gynecology*, 155: 14–19.

Langer, M., M. Ringler and E. Reinold (1988) 'Psychological effects of ultrasound examinations: Changes of body perception and child image in pregnancy.' *Journal of Psychosomatic Obstetrics and Gynecology*, 8: 199–208.

Lavie, P. (1996) *The Enchanted World of Sleep*. New Haven, Conn.: Yale University Press.

Lecanuet, J.P., C. Granier-Deferre and M.C. Busnel (1989) 'Sensorialiteé foetale. Ontogenèse des systèmes sensoriels, conséquences de leur functionnement foetal.' In: J.P. Relier, J. Laugier and B. Louis-Salle (eds) *Médecine Périnatale*. Paris: Flammarion.

Lecanuet, J.P. *et al.* (1995) *Fetal Development: A Psychobiological Perspective*. Hillsdale, N.J.: Lawrence Erlbaum Associates.

Lederman, R.P. *et al.* (1978) 'The relationship of maternal anxiety, plasma catecholamines and plasma cortisol to progress in labor.' *American Journal of Obstetrics and Gynecology*, 132: 495–500.

—— (1979) 'Relationship of psychological factors in pregnancy to progress in labor.' *Nursing Research*, 28: 94–97.

—— (1981) 'Maternal psychological and physiological correlates of fetal–newborn health status.' *American Journal of Obstetrics and Gynecology*, 139: 956–958.

LeDoux, J. (1996) *The Emotional Brain*. New York: Simon and Schuster.

Leifer, M. (1977) 'Psychological changes accompanying pregnancy and motherhood.' *Genetic Psychology Monographs*, 95: 55–96.

Leon, I.G. (1986) 'Psychodynamics of perinatal loss.' *Psychiatry*, 9: 312–324.

Lerum, C.W., N.C. Major and G. LoBiondo-Wood (1989) 'The relationship of maternal age, quickening, and physical symptoms of pregnancy to the development of maternal–fetal attachment.' *Birth*, 16: 13–17.

Lester, B.M. and E. Tronick (eds) (1990) *Clinics in Perinatology*. Vol. 17: *Stimulation and the Preterm Infant: The Limits of Plasticity*. Philadelphia, Pa.: W.B. Saunders.

Levi, S. (1976) 'Ultrasonic assessment of the high rate of human multiple pregnancy in the first trimester.' *Journal of Clinical Ultrasound*, 4: 3–5.

Lévi-Strauss, C. (1991) *Histoire de Lynx*. Paris: Plon.

Levy, G.D. and R.A. Haaf (1994) 'Detection of gender-related categories by 10-month-old infants.' *Infant Behavior and Development*, 17: 457–459.

Lewin, B. (1997) *Genes VI*. Oxford: Oxford University Press.

Lewis, B.A. and L.A. Thompson (1992) 'A study of developmental speech and language disorder in twins.' *Journal of Speech and Hearing Research*, 35: 1086–1094.

Lewis, E. (1976) 'Management of stillbirth. Coping with an unreality.' *Lancet*, ii: 619–620.

—— (1979) 'Inhibition of mourning by pregnancy: Psychopathology and management.' *Archives of Diseases in Childhood*, 54: 303–305.

Lewis, E. and A. Page (1978) 'Failure to mourn a stillbirth: An overlooked catastrophe.' *British Journal of Medical Psychology*, 51: 237–240.

Lewis, M. (1987) 'Social development in infancy and early childhood.' In: J. Osofsky (ed.) *Handbook of Infant Development* (2nd edn). New York: John Wiley.

Lewis, M. *et al.* (1975) 'The beginning of friendship.' In: M. Lewis and L.A. Rosenblum (eds) *Friendship and Peer Relations*. New York: Wiley.

Lewontin, R.C., S. Rose and L.J. Kamin (1984) *Not In Our Genes*. New York: Random House.

Liebermann, J., N.O. Borani and M. Feinleib (1978) 'Twinning as a heterozygote advantage for a1 antitrypsin deficiency.' In: W.E. Nance (ed.) *Twin Research: Biology and Epidemiology. Progress in Clinical Biological Research*, 24B.

Liebmann-Smith, J. (1987) *In Pursuit of Pregnancy*. New York: New Market Press.

Liley, A.W. (1972) 'The fetus as a personality.' *Australia and New Zealand Journal of Psychiatry*, 6: 99–105.

Linney, J. (1983) *Multiple Births. Preparation, Birth, Managing Afterwards*. Chichester: John Wiley.

Little, J. and E.M. Bryan (1988) 'Congenital anomalies in twins.' In: I. MacGillivray, D.M. Campbell and B. Thompson (eds) *Twinning and Twins*. Chichester: John Wiley.

Little, J. and B. Thompson (1988) 'Descriptive epidemiology.' In: I. MacGillivray, D.M. Campbell and B. Thompson (eds) *Twinning and Twins*. Chichester: John Wiley.

Loehlin, J.C. and R.C. Nichols (1976) *Heredity, Environment and Personality: A Study of 850 Sets of Twins*. Austin: University of Texas Press.

Longo, L.D. and S.M. Yellon (1988) 'Biological timekeeping during pregnancy and the role of circadian rhythms in parturition.' In: W. Kunzel and A. Jensen (eds) *The Endocrine Control of the Fetus*. New York: Springer-Verlag.

Lopez-Zeno, J.A. and J. Navarro-Pando (1995) 'The intrauterine demise of one fetus.' In: L.G. Keith *et al.* (eds) *Multiple Pregnancy: Epidemiology, Gestation and Perinatal Outcome*. New York: The Parthenon Publishing Group.

Lopriore, E., F.P.H.A. Vandenbussche and E.S.M. Tiersma (1995) 'Twin-to-twin transfusion syndrome: New perspectives.' *Journal of Pediatrics*, 127: 675–680.

Luria, A.R. and F.I. Yudovitch (1959) *Speech and the Development of Mental Processes in the Child*. London: Staples Press.

Lykken, D.T. *et al.* (1992) 'Emergenesis: Genetic traits that may not run in families.' *American Psychologist*, 47: 1565–1577.

Lytton, H. (1980) *Parent–Child Interaction. The Socialization Process Observed in Twin and Singleton Families*. New York: Plenum Press.

Lytton, H., D. Conway and R. Suavé (1977) 'The impact of twinship on parent–child interaction.' *Journal of Personality and Social Psychology*, 35: 97–107.

Lytton, H. and D.M. Romney (1991) 'Parents' differential socialization of boys and girls: A meta-analysis.' *Psychological Bulletin*, 109: 267–296.

Maccoby, E.E. (1994) 'Commentary: Gender segregation in childhood.' In: C. Leaper (ed.) *Childhood Gender Segregation: Causes and Consequences*. New Directions for Child Development No. 65. San Francisco, Calif.: Jossey-Bass.

Maccoby, E.E. and C.N. Jacklin (1987) 'Gender segregation in childhood.' *Advances in Child Development and Behavior*, 20: 239–287.

McEvoy, S. and B. Dodd (1992) 'The communication abilities of 2- to 4-year-old twins.' *European Journal of Disorders of Communication*, 27: 72–88.

Macfarlane, A.J., F.V. Price and E.G. Daw (1990) 'Infertility drugs and procedures.' In: B.J. Blotting, A.J. Macfarlane and F.V. Price (eds) *Three, Four and More*. London: HMSO.

MacFarlane, A. (1975) 'Olfaction in the development of social preferences in the human neonate.' In: *Parent–Infant Interaction. Ciba Foundation Symposium 33*. New York: Elsevier.

—— (1977) *The Psychology of Childbirth*. London: Fontana Open Books.

MacGillivray, I. (1986) 'Epidemiology of twin pregnancy.' *Seminars in Perinatology*, 10 (1): 4–8.

MacGillivray, I. and D.M. Campbell (1988) 'Management of twin pregnancies.' In:

I. MacGillivray, D.M. Campbell and B. Thompson (eds) *Twinning and Twins*. Chichester: John Wiley.

MacGillivray, I., M. Samphier and J. Little (1988) 'Factors affecting twins.' In: I. McGillivray, D.M. Campbell and B. Thompson (eds) *Twinning and Twins*. Chichester: John Wiley.

Machin, G.A. (1993) 'Pathology of twinning.' In: J.W. Keeling (ed.) *Fetal and Neonatal Pathology* (2nd edn). London: Springer-Verlag.

—— (1996) 'Some causes of genotypic and phenotypic discordance in monozygotic twin pairs.' *American Journal of Medical Genetics*, 61: 216–228.

Machin, G.A., K. Still and T. Lalani (1996) 'Correlations of placental vascular anatomy and clinical outcomes in 69 monochorionic twin pregnancies.' *American Journal of Medical Genetics*, 61: 229–236.

Machin, G.A. and L.G. Keith (1999) *An Atlas of Multiple Pregnancy. Biology and Pathology*. New York: The Parthenon Publishing Group.

McLaren, A. (1976) *Mammalian Chimeras*. Cambridge: Cambridge University Press.

McNaughton, N. (1989) *Biology and Emotion. Problems in the Behavioural Sciences No. 8*. Cambridge: Cambridge University Press.

Mahler, M.S., F. Pine and A. Bergman (1975) *The Psychological Birth of the Human Infant*. London: Hutchinson.

Mahony, B.S. *et al.* (1990) 'The "stuck twin" phenomenon: ultrasonographic findings, pregnancy outcome, and management with serial amniocenteses.' *American Journal of Obstetrics and Gynecology*, 163: 1513–1522.

Main, M., N. Kaplan and J. Cassidy (1985) 'Security in infancy, childhood and adulthood: A move to the level of representation.' In: I. Bretherton and E. Waters (eds) *Growing Points of Attachment Theory and Research, SRCD Monographs No. 209. 50* (1–2): 66–104.

Majiskys, A. and M. Kout (1982) 'Another case of occurrence of two different fathers of twins by HLA typing.' *Tissue Antigens*, 20: 305.

Makin, J.W. and R.H. Porter (1989) 'Attractiveness of lactating females' breast odors to neonates.' *Child Development*, 60: 803–810.

Malter, H.E. and J. Cohen (1989) 'Blastocyst formation and hatching in vitro following zona drilling of mouse and human embryos.' *Gamete Research*, 24: 67–80.

Manning, F.A. (1995) 'Fetal movement and tone' In: F.A. Manning, *Fetal Medicine. Principles and Practice*. Norwalk, Conn.: Appleton and Lange.

Manning, F.A., L.D. Platt and L. Sipos (1979) 'Fetal movements in human pregnancies in the third trimester.' *Obstetrics and Gynecology*, 54: 699–702.

—— (1980) 'Antepartum fetal evaluation: Development of a fetal biophysical score.' *American Journal of Obstetrics and Gynecology*, 136: 787–792.

Marie Claire USA (1998) 'I had a face-lift to look more like my twin.' October: 129–133.

Martin, N.G., J.L. Beaini and M.E. Olsen (1984) 'Gonadotropin levels in mothers who have had two sets of twins.' *Acta Geneticae Medicae et Gemellologiae*, 33: 131–137.

Martin, P. and P. Bateson (1992) *Measuring Behaviour*. Cambridge: Cambridge University Press.

Maudry, M. and M. Nekula (1939) 'Special relations between children of the same age during the first two years of age.' *Journal of Genetic Psychology*, 54: 193–215.

Mazor, M. and H.F. Simons (1984) *Infertility: Medical, Emotional and Social Considerations*. New York: Human Sciences Press.

Meltzoff, A. and M.K. Moore (1977) 'Imitation of facial and manual gestures by human neonates.' *Science*, 198: 75–78.

—— (1983a) 'Newborn infants imitate adult facial gestures.' *Child Development*, 54: 702–709.

—— (1983b) 'The origins of imitation in infancy: Paradigm, phenomena and theories.' In: L.P. Lipsitt and C. Rovee-Collier (eds) *Advances in Infancy Research*, Vol. 2. Norwood: Ablex.

Mercer, R.T. *et al.* (1988) 'Further exploration of maternal and paternal fetal attachment.' *Research in Nursing and Health*, 11: 83–95.

Merenkov, K.E. (1995) 'Psychiatric considerations after the birth of multiples.' In: L.G. Keith *et al.* (eds) *Multiple Pregnancy: Epidemiology, Gestation and Perinatal Outcome*. New York: Parthenon Publishing Group.

Michel, G. and C. Moore (1995) *Developmental Psychobiology*. Cambridge, Mass.: MIT Press.

Miles, M.B. and A.M. Huberman (1984) *Qualitative Data Analysis. A Sourcebook of New Methods*. London: Sage.

Milham S. Jr. (1964) 'Pituitary gonadotropin and dizygotic twinning.' *Lancet*, ii: 566–567.

Miller, L., M. Rustin and J. Shuttelworth (eds) (1989) *Closely Observed Infants*. London: Duckworth.

Minde, K. (1993) 'Prematurity and serious medical illness in infancy: implications for development and intervention.' In: C.H. Zeanah Jr. (ed.) *Handbook of Infant Mental Health*. New York: The Guilford Press.

Minde, K., M. Perrotta and C. Corter (1982) 'The effect of neonatal complications in same-sexed premature twins on their mother's performance.' *Journal of the American Academy of Child Psychiatry*, 21: 446–452.

Minde, K. *et al.* (1990) 'Maternal preference between premature twins up to the age of four.' *Journal of the American Academy of Child and Adolescent Psychiatry*, 29: 367–374.

Mistretta, C.M. and R.M. Bradley (1986) 'Development of the sense of taste.' In: M.E. Blass (ed.) *Handbook of Behavioral Neurobiology*. Vol. 8: *Developmental Psychobiology and Developmental Neurobiology*. New York: Plenum Press.

Mittler, P. (1970) 'Biological and social aspects of language development in twins.' *Developmental Medicine and Child Neurology*, 12: 741–757.

—— (1971) *The Study of Twins*. Harmondsworth, Middlesex: Penguin.

Moessinger, A.C. (1983) 'Fetal akinesia deformation sequence: An animal model.' *Pediatrics*, 72: 857–863.

Mogford-Bevan, K. (1999) 'Twins and language development.' In: A. Sandbank (ed.) *Twin and Triplet Psychology*. London: Routledge.

Moilanen, I. (1987) 'Dominance and submissiveness between twins: consequences for mental health.' *Acta Geneticae Medicae et Gemellologiae*, 36: 257–265.

Moll, W. (1988) 'Placental hormone transfer.' In: W. Kunzel and A. Jensen (eds) *The Endocrine Control of the Fetus*. New York: Springer-Verlag.

Monga, M. and R.L. Reid (1992) 'Superfoetation in the human: a case report.' *Journal of the Canadian Society of Obstetrics and Gynecology*, 14 (2): 81–84.

Monteagudo, A., K. Murphy and I.E. Timor-Tritsch (1997) 'Epidemiology of twins.' In: A. Monteagudo and I.E. Timor-Tritsch (eds) *Ultrasound and Multifetal Pregnancy*. New York: The Parthenon Publishing Group Inc.

Moore, K.L. (1996) *Clinically Oriented Embryology*. Philadelphia, Pa.: W.B. Saunders.

Moore, K.L. and T.V.N. Persaud (1993) *Essentials of Embryology and Birth Defects*. Philadelphia, Pa.: W.B. Saunders.

—— (1998) *The Developing Human. Clinically Oriented Embryology* (6th edn). Philadelphia, Pa.: W.B. Saunders.

Morris, D. (1977) *Manwatching*. London: Jonathan Cape.

—— (1985) *Bodywatching*. London: Jonathan Cape.

Morton, J. and M.H. Johnson (1991) 'CONSPEC and CONLERN: A two-process theory of infant face recognition.' *Psychological Review*, 98: 164–181.

Moyer, J.A., L.R. Herrenkol and D.M. Jacobowitz (1978) 'Stress during pregnancy: Effect on catecholamines in discrete brain regions of offspring as adult.' *Brain Research*, 144: 173–178.

Mueller, E. and J. Brenner (1977) 'The origins of social skills and interaction among play-group toddlers.' *Child Development*, 48: 854–861.

Mulder, E.J.H. and G.H.A. Visser (1987) ' "Braxton Hicks" contractions and motor behavior in the near term fetus.' *American Journal of Obstetrics and Gynecology*, 156: 543–549.

Muller, A., J. Grouchy, M. Garretta, J. André, M. Roubin and J. Moullec (1974) 'Chimere sanguine chez des jumeaux dizygotes.' *Annales de Genetique*, 17: 23–28.

Murray, L. and P.J. Cooper (1997) *Postpartum Depression and Child Development*. New York: The Guilford Press.

Murray, L. and C. Trevarthen (1986) 'The infant's role in mother–infant communication.' *Journal of Child Language*, 13: 15–29.

Murray Parkes, C., J. Stevenson-Hinde and P. Marris (1991) *Attachment Across the Life Cycle*. London: Routledge.

Myrianthopolous, N.C. (1975) 'Congenital malformations in twins.' *Birth Defects*, 11 (8): 1–39.

Naeye, R.L. (1992) *Disorders of the Placenta, Fetus and Neonate*. St Louis, Mo.: Mosby Year Book.

Nakamura I. and T. Miura (1987) 'Seasonality of birth in mothers of like-sexed and unlike-sexed twins.' *Progress in Biometerology*, 5: 51–60.

Nasello-Patterson, C., R. Natale and G. Conners (1988) 'Ultrasonic evaluation of fetal body movements over 24 hours in the human fetus at 24 to 28 weeks gestation.' *American Journal of Obstetrics and Gynecology*, 158: 312–314.

Nathanielsz, P.W. (1992) *Life Before Birth. A Time To Be Born*. Ithaca, N.Y.: Promethean Press.

Nelson, C.A. (1994) 'Neural correlates of recognition memory in the first year of postnatal life.' In: G. Dawson and K.W. Fisher (eds) *Human Behavior and the Developing Brain*. New York: Guilford Press.

Newton, C.R. (1990) 'Psychological assessment and follow-up after in vitro fertilization. Assessing the impact of failure.' *Fertility and Sterility*, 54: 879–886.

Nijhuis, J.G. (1999) 'Maturation of the brain and behavioral states.' In: C.H. Rodeck and M.J. Whittle (eds) *Fetal Medicine: Basic Science and Clinical Practice*. London: Churchill Livingstone.

Nijhuis, J.G., C.B. Martin and H.F.R. Prechtl (1984) 'Behavioral states in the human fetus.' In: H.F.R. Prechtl (ed.) *Continuity of Neural Functions from Prenatal to Postnatal Life*. London: Mac Keith Press.

Nijhuis, J.G., H.F.R. Prechtl and C.B. Martin (1982) 'Are there behavioral states in the human fetus?' *Early Human Development*, 6: 177–195.

Noble, E. (1995) 'Psychophysiological adaptation to multiple pregnancy.' In: L.G. Keith *et al.* (eds) *Multiple Pregnancy: Epidemiology, Gestation and Perinatal Outcome*. New York: The Parthenon Publishing Group.

Nussbaum, M.C. and C.R. Sunstein (1997) *Clones and Clones*. New York: W.W. Norton and Company.

Nylander, P.P.S. (1971) 'Biosocial aspects of multiple births.' *Journal of Biosocial Sciences*, 3: 29–38.

—— (1973) 'Serum levels of gonadotropins in relation to multiple pregnancy in Nigeria.' *Journal of Obstetrics and Gynecology of the British Commonwealth*, 80: 651–658.

—— (1975) 'The causation of twinning.' In I. MacGillivray, P.P.S. Nylander and G. Corney (eds) *Human Multiple Reproduction*. Philadelphia, Pa.: W.B. Saunders.

—— (1978) 'Causes of high twinning frequencies in Nigeria.' In: W.E. Nance, G. Allen and P. Parisi (eds) *Twin Research: Biology and Epidemiology*. New York: Allan Liss.

O'Hara, M.W. (1994) *Postpartum Depression: Causes and Consequences*. New York: Springer-Verlag.

O'Kusky, J. and M. Colonnier (1982) 'Postnatal changes in the number of neurons and synapses in the visual cortex (area 17) of the Macaca monkey: A stereological analysis in normal and monocularly deprived animals.' *Journal of Comparative Neurology*, 210: 291–306.

Olson, G.M. and T. Sherman (1983) 'Attention, learning and memory in infants.' In: P.H. Mussen (ed.) *Handbook of Child Psychology.* Vol. 2: *Infancy and Developmental Psychobiology* (4th edn). [M.M. Haith and J.J. Campos vol. eds]. New York: Wiley.

Oppenheim, R.W. (1981) 'Ontogenetic adaptations and retrogressive processes in the development of the nervous system and behavior: A neuroembryological perspective.' In: K.J. Connolly and H.F.R. Prechtl (eds) *Maturation and Development: Biological and Psychological Perspectives.* Philadelphia, Pa.: Lippincott.

—— (1984) 'Ontogenetic adaptations in neural development: Toward a more "ecological" developmental psychobiology.' In: H.F.R. Prechtl (ed.) *Continuity of Neural Functions from Prenatal to Postnatal Life.* London: Mac Keith Press.

—— (1991) 'Cell death during development of the nervous system.' *Annual Review of Neurosciences,* 14: 453–501.

Otake, M. and W.J. Schull (1984) 'In utero exposure of A-bomb radiation and mental retardation.' *British Journal of Radiology,* 57: 409–414.

Papiernick, E. (1991) 'Cost of multiple pregnancies.' In: D. Harvey and E. Bryan (eds) *The Stress of Multiple Births.* London: Multiple Birth Foundation.

Papiernick-Berkauer, E. and A. Richards (1991) 'Le moment optimal de la naissance des jumeaux.' In: E. Papiernick-Berkhauer and J.C. Pons (eds) *Les Grossesses Multiples.* Paris: Doin.

Papousek, H. and M. Papousek (1975) 'Cognitive aspects of preverbal social interaction between human infants and adults.' In: M. Hofer (ed.) *Parent–Infant Interaction.* Amsterdam: Elsevier.

—— (1993) 'Apprentissage chez le nourisson: un point de vue synthétique.' In: V. Poutas and F. Jouen (eds) *Les comportements du bébé: expression de son savoir?* Liège: Pierre Mardaga.

Parisi, P. *et al.* (1983) 'Familial incidence of twinning.' *Nature,* 304: 626–628.

Parke, R.D. (1996) *Fatherhood.* Cambridge, Mass.: Harvard University Press.

Parke, R.D. and B.J. Tinsley (1987) 'Family interaction in infancy.' In: J. Osofsky (ed.) *Handbook of Infant Development* (2nd edn). New York: John Wiley.

Parkes, M.J. (1991) 'Sleep and wakefulness – do they occur in utero?' In: M.A. Hanson (ed.) *Fetal and Neonatal Brain Stem.* Cambridge: Cambridge University Press.

Parmelee, A.H. and E. Stern (1972) 'Development of states in infants.' In: C. Clemente, D. Purpura and F. Meyer (eds) *Sleep and the Maturing Nervous System.* New York: Academic Press.

Parmelee, A.H. *et al.* (1969) 'A periodic cerebral rhythm in newborn infants.' *Experimental Neurology,* 25: 575–584.

Parmelee, A.H. *et al.* (1968) 'Maturation of EEG activity during sleep in premature infants.' *Electroencephalography and Clinical Neurophysiology,* 24: 319–329.

Patrick, J. *et al.* (1980a) 'Patterns of human fetal breathing during the last 10 weeks of pregnancy.' *Obstetrics and Gynecology,* 56: 24–30.

—— (1980b) 'Circadian rhythms in maternal plasma cortisol and estriol concentrations at 30 to 31, 34 to 35, and 38 to 39 weeks gestational age.' *American Journal of Obstetrics and Gynecology,* 136: 325–334.

—— (1982) 'Patterns of gross fetal body movements over 24-hour observation intervals during the last 10 weeks of pregnancy.' *American Journal of Obstetrics and Gynecology,* 142: 363–371.

Patten, R.M. *et al.* (1989) 'Twin embolization syndrome: prenatal sonographic detection and significance.' *Radiology,* 173: 685–689.

Patton, M.Q. (1990) *Qualitative Evaluation and Research Methods.* Newbury Park, Calif.: Sage.

Peck, J.E. (1995) 'Development of hearing. Part III: Postnatal development.' *Journal of the American Academy of Audiology,* 6: 113–123.

Pedersen, F.A. (ed.) (1980) *The Father–Infant Relationship: Observational Studies in the Family Setting*. New York: Praeger.

Pedersen, I.K. *et al.* (1980) 'Monozygotic twins with dissimilar phenotypes and chromosome complements.' *Acta Obstetrica et Gynecologica Scandinavica*, 4: 99–105.

Pedersen, N.L. *et al.* (1988) 'Neuroticism, extraversion and related traits in adult twins reared apart and reared together.' *Journal of Gerontology*, 44 (4): 100–105.

Pedersen, P.E., C.A. Greer and G.M. Shepherd (1986) 'Early development of olfactory function.' In: E. Blass (ed.) *Handbook of Behavioral Neurobiology*. Vol. 8: *Developmental Psychobiology and Developmental Neurobiology*. New York: Plenum Press.

Pedersen, P.E. *et al.* (1983) 'Evidence for olfactory function in utero.' *Science*, 221: 478–480.

Peiper, A. (1963) *Cerebral Function in Infancy and Childhood. The International Behavioral Sciences Series* (J. Wortis, ed.). New York: Consultants Bureau.

Perlman, E.J. *et al.* (1990) 'Sexual discordance in monozygotic twins.' *American Journal of Medical Genetics*, 37: 551–557.

Peters, D.A.V. (1984) 'Prenatal stress: effect on development of rat brain adrenergic receptors.' *Pharmacology, Biochemistry and Behavior*, 21: 417–422.

—— (1986) 'Prenatal stress: effect on development of rat brain serotonergic neurons.' *Pharmacology, Biochemistry and Behavior*, 24: 1377–1382.

Petterson, B., F. Stanley and D. Henderson (1990) 'Cerebral palsy in multiple births in Western Australia.' *American Journal of Medical Genetics*, 37: 346–351.

Philips, C.J. and M. Watkinson (1981) 'Characteristics of the families and similarity of environment within twin pairs.' In: C.J. Philips (ed.) *Twins Research: Birmingham 1968–(1972)*, Vol. 2, Part 1. Birmingham: Centre for Child Study, University of Birmingham.

Piaget, J. (1923) *Le langage et la pensée chez l'enfant*. Neuchatel: Delachaux et Niestlé.

Pinker, S. (1984) *Language Learnability and Language Development*. Cambridge, Mass.: Harvard University Press.

—— (1994) *The Language Instinct*. New York: Harper and Collins.

Piontelli, A. (1989) 'A study on twins before and after birth.' *International Review of Psycho-Analysis*, 68: 453–463.

—— (1992) *From Fetus to Child*. London: Routledge.

—— (1995) 'Non-shared intra-uterine environmental factors: pre and post natal observations of twins.' Invited Address, Fifteenth Annual Spring Meeting of the American Psychological Association (Division 39). Santa Monica, California, 25–30 April.

—— (1998) 'L'observation des jumeaux avant la naissance.' In: R. Frydman and M. Szeyer (eds) *Le Bébé dans tous ses états*. Paris: Odile Jacob.

—— (1999) 'Twins in utero.' In: A. Sandbank (ed.) *Twin and Triplet Psychology*. London: Routledge.

—— (2000) 'Is there something wrong? The impact of technology in pregnancy.' In: J. Raphael-Leff (ed.) *Perinatal Loss and Breakdown*. London: IPA Publications.

Piontelli, A. *et al.* (1997) 'Patterns of evoked behavior in twin pregnancies during the first 22 weeks of gestation.' Special Issue H.F.R. Prechtl (ed.), *Early Human Development*, 50: 39–46.

Piontelli, A. *et al.* (1999) 'Differences and similarities in the intra-uterine behavior of Monozygotic and Dizygotic twins.' *Twin Research*, 2 (4): 264–273.

Pison, G. (1991) 'Mythes et rituels autour de la gémellité en Afrique.' E. Papiernik-Berkhauer and J. Pons (eds) *Les Grossesses Multiples*. Paris: Doin.

Playfair, G. (1999) 'Telepathy and identical twins.' *Journal of the Society for Psychological Research*, 63 (854): 86–89.

Plomin, R. (1990) 'The role of inheritance in behavior.' *Science*, 248: 183–188.

Plomin, R. and D. Daniels (1987) 'Why are children in the same family so different from one another?' *Behavioral and Brain Sciences*, 10: 1–60.

Plomin, R. and J. Dunn (1986) *The Study of Temperament: Changes, Continuities and Challenges*. Hillsdale, N.J.: Lawrence Erlbaum Associates.

Plomin, R. *et al.* (1980) 'EAS temperaments during the last half of the life span: twins reared apart and twins reared together.' *Psychology and Aging*, 3 (1): 43–50.

Plutchik, R. (1990) 'Evolutionary bases of empathy.' In: N. Eisenberg and J. Strayer (eds) *Empathy and its Development*. Cambridge Studies in Social and Emotional Development Series. Cambridge: Cambridge University Press.

Polishuk, W.Z., N. Laufer and E. Sadowsky (1975) 'Fetal reaction to external light.' *Harefuah*, 89: 397–395.

Porter, R.H. (1987) 'Kin recognition: Function and mediating mechanisms.' In: C. Crawford, M. Smith and D. Krebs (eds) *Sociobiology and Psychology: Ideas, Issues and Applications*. Hillsdale, N.J.: Erlbaum.

Porter, R.H., J.M. Cernoch and R.D. Balogh (1985) 'Odor signatures and kin recognition.' *Physiology and Behavior*, 34: 445–448.

Porter, R.H., J.A. Matochick and J.W. Makin (1986) 'Discrimination between full-sibling spiny mice (Acomys cahirinius) by olfactory signatures.' *Animal Behavior*, 34: 1182–1188.

Porter, R.H., S.A. McFayden-Ketchum and G.A. King (1989) 'Underlying bases of recognition signatures in spiny mice (Acomys cahirinius).' *Animal Behavior*, 37: 638–644.

Porter, R.H. and J.D. Moore (1981) 'Human kin recognition by olfactory cues.' *Physiology and Behavior*, 27: 493–495.

Poznanski, E.O. (1972) 'The "replacement child": A saga of unresolved parental grief.' *Journal of Pediatrics*, 81: 1190–1197.

Prechtl, H.F.R. (1974) 'The behavioral states of the newborn infant. A review.' *Brain Research*, 76: 185–212.

—— (1981) 'The study of neural development as a perspective of clinical problems.' In: K.J. Connolly and H.F.R. Prechtl (eds) *Clinics in Developmental Medicine*, Nos 77–78. London: Heinemann.

—— (1984) 'Continuity and change in early neural development.' In: H.F.R. Prechtl (ed.) *Continuity of Neural Functions from Prenatal to Postnatal Life*. London: Mac Keith Press.

—— (1985) 'Ultrasound studies of human fetal behavior.' *Early Human Development*, 12: 91–98.

—— (1989) 'Fetal behavior.' In: A. Hill and J.J. Volpe (eds) *Fetal Neurology*. New York: Raven Press.

Preedy, P. (1999) 'Meeting the educational needs of pre-school and primary aged twins and higher multiples.' In: A. Sandbank (ed.) *Twin and Triplet Psychology*. London: Routledge.

Price, B. (1950) 'Primary biases in twin studies.' *American Journal of Human Genetics*, 2: 293–352.

Pridjian, G. and L. Chin-Chu (1993) 'Multifetal gestation.' In: L. Chin-Chu, M.S. Verp and R.E. Sabbagha (eds) *The High-Risk Fetus*. New York: Springer-Verlag.

Prins, R.P. (1994) 'The second-born twin: Can we improve outcomes?' *American Journal of Obstetrics and Gynecology*, 170: 1649–1656.

Provine, R.R. (1986) 'Behavioral neuroembryology: Motor perspectives.' In: W.T. Greenough and J.M. Juraska (eds) *Developmental Neuropsychology*. Orlando, Fla.: Academic Press.

—— (1993) 'Prenatal behavior development: ontogenetic adaptations and non-linear processes.' In: G.J.P. Savelsbergh (ed.) *The Development of Coordination in Infancy*. New York: Elsevier.

Provis, J.M. *et al.* (1985) 'Human fetal optic nerve: Overproduction and elimination of retinal axons during development.' *Journal of Comparative Neurology*, 238: 92–101.

Purves, D. (1988) *Body and Brain. A Trophic Theory of Neural Connections*. Cambridge, Mass.: Harvard University Press.

Rabinovich, J., G. Barkai and B. Reichman (1987) 'Randomized management of the second nonvertex twin: Vaginal delivery or Cesarean section.' *American Journal of Obstetrics and Gynecology,* 156: 52–56.

Radke-Yarrow, M., C. Zahn-Walker and M. Chapman (1983) 'Children's prosocial dispositions and behavior.' In: P.H. Mussen (ed.) *Handbook of Child Psychology.* Vol. IV: *Socialization, Personality and Social Development* (4th edn). New York: John Wiley.

Rakic, P. (1978) 'Neuronal migration and contact interaction in primate telencephalon.' *Postgraduate Medical Journal,* 54: 25–40.

—— (1988) 'Defects of neuronal migration and pathogenesis of cortical malformations.' *Progess in Brain Research,* 73: 15–37.

—— (1991) 'Plasticity of cortical development.' In: S.E. Brauth, W.S. Hall and R.J. Dooling (eds) *Plasticity of Development.* Cambridge, Mass.: MIT Press.

Rakic, P. *et al.* (1986) 'Concurrent overproduction of synapses in diverse regions of the primate cerebral cortex.' *Science,* 232: 232–235.

Raphael-Leff, J. (1991) *Psychological Processes of Childbearing.* London: Chapman and Hall.

—— (1996) *Pregnancy. The Inside Story.* New York: Aronson.

Reading, A. (1983) 'The influence of maternal anxiety on the course and outcome of pregnancy: A review.' *Health Psychology,* 2 (2): 187–202.

Reading, A. *et al.* (1984) 'Psychological changes over the course of pregnancy: A study of attitudes towards the fetus/neonate.' *Health Psychology,* 3: 211–221.

Redshaw, J. and M. Rutter (1991) 'Growing up as a twin: Twin–singleton differences in psychological development.' In: D. Harvey and E. Bryan (eds) *The Stress of Multiple Births.* London: The Multiple Births Foundation.

Rehmann, J.T. (1979) 'A study of the conjoint drawings of identical and fraternal twins: A pilot study.' *Art Psychotherapy,* 6: 109–117.

Reisner, D.P., B.S. Mahony and C.N. Petty (1993) 'Stuck twin syndrome: Outcome of thirty-seven consecutive cases.' *American Journal of Obstetrics and Gynecology,* 169: 991–995.

Richards, M.P.M. (1974) *The Integration of a Child into a Social World.* Cambridge: Cambridge University Press.

—— (1978) 'Possible effects of early separation on later development in children.' In: F.S. Brimblecombe, M.P.M. Richards and N.R.C. Roberton (eds) *Early Separation and Special Care Nurseries.* London: Heinemann Medical Books.

—— (1979) 'Effects on development of medical interventions and the separation of newborns from their parents.' In: D. Shaffer and J. Dunn (eds) *The First Year of Life: Psychological and Medical Implications of Early Experience.* Chichester: John Wiley.

—— (1983) 'Parent–child relationships: Some general considerations.' In: A.J. Davies, M.P.M. Richards and N.R.C. Roberton (eds) *Parent–Baby Attachment in Premature Infants.* London: Croom Helm.

—— (1989) 'The social and emotional needs of the parents and baby.' In: D. Harvey, R.W.I. Cooke and G.A. Levitt (eds) *The Baby Under 1000g.* London: Butterworth.

Rich-Harris, J. (1998) *The Nurture Assumption.* New York: The Free Press.

Richman, J.A., V.D. Raskin and C. Gaines (1991) 'Gender roles, social support, and postpartum depressive symptomatology: The benefits of caring.' *Journal of Nervous and Mental Diseases,* 179: 139–147.

Riese, M.L. (1990) 'Neonatal temperament in monozygotic and dizygotic twin pairs.' *Child Development,* 61: 1230–1237.

—— (1998) 'Predicting infant temperament from neonatal reactivity for AGA/SGA twin pairs.' *Twin Research,* 1: 65–70.

Rizzardo, R. *et al.* (1985) 'Psychosocial aspects during pregnancy and obstetrical complications.' *Journal of Psychosomatic Obstetrics and Gynaecology,* 4: 11–22.

Roberts, A.B., D. Little and S. Campbell (1978) '24-hour studies of fetal respiratory movements and fetal body movements: relationship to glucose, catecolamine, oestriol, and cortisol levels.' In: A. Kujak (ed.) *Recent Advances in Ultrasound Diagnosis*. Amsterdam: Excerpta Medica.

Robertson, S.S. (1988) 'Mechanism and function of cyclicity in spontaneous movement.' In: W.P. Smootherman and S.C. Robinson (eds) *Behavior of the Fetus*. Caldwell, N.J.: Telford Press.

Robertson, S.S. *et al.* (1982) 'Human fetal movement: Spontaneous oscillations near one cycle per minute.' *Science*, 218: 1327–1330.

Robin, M., D. Josse and C. Tourrette (1988) 'Early mother–twins interaction.' *Acta Geneticae Medicae et Gemellologiae*, 37: 151–159.

—— (1991) 'Forms of family reorganization following the birth of twins.' *Acta Geneticae Medicae et Gemellologiae*, 40: 67–80.

Robinson, H.P. and J.S. Caines (1977) 'Sonar evidence of early pregnancy failure in patients with twin conceptions.' *British Journal of Obstetrics and Gynecology*, 84: 22–25.

Robinson, S.R. and W.P. Smootherman (1987) 'Environmental determinants of behavior in the rat fetus. II. The emergence of sychronous movement.' *Animal Behavior*, 35: 1652–1662.

Roffwarg, H., J. Muzio and W. Dement (1966) 'Ontogenic development of the human sleep–dream cycle.' *Science*, 152: 604–607.

Rogers, J.G., L. Voullaire and H. Gould (1982) 'Monozygotic twins discordant for Trisomy 21.' *American Journal of Medical Genetics*, 11: 143–146.

Rolbin, S.H. and E.M. Hew (1991) 'Uterine relaxation can be life saving.' *Canadian Journal of Anesthesiology*, 38: 939–943.

Rophie, H. and E. Galenson (1981) *Infantile Origins of Sexual Identity*. New York: International Universities Press.

Rossignol, S., G.P. Lund and T. Drew (1988) 'The role of sensory inputs in regulating patterns of rhythmical movements in higher vertebrates: A comparison between locomotion, respiration and mastication.' In: A.H. Cohen, S. Rossignol and S. Grillner (eds) *Neural Control of Rhythmic Movements in Vertebrates*. New York: Wiley.

Rovee-Collier, C. (1987) 'Learning and memory.' In: J.D. Osofsky (ed.) *Handbook of Infant Development*. New York: Wiley.

Rovee-Collier, C. and D. Dufault (1991) 'Multiple contexts and memory retrieval at 3 months.' *Developmental Psychobiology*, 24: 39–50.

Rovee-Collier, C. *et al.* (1980) 'Reactivation of infant memory.' *Science*, 208: 1159–1161.

Rowland, C. (1991) 'Family relationships.' In: D. Harvey and E.M. Bryan (eds) *The Stress of Multiple Births*. London: Multiple Births Foundation.

Rubenstein, J. and C. Howes (1976) 'The effects of peers on toddler interaction with mother and toys.' *Child Development*, 47: 597–605.

Ruble, D.N. and C. Martin (1998) 'Gender development.' In: N. Eisenberg (ed.) *Handbook of Child Psychology*. Vol. 3: *Personality and Social Development* (5th edn). New York: Wiley.

Rutter, M. (1971) 'Parent–child separation: Psychological effects on the children.' *Journal of Child Psychology and Psychiatry*, 2: 435–450.

—— (1981) *Maternal Deprivation Reassessed* (2nd edn). London: Penguin Books.

—— (1988) *Studies of Psychosocial Risk: the Power of Longitudinal Data*. Cambridge: Cambridge University Press.

Rutter, M. and J. Redshaw (1991) 'Annotation: growing up as a twin: Twin–singleton differences in psychological development.' *Journal of Child Psychology and Psychiatry*, 32: 885–895.

Rutter, M. and E. Schopler (1987) 'Autism and pervasive developmental disorders: Concepts and diagnostic issues.' *Journal of Autism and Developmental Disorders*, 17: 159–186.

Rutter, M., E. Simonoff and J. Silberg (1993) 'How informative are twin studies of child pyschopathology?' In: T.J. Bouchard Jr. and P. Propping (eds) *Twins as a Tool of Behavioral Genetics*. Chichester: Wiley.

Rydstrom, H. (1990) 'The effects of maternal age, parity and sex of the twins on twin perinatal mortality: A population based study.' *Acta Geneticae Medicae et Gemellologiae*, 39: 401–408.

Saarikoski, S. (1974) 'Fate of noradrenaline in the human foeto-placental unit.' *Acta Physiologica Scandinavica*, 421: 1–82.

Sandbank, A.C. (1988) 'The effect of twins on family relationships.' *Acta Geneticae Medicae et Gemellologiae*, 39: 497–500.

—— (1991) *Twins and The Family*. South Wirral, UK: TAMBA.

Sandbank, A.C. and G.A. Brown (1990) 'An examination of the psychological and behavioral factors in the development of language retardation in twins.' *Acta Geneticae Medicae et Gemellologiae*, 39: 497–500.

Saunders, N.J., R.J.M. Snijers and K.H. Nicolaides (1992) 'Therapeutic amniocentesis in twin–twin transfusion syndrome appearing in the second trimester of pregnancy.' *American Journal of Obstetrics and Gynecology*, 166: 820–824.

Savary, C. and C. Gros (1995) *Des Jumeaux et des autres*. Geneva: Musée d'Ethnographie.

Savic, S. (1980) *How Twins Learn to Talk. A Study of Speech Development of Twins*. London: Academic Press.

Scardo, J.A., J.M. Ellings and R.B. Newman (1995) 'Prospective determination of chorionicity, amnionicity, and zygosity in twin gestations.' *American Journal of Obstetrics and Gynecology*, 173: 1376–1380.

Scarr, S. (1968) 'Environmental bias in twin studies.' *Eugenetic Quarterly*, 15: 34–40.

Scarr, S. and K. McCartney (1983) 'How people make their own environments: A theory of genotype–environment effects.' *Child Development*, 54: 424–435.

Schaall, B. (1988) 'Olfaction in infants and children: Developmental and functional perspectives.' *Chemical Senses*, 13: 145–190.

Schaall, B. *et al.* (1980) 'Les stimulations olfactives dans les relations entre l'enfant et la mère.' *Reproduction, Nutrition et Développement*, 20: 843–858.

Schaffer, H.R. (ed.) (1977) *Studies in Mother–Infant Interaction*. New York: Academic Press.

Schaffer, H.R. and C. Liddell (1984) 'Adult–child interaction under dyadic and polyadic conditions.' *British Journal of Developmental Psychology*, 2: 33–42.

Schmidt, H.J. and G.K. Beauchamp (1988) 'Adult-like odor preferences and aversions in three-year-old children.' *Child Development*, 59: 1136–1143.

Schore, A.N. (1994) *Affect Regulation and the Origin of the Self*. Hillsdale, N.J.: Lawrence Erlbaum Associates.

Schwartz, M.R. *et al.* (1980) 'The use of menopausal and chorionic gonadotrophins for induction of ovulation.' *American Journal of Obstetrics and Gynecology*, 138: 801–807.

Schwarz, J.C. (1972) 'Effects of peer familiarity on the behavior of preschoolers in a novel situation.' *Journal of Personality and Social Psychology*, 24: 276–284.

Segal, N.L. (1984) 'Cooperation, competition and altruism within twin sets: A reappraisal.' *Ethology and Sociobiology*, 5: 163–177.

—— (1999) *Entwined Lives: Twins and What They Tell Us About Human Behavior*. New York: Dutton.

Segal, N.L. and S.L. Ream (1998) 'Decrease in grief intensity for deceased twin and non-twin relatives.' *Personality and Individual Differences*, 25: 317–325.

Segal, N.L. and J.M. Russell (1992) 'Twins in the classroom: School policy issues and recommendations.' *Journal of Educational Psychology Consultations*, 3: 69–84.

Sepulveda, W. *et al.* (1996) 'The lambda sign at 10–14 weeks of gestation as a predictor of chorionicity in twin pregnancies.' *Ultrasound in Obstetrics and Gynecology*, 7: 421–423.

Serbin, L.A. *et al.* (1994) 'The emergence of segregation in toddler playgroups.' In: C. Leaper (ed.) *Childhood Gender Segregation: Causes and Consequences*. New Directions for Child Development No. 65. San Francisco, Calif.: Jossey-Bass.

Sergent, B. (1992) 'De quelques jumeaux indo-européens.' *Topique*, 50: 205–238.

Sharma, S. *et al.* (1995) 'Detection of twin–twin transfusion syndrome by first trimester ultrasonography.' *Journal of Ultrasound Medicine,* 14: 635–637.

Shatz, M. (1983) 'Communication.' In: P.H. Mussen (ed.) *Child Psychology.* Vol. III: *Cognitive Development.* [J.H. Flavell and E.M. Markman vol. eds]. New York: John Wiley.

Sidman, R.L. and P. Rakic (1982) 'Development of the human central nervous system.' In: W. Haymeker and R.D. Adams (eds) *Histology and Histopathology of the Nervous System.* Springfield, Ill.: C.C. Thomas.

Simner, M.L. (1971) 'Newborn's response to the cry of another infant.' *Developmental Psychology,* 5: 136–150.

Skupski, D.W. and F.A. Chervanek (1996) 'Maternal complications.' In: S.A. Gall (ed.) *Multiple Pregnancy and Delivery.* St Louis, Mo.: Mosby Year Book.

Slotkin, T.A. and F.J. Seidler (1989) 'Catecholamines and stress in the newborn.' In: S. Breznitz and O. Zinder (eds) *Molecular Biology of Stress.* New York: Alan R. Liss.

Smootherman, W.P. and R.R. Robinson (1988) 'The uterus as environment: The ecology of fetal behavior.' In: E.M. Blass (ed.) *Handbook of Behavioral Neurobiology.* Vol. 9: *Developmental Psychobiology and Behavioral Ecology.* New York: Plenum Press.

—— (1989) 'The prenatal origins of behavioral organization.' *Psychological Science,* 1: 97–106.

Snowden, R. and G.D. Mitchell (1981) *The Artificial Family.* London: Allen and Unwin.

Snowden, R., G.D. Mitchell and E.M. Snowden (1983) *Artificial Reproduction: A Social Investigation.* London: Allen and Unwin.

Sommer, R., H. Osmond and L. Pancyr (1961) 'Selection of twins for ESP experimentation.' *International Journal of Parapsychology,* 3: 55–73.

Spillman, J.R. (1985) ' "You have a little bonus my dear". The effect on mothers of the diagnosis of multiple pregnancy.' *Bulletin of the British Society of Medical Ultrasound,* 39: 6–9.

—— (1992) 'A study of maternity provision and multiple births in the UK.' *Acta Geneticae Medicae et Gemellologiae,* 41 (4): 353–364.

—— (1993) 'Multiple pregnancy: Effects of caesarean section and epidural anaesthesia on postnatal health.' *Proceeding of the 23rd International Congress of Midwives, Vancouver,* IV: 1766–1776.

—— (1999) 'Antenatal and postnatal influences in family relationships.' In: A.C. Sandbank (ed.) *Twin and Triplet Psychology.* London: Routledge

Stainton, M.C. (1985) 'The fetus: A growing member of family.' *Family Relations,* 34: 321–326.

Stern, D.N. (1974) 'The goal and structure of mother–infant play.' *Journal of the Academy of Child Psychiatry,* 13: 402–421.

—— (1977) *The First Relationship: Infant and Mother.* Cambridge, Mass.: Harvard University Press.

—— (1985) *The Interpersonal World of the Infant.* New York: Basic Books.

Stern, D.N. and N. Bruschweiler-Stern (1998) *The Birth of a Mother.* New York: Basic Books.

Stern, D.N. *et al.* (1983) 'The prosody of maternal speech: Infant age and context-related changes.' *Journal of Child Language,* 10: 1–15.

Storlazzi, E. *et al.* (1987) 'Ultrasonic diagnosis of discordant fetal growth in twin gestations.' *Obstetrics and Gynecology,* 69: 363–368.

Storrs, E.E. and R.J. Williams (1968) 'A study of monozygous quadruplet armadillos in relation to mammalian inheritance.' *Proceedings of the National Academy of Science (USA),* 60: 910–914.

Sumethkul, V., S. Jirasiritham and T. Sura (1994) 'Renal transplantation between identical twins: The application of reciprocal full-thickness skin grafts as a guideline for anti-rejection therapy.' *Transplant Procedures,* 26: 2141–2142.

Talbert, D.G., P. Benson and J. Dewhurst (1982) 'Fetal response to maternal anxiety: A factor in antepartum heart rate monitoring.' *Journal of Obstetrics and Gynaecology*, 3: 34–38.

Tchobroutsky, C. (1991) 'Retard de croissance intra-utérin et grossesse gémellaire.' In: E. Papiernick-Berkhauer and J.C. Pons (eds) *Les Grossesses Multiples*. Paris: Doin.

Teraski, P.I. *et al.* (1978) 'Twins with two different fathers identified by HLA.' *New England Journal of Medicine*, 299: 590–592.

Tesla, C. and J. Dunn (1992) 'Getting along or getting your way: The development of young children's argument in conflicts with mother and siblings.' *Social Development*, 1: 107–121.

Thelen, E. (1990) 'Dynamical systems and the generation of individual differences.' In: J. Colombo and J. Fagen (eds) *Individual Differences in Infancy: Reliability, Stability, Prediction*. Hillsdale, N.J.: Erlbaum.

Thelen, E. and L.B. Smith (1994) *A Dynamic System Approach to the Development of Cognition and Action*. Cambridge, Mass.: MIT Press.

Thornburgh, K.L. (1991) 'Fetal response to intrauterine stress.' In: *The Childhood Environment and Adult Disease*. Ciba Foundation Symposium 156. Chichester: Wiley.

Thorpe, K. *et al.* (1991) 'Comparison of prevalence of depression in mothers of twins and mothers of singletons.' *British Medical Journal*, 302: 875–878.

Timor-Tritsch, I.E. (1986) 'The effect of external stimuli on fetal behaviour.' *European Journal of Obstetrics, Gynecology and Reproductive Biology*, 21: 321–329.

Trehub, S.E. and B. Schneider (1985) *Auditory Development in Infancy*. New York: Plenum Press.

Trevarthen, C.B. (1976) 'Descriptive analyses of infant communicative behaviour.' In: H.R. Schaffer (ed.) *Studies in Mother–Infant Interaction*. London: Academic Press.

—— (1979) 'Communication and cooperativity in early infancy: A description of primary intersubjectivity.' In: M. Bollowa (ed.) *Before Speech*. Cambridge: Cambridge University Press.

Trevarthen, C. *et al.* (1996) *Children with Autism: Diagnosis and Interventions to Meet Their Needs*. London: Kingsley.

Trevarthen, C. and H. Marwick (1986) 'Signs of motivation for speech in infants and the nature of a mother's support for development of language.' In: B. Lindblom and R. Zetterstrom (eds) *Precursors of Early Speech*. Basingstoke: Macmillan.

Tronick, E.Z. and T. Field (1987) *Maternal Depression and Infant Disturbance*. San Francisco, Calif.: Jossey-Bass.

Trowell, J. (1982) 'Possible effects of emergency caesarian section on the mother–child relationship.' *Early Human Development*, 7: 41–51.

Tyschen, L. (1994) 'Vision in infants: Development and testing.' In: S.J. Isenberg (ed.) *The Eye in Infancy* (2nd edn). St Louis, Mo.: Mosby Year Book.

Urig, M.A., W.H. Clewell and J.P. Elliott (1990) 'Twin–twin transfusion syndrome.' *American Journal of Obstetrics and Gynecology*, 163: 1522–1526.

Uzgiris, I.C. (1981) 'Two functions of imitation during infancy.' *International Journal of Behavioural Development*, 4: 1–12.

—— (1984) 'Imitation in infancy: Its interpersonal aspects.' In: M. Perlemutter (ed.) *Minnesota Symposium on Child Psychology*, Vol. 17. New York: Lawrence Erlbaum Associates.

—— (1990) 'The social context of infant imitation.' In: M. Lewis and S. Feinman (eds) *Social Influences and Socialization in Infancy*. New York: Plenum Press.

—— (1993) 'L'imitation dans les interactions précoces.' In: V. Poutas and F. Jouen (eds) *Les Comportements du bébé: expression de son savoir?* Liège: Pierre Mardaga.

Vandell, D.L. (1980) 'Sociability with peer and mother during the first year.' *Developmental Psychology*, 16: 355–361.

Vandell, D.L. *et al.* (1988) 'Social development in infant twins: Peer and mother child relationships.' *Child Development*, 59: 168–177.

Van den Bergh, B.R.H. (1992) 'Maternal emotions during pregnancy and fetal and neonatal behavior.' In: J.H. Nijhuis (ed.) *Fetal Behavior: Developmental and Perinatal Aspects.* Oxford: Oxford University Press.

Van den Bergh, B.R.H. *et al.* (1989) 'The effect of (induced) maternal emotions on fetal behavior: A controlled study.' *Early Human Development,* 19: 9–19.

Villeneuve, C., C. Laroche and A. Lippman (1987) 'Psychological aspects of ultrasound imaging during pregnancy.' *Canadian Journal of Psychiatry,* 33: 530–535.

Visser, G.H.A. *et al.* (1983) 'External physical stimulation of the human fetus during episodes of low heart rate variation.' *American Journal of Obstetrics and Gynecology,* 145: 579–584.

Volling, B.L., L.M. Youngblade and J. Belski (1997) 'Young children's social relationships with siblings and friends.' *American Journal of Orthopsychiatry,* 67: 102–111.

Volpe, J.J. (1987) 'Neuronal proliferation, migration, organization and myelination.' In: J.J. Volpe, *Neurology of the Newborn* (2nd edn). Philadelphia, Pa.: W.B. Saunders.

Voss, D.H. (1996) 'Outcome.' In: S.A. Gall (ed.) *Multiple Pregnancy and Delivery.* St Louis, Mo.: Mosby Year Book.

Vries, J.I.P. de (1992a) 'The first trimester.' In: J.G. Nijhuis (ed.) *Fetal Behavior. Developmental and Perinatal Aspects.* Oxford: Oxford University Press.

—— (1992b) 'The second trimester.' In: J.G. Nijhuis (ed.) *Fetal Behavior. Developmental and Perinatal Aspects.* Oxford: Oxford University Press.

—— (1992c) 'The third trimester.' In: J.G. Nijhuis (ed.) *Fetal Behavior. Developmental and Perinatal Aspects.* Oxford: Oxford University Press.

Vries, J.I.P. de, G.H.A. Visser and H.F.R. Prechtl (1982) 'The emergence of fetal behavior. I: Qualitative aspects.' *Early Human Development,* 7: 301–322.

—— (1984) 'The emergence of fetal behavior. II: Quantitative aspects.' *Early Human Development,* 16: 85–103.

—— (1988) 'The emergence of fetal behavior. III: Individual differences and consistencies.' *Early Human Development,* 16: 85–103.

Wahlsten, D. (1990) 'Insensitivity of the analysis of variance to heredity–environment interactions.' *Behavioral and Brain Sciences,* 13: 109–161.

Wallace, M. (1986) *The Silent Twins.* Harmondsworth, Middlesex: Penguin Books.

Wallace, P. (1977) 'Individual discrimination of humans by odors.' *Physiology and Behavior,* 19: 577–579.

Wax, J.R., K.J. Blakemore and P. Blohm (1991) 'Stuck twin with co-twin nonimmune hydrops: Successful treatment by amniocentesis.' *Fetal Diagnosis and Therapy,* 9: 283–290.

Weaver, R.H. and M.S. Cranley (1983) 'An exploration of paternal–fetal attachment.' *Nursing Research,* 32: 68–72.

Weiner, C.P. and A. Ludomirski (1994) 'Diagnosis, pathophysiology, and treatment of chronic twin to twin transfusion.' *Fetal Diagnosis and Therapy,* 9: 283–290.

Welburn, V. (1980) *Postnatal Depression.* London: Fontana.

Wenstrom K.D. and S.A. Gall (1988) 'Incidence, morbidity and mortality, and diagnosis of twin gestations.' *Clinics in Perinatology,* 15 (1): 1–11.

White, D.G. and A. Wollett (1987) 'The father role in the neonatal period.' In: D. Harvey (ed.) *Parent–Infant Relationships.* Series on Perinatal Practice, Vol. 4. Chichester: Wiley.

Williams, L. (1988) 'It's going to work for me: Responses to failure of IVF.' *Birth,* 15: 153–156.

Wilmut, I. *et al.* (1997) 'Viable offspring derived from fetal and adult mammalian cells.' *Nature,* 385: 810–813.

Wilson, R. (1974) 'Twins: Mental development in the preschool years.' *Developmental Psychology,* 10: 580–588.

—— (1975) 'Twins: Patterns of cognitive development.' *Developmental Psychology,* 11: 126–134.

—— (1986) 'Twins: Genetic influence on growth.' In: R.M. Malina and C. Bouchard (eds) *Sports and Human Genetics*. Champaign, Ill.: Human Kinetics.

Wilson, R.S. and E.B. Harpring (1972) 'Mental and motor development in infant twins.' *Developmental Psychology*, 7: 277–287.

Wing, L. (1988) 'Possible clues to the underlying pathology. 1. Clinical facts.' In: L. Wing (ed.) *Aspects of Autism: Biological Research*. London: Gaskell.

Wing, L. and J. Gould (1979) 'Severe impairments of social interaction and associated abnormalities in children: Epidemiology and classification.' *Journal of Autism and Developmental Disorders*, 9: 11–30.

Wohlreich, M.M. (1986) 'Psychiatric aspects of high-risk pregnancies.' *Psychiatric Clinics of North America*, 10: 53–68.

Wolkind, S. (1981) 'Pre-natal emotional stress: Effects on the fetus.' In: S. Wolkind and E. Zajiecek (eds) *Pregnancy: A Psychological and Social Study*. London: Academic Press.

Wollf, P.H. (1963) 'Observations on the early development of smiling.' In: B.M. Foss (ed.) *Determinants of Infant Behavior*, Vol. 2. London: Methuen.

—— (1966) 'The causes, controls and organization of behavior in the neonate.' *Psychological Issues*, 5: 1–105.

—— (1969) 'The natural history of crying and other vocalizations in early infancy.' In: B.M. Foss (ed.) *Determinants of Infant Behavior*, Vol. 4. London: Methuen.

—— (1973) 'The organization of behavior in the first three months of life.' *Research Publications of the Association for Research in Nervous and Mental Diseases*, 51: 132–153.

—— (1984) 'Discontinuous changes in human wakefulness around the end of the second month of life: A developmental perspective.' In: H.F.R. Prechtl (ed.) *Continuity of Neural Functions from Prenatal to Postnatal Life*. London: Mac Keith Press.

Wolpert, L. (1991) *The Triumph of the Embryo*. Oxford: Oxford University Press.

—— (1994) 'Do we understand development?' *Science*, 266: 571–572.

Wolpert, L. *et al.* (1998) *Principles of Development*. Oxford: Oxford University Press.

Wood, S.L. *et al.* (1996) 'Evaluation of the twin peak or lambda sign in determining chorionicity in multiple pregnancy.' *Obstetrics and Gynecology*, 88: 6–9.

Woodward, J. (1998) *The Lone Twin. Understanding Twin Bereavement and Loss*. London: Free Association Books.

Woollett, A. (1986) 'The influence of older siblings on the language environment of young children.' *British Journal of Developmental Psychology*, 4 (3): 235–245.

Wright, L. (1997) *Twins: Genes, Environment and the Mystery of Identity*. London: Weidenfeld and Nicolson.

Wyshak, G. (1978a) 'Statistical findings on the effects of fertility drugs on plural births.' In: W.E. Nance (ed.) *Twin Research: Biology and Epidemiology. Progress in Clinical Biological Research*, 24B: 17–33.

—— (1978b) 'Menopause in mothers of multiple births and mothers of singletons only.' *Social Biology*, 25: 52–61.

—— (1981) 'Reproductive and menstrual characteristics of mothers of multiple births and mothers of singletons only: a discriminative analysis.' In: W.E. Nance (ed.) *Twin Research 3: Twin Biology and Multiple Pregnancy*. New York: Alan R. Liss.

Yokata, Y., A. Akane and N. Fujino (1994) 'Monozygotic twins of different apparent sex.' *American Journal of Medical Genetics*, 53: 52–55.

Zazzo, R. (1960) *Les Jumeaux, le Couple et la Personne*. Paris: Presses Universitaires de France.

—— (1975) 'Des jumeaux devant le miroir: questions de méthode.' *Journal de Psychologie Normale et Pathologique*, 4: 389–413.

—— (1979a) 'The twin condition and the couple effects on personality development.' *Acta Geneticae Medicae et Gemellologiae*, 25: 343–352.

—— (1979b) 'Des enfants, des singes et des chiens devant le miroir.' *Revue de Psychologie Appliquée*, 29: 235–246.

—— (1984) *Le Paradoxe des Jumeaux*. Paris: Stock-Laurance Pernoud.

—— (1993) *Reflets de Miroir et Autres Doubles*. Paris: Presses Universitaires de France.

Zeanah, C.H. (1989) 'Adaptation following perinatal loss: A critical review.' *Journal of the American Academy of Child and Adolescent Psychiatry*, 28: 467–480.

Zeanah, C.H., O.K. Mannen and A.F. Liebermann (1993) 'Disorders of attachment.' In: C.H. Zeanah (ed.) *Handbook of Infant Mental Health*. New York: The Guilford Press.

Zecevich, N. and P. Rakic (1991) 'Synaptogenesis in monkey somatosensory cortex.' *Cerebral Cortex*, 1: 510–523.

Zimmerman, L. and L. McDonald (1995) 'Emotional availability in infants' relationships with multiple caregivers.' *American Journal of Orthopsychiatry*, 65: 147–152.

INDEX

Note: Figures are indicated by *italic page numbers*